Phlebotomy
Worktext and Procedures Manual

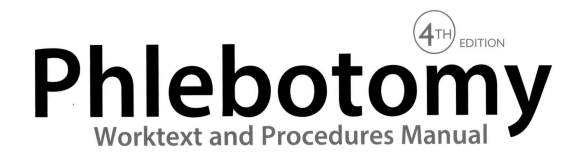

Phlebotomy

Worktext and Procedures Manual

4TH EDITION

Robin S. Warekois, MT(ASCP)

Avee Laboratory
Clearwater, Florida

Richard Robinson, NASW

Sherborn, Massachusetts

Consulting Educator

Pamela B. Primrose, PhD, MLS(ASCP)

Program Chair of Medical Laboratory Technology
Professor of Medical Laboratory Technology/Life Sciences
Ivy Tech Community College
South Bend, Indiana

ELSEVIER

ELSEVIER

3251 Riverport Lane
St. Louis, Missouri 63043

Notices

Knowledge and best practice in this field are constantly changing. As new research and experience broaden our understanding, changes in research methods, professional practices, or medical treatment may become necessary.

Practitioners and researchers must always rely on their own experience and knowledge in evaluating and using any information, methods, compounds, or experiments described herein. In using such information or methods they should be mindful of their own safety and the safety of others, including parties for whom they have a professional responsibility.

With respect to any drug or pharmaceutical products identified, readers are advised to check the most current information provided (i) on procedures featured or (ii) by the manufacturer of each product to be administered, to verify the recommended dose or formula, the method and duration of administration, and contraindications. It is the responsibility of practitioners, relying on their own experience and knowledge of their patients, to make diagnoses, to determine dosages and the best treatment for each individual patient, and to take all appropriate safety precautions.

To the fullest extent of the law, neither the Publisher nor the authors, contributors, or editors, assume any liability for any injury and/or damage to persons or property as a matter of products liability, negligence or otherwise, or from any use or operation of any methods, products, instructions, or ideas contained in the material herein.

International Standard Book Number: 978-0-323-27940-6

Content Strategist: Kristin Wilhelm
Content Development Manager: Ellen Wurm-Cutter
Publishing Services Manager: Jeff Patterson
Senior Project Manager: Mary Stueck
Design Direction: Margaret Reid

Printed in Canada

Last digit is the print number: 9   8   7   6   5   4   3

Contributors

MOCK CERTIFICATION EXAM

Rachel Houston
CMA(AAMA)
Program Director, Medical Assistant Program
Cabarrus College of Health Sciences
Concord, North Carolina

TEST BANK

Nicole Palmieri
BSN, RN
Medical Assistant Instructor
Advantage Career Institute, Inc.
Eatontown, New Jersey

Reviewers

Belinda Beeman
MEd, CAM(AAMA), PBT(ASCP)
Medical Assisting and Phlebotomy Instructor
Eastern New Mexico University
Roswell, New Mexico

Sylvia R. Crawford
PBT(ASCP)
Phlebotomy Instructor
Bellevue College
Bellevue, Washington

Susanna M. Hancock
AAS-MOM, RMA, CMA, RPT, COLT
Medical Program Consultant
Retired Medical Assistant Program Director
American Institute of Health Technology
Boise, Idaho

Julian A. Kiler
MD(FMG), MPH, ATI(AMT), RMA(AMT)
Medical Clinical Administrative Program Instructor
School of Career Education
Riverside County Office of Education
Riverside, California

Julie S. Monsegur
RN, MSN-Ed
Health Programs Laboratory Assistant
Pasco-Hernando Community College
New Port Richey, Florida

Anne O'Neil
MT(ASCP)
Retired MLT Program Director
Lakewood, Washington

Kathleen Park
MA, MT(ASCP)
Associate Professor
Austin Community College
Medical Laboratory Technology Program
Round Rock, Texas

Pamela B. Primrose
PhD, MLS(ASCP)
Program Chair of Medical Laboratory Technology
Professor of Medical Laboratory Technology/Life Sciences
Ivy Tech Community College
South Bend, Indiana

Karen Marie Ragusa
PBT(ASCP)
Adult Educator
Monroe 2 Orleans BOCES
Rochester, New York

Mary Stassi
RN
Health Occupations Coordinator
St. Charles County Community College
St. Charles, Missouri

Margie West
Phlebotomy Instructor
Petra Allied Health
Springdale, Arkansas

Carole Stemple Zeglin
MSEd, BSMT, RMA(AMT)
Associate Professor
Director Clinical Laboratory Programs & Medical Assisting
Westmoreland County Community College
Youngwood, Pennsylvania

Acknowledgments

We are grateful to the many people who have contributed their time and expertise to help make this fourth edition of *Phlebotomy: Worktext and Procedures Manual* a valuable teaching tool. Our reviewers continue to provide important insights into the best ways to communicate concepts based on their own classroom experience. Pam Primrose and Kristin Wilhelm offered valuable help, each in her own way, in bringing this edition forward. As we have in the past, we offer our deepest gratitude to Ellen Wurm-Cutter, whose continued dedication to this text and unflappable good cheer have made our jobs easier and our book better.

Robin S. Warekois
Richard Robinson

Preface

The successful practice of phlebotomy requires a combination of highly skilled technique, wide knowledge of the current health care environment, and a sympathetic approach to patients of all ages, backgrounds, and medical conditions. We have designed *Phlebotomy: Worktext and Procedures Manual,* 4th edition, to provide a complete introduction to the practice of phlebotomy in all its aspects. We believe its emphasis on procedures, its up-to-date and thorough professional information, and its comprehensive approach to the many situations encountered by the modern phlebotomist make it a unique and valuable offering in the field of phlebotomy training.

WHO WILL BENEFIT FROM THIS BOOK?

Phlebotomy: Worktext and Procedures Manual, 4th edition, is suitable for phlebotomy certification programs, medical technologist and medical laboratory technician programs, medical assisting programs, and nurse training. No prior training in phlebotomy is assumed. The text may also be used by experienced phlebotomists, allied health professionals, or nurses seeking to expand or update their training in phlebotomy.

WHY IS THIS BOOK IMPORTANT TO THE PROFESSION?

Students, above all, learn by doing. Teaching phlebotomy technique is at the heart of this book, and we have therefore designed it as a worktext for both the classroom and the laboratory. Each major skill in phlebotomy, from handwashing to venipuncture to preparing a blood smear, is shown and described in step-by-step, fully illustrated procedures. We believe these will provide the student with an invaluable visual tool for understanding the essentials of the techniques before, during, and after their practical laboratory experience.

In addition to thorough training in the skills of phlebotomy, this text provides an introduction to development of skills beyond blood collection with a chapter on point-of-care testing. In this way, phlebotomy students can begin their training as multiskilled health professionals ready for the challenges of the modern health care workplace.

ORGANIZATION

The text is divided into five units. Unit 1 provides an introduction and general information needed for working in a health care facility. Unit 2 covers the basics needed to study phlebotomy, from medical terminology to anatomy and physiology. Unit 3 features the various methods of specimen collection, including venipuncture, dermal puncture, arterial blood collection, and special procedures. Unit 4 presents specimen handling, processing, and point-of-care testing. Unit 5 concludes the text with a section on professional issues. Individual units and chapters may be taught in the sequence chosen by the instructor. Numerous *Flash Forward* and *Flashback* notes help the student connect and recall material from different chapters. A comprehensive index is provided to allow quick access to any topic.

DISTINCTIVE FEATURES AND LEARNING AIDS

Phlebotomy courses are offered in a variety of settings. *Phlebotomy: Worktext and Procedures Manual,* 4th edition, provides the essential learning tools students need to succeed in each of them. Because we believe that students learn best when they know the "why" as well as the "how," we explain the reasoning behind the clinical information they must learn to become successful phlebotomists.

This approach is strengthened by key features of each chapter, including the following:

- Detailed **Objectives, Key Terms, Abbreviations**, and **Study Questions** serve as a study guide for students and provide instructors with the framework for regular assignments.

- **Review for Certification and Certification Exam Preparation** allow students to assess their progress toward preparedness for the certification exam.

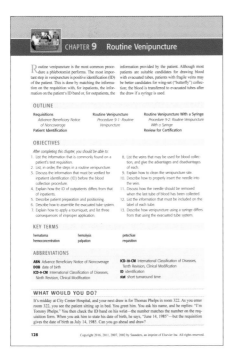

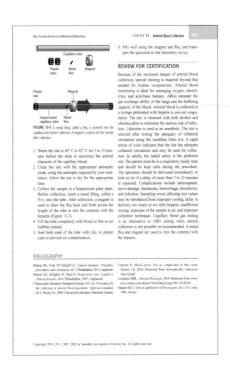

- **Boxes, Tables,** and **Figures** summarize key information and illustrate difficult concepts.
- Each major skill in phlebotomy is shown and described in step-by-step, fully illustrated **Procedures.**

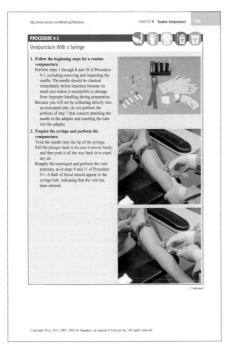

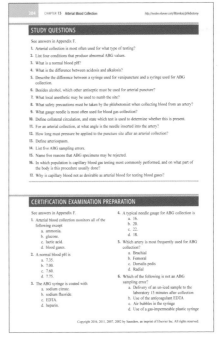

- **Flashbacks and Flash Forwards** directly link students to material they have encountered before or will cover in more depth in the future.

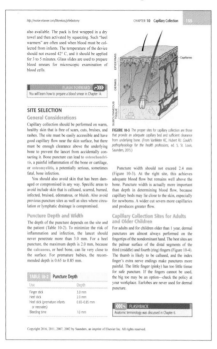

- **Clinical Tips** offer students pearls of wisdom they can use in the clinical setting.
- **What Would You Do?** boxes offer students real-life scenarios that challenge them to apply what they are learning to difficult workplace situations. We believe these scenarios will resonate with students as they learn about the nuances of their profession and will provide the grist for lively discussions in class.

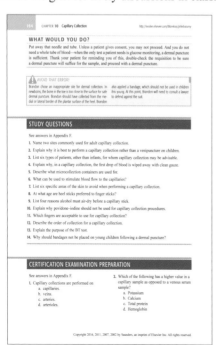

- In addition to these chapter features, a comprehensive **Glossary** is found at the end of the book, along with appendices, including one listing **Spanish phrases** important in phlebotomy. Finally, a **Mock Certification Exam** provides students with the opportunity to test themselves at the end of the course as they prepare for certification.

NEW TO THIS EDITION

A new edition offers the opportunity to both update and improve. We have taken advantage of this opportunity in *Phlebotomy: Worktext and Procedures Manual,* 4th edition. Every chapter has been reviewed and updated as needed while maintaining the approach and features that made earlier editions successful.

- **Safety protocols and equipment** undergo continual change. For this edition, we have captured those changes, with revised procedures, discussions, illustrations, and guidelines throughout the book to reflect the most current guidelines from OSHA, CLSI, and other governmental and professional organizations.
- **New photographs** of procedures and equipment show the latest equipment and safety practices so that students receive the most current information in the field.
- **Avoid That Error!** boxes provide students with additional clinical scenarios that challenge their understanding, encourage them to think about how to avoid errors, and what to do when errors are made.
- **Procedural Videos** accessed through the Evolve website include 27 videos that show important skills, including venipuncture and capillary collection.

ANCILLARIES

For the Instructor

With the fourth edition, we are offering several assets.

TEACH

- **TEACH Lesson Plan Manual,** available via Evolve: Provides instructors with customizable lesson plans and lecture outlines based on learning objectives. With these valuable resources, instructors will save valuable preparation time and create a learning environment that fully engages students in classroom preparation. The lesson plans are keyed chapter-by-chapter and are divided into

50-minute units. In addition to the lesson plans, instructors will have unique lecture outlines in PowerPoint with lecture notes, thought-provoking questions, and unique ideas for lectures.

Evolve Website

- **Test Bank:** An ExamView test bank of approximately 500 multiple-choice questions that feature rationales, cognitive levels, and page number references to the text. The test bank can be used for class reviews, quizzes, or exams.
- **Image Collection:** All of the images from the book are available as .jpg files and can be downloaded into PowerPoint presentations. These can also be used during lecture to illustrate important concepts.
- **Competency Checklists:** All of the competency checklists from the book are available as PDFs to be printed and used electronically.

- **TEACH assets** containing all TEACH resources.

For the Student

The following assets are available via the Evolve Website:

- **New Procedural Videos:** 27 video clips showing "real-life" examples of how to perform a variety of skills such as venipuncture, capillary collection, and hematologic testing.
- **Mock Certification Exam:** Provides additional practice with an electronic, timed version of the exam.
- **Audio Glossary:** Definitions of the key terms in the text, with audio pronunciations.
- **Interactive Exercises:** Drag-and-drop exercises and flashcards to help reinforce new vocabulary.

Procedure Photo Credits

Procedure 4-1

Steps 1, 3, 4, 5, 6. from Proctor DB, Adams AP: *Kinn's the medical assistant: An applied learning approach,* ed. 12, St. Louis, 2014, Saunders.

Step 2 from Chester GA: *Modern medical assisting,* Philadelphia, 1999, Saunders.

Procedure 10-2

Step 1 from Stepp CA, Woods MA: *Laboratory procedures for medical office personnel,* Philadelphia, 1998, Saunders.

Procedure 13-2

Steps 3, 4 from Potter P, Perry A: *Fundamentals of nursing,* ed. 6, St. Louis, 2005, Mosby.

Step 6 from Stepp CA, Woods MA: *Laboratory procedures for medical office personnel,* Philadelphia, 1998, Saunders.

Procedure 14-1

Step 1 from Leahy JM, Kizilay PE: *Foundations of nursing practice: A nursing process approach,* Philadelphia, 1998, Saunders.

Procedure 15-1

Steps 1, 2, 3 from Stepp CA, Woods MA: *Laboratory procedures for medical office personnel,* Philadelphia, 1998, Saunders.

Procedure 15-2

Step 1 from Bonewit-West K: *Clinical procedures for medical assistants,* ed. 9, St. Louis, 2015, Saunders.

Procedure 17-1

Step 1 courtesy Zack Bent. From Garrels M, Oatis CS: *Laboratory testing for ambulatory settings,* Philadelphia, 2006, Saunders.

Step 2 from Chester GA: *Modern medical assisting,* Philadelphia, 1999, Saunders.

Icons Used in This Book

The Occupational Safety and Health Administration (OSHA) standards must be followed when performing most of the procedures presented in this text. Icons have been incorporated into the procedures to assist in following these standards. An illustration of each icon, along with its description, is given here.

HAND HYGIENE is an important medical aseptic practice and is crucial in preventing the transmission of pathogens in the medical office. The phlebotomist should perform hand hygiene frequently, using the proper technique. When performing venipuncture procedures, the hands should always be cleaned before and after patient contact, before applying and after removing gloves, and after contact with blood or other potentially infectious materials. In some institutions, an alcohol-based agent may be preferred, but CLSI guidelines indicate that it should not be used as a substitute for hand washing.

Clean disposable *GLOVES* should be worn if the phlebotomist anticipates hand contact with blood and other potentially infectious materials, mucous membranes, and contaminated articles or surfaces.

Appropriate *PROTECTIVE CLOTHING* such as gowns, aprons, and laboratory coats should be worn when gross contamination can reasonably be anticipated during performance of a task or procedure.

FACE SHIELDS or *MASKS,* in combination with *EYE PROTECTION DEVICES,* must be worn whenever splashes, spray, spatter, or droplets of blood or other potentially infectious materials may be generated, posing a hazard through contact with eyes, nose, or mouth.

Infectious waste must be placed in *BIOHAZARD CONTAINERS* that are closeable, leak-proof, and suitably constructed to contain the contents during handling, storage, transport, or shipping. The containers must be labeled or color coded and closed before removal to prevent the contents from spilling.

Used disposable syringes, needles, lancets, and other sharp items must be placed in puncture-resistant *SHARPS CONTAINERS* located as close as practical to the area in which the items were used.

Contents

UNIT 1
Introduction to Phlebotomy

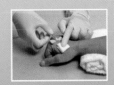

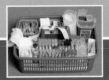

CHAPTER 1   Introduction to Phlebotomy

The modern phlebotomist is a professional trained to draw blood who has a variety of job skills and personal characteristics, including communication skills, organizational skills, and compassion. After initial training, the phlebotomist may become certified by one or more professional organizations. Continuing education courses keep the phlebotomist up to date on the latest changes in techniques and regulations in the field. The phlebotomist must also be aware of important legal issues, including patient confidentiality, informed consent, and Health Insurance Portability and Accountability Act (HIPAA) regulations.

OUTLINE

What Is Phlebotomy?
Modern Phlebotomy
  Job Skills
  Job Duties
  Personal Characteristics

Professional Organizations and
  Standards
  Accreditation
  Certification
  State Licensure
  Continuing Education

Legal Issues in Phlebotomy
  Informed Consent
  Confidentiality
  HIPAA
Review for Certification

OBJECTIVES

After completing this chapter, you should be able to:

1. Define phlebotomy.
2. List at least five job skills that are important for phlebotomists to have, and explain why each is important.
3. Describe the major duty of phlebotomists, and discuss four other responsibilities that are important.
4. List six personal qualities that characterize a professional, and explain how phlebotomists demonstrate these qualities.
5. Differentiate accreditation and certification.
6. Identify professional organizations with an interest in phlebotomy.
7. Explain why informed consent and confidentiality are important legal issues for phlebotomists.

KEY TERMS

accreditation
approval
certification

continuing education units
  (CEUs)
informed consent

phlebotomy
protected health
  information

standards

ABBREVIATIONS

ACA American Certification Agency for Healthcare Professionals
AMT American Medical Technologists
ASCLS American Society for Clinical Laboratory Science

ASCP American Society for Clinical Pathology
ASPT American Society of Phlebotomy Technicians
CEUs continuing education units
CPT certified phlebotomy technician

HIPAA Health Insurance Portability and Accountability Act

NAACLS National Accrediting Agency for Clinical Laboratory Sciences

NHA National Healthcareer Association

NPA National Phlebotomy Association

PBT phlebotomy technician by AMT

PHI Protected health information

RPT registered phlebotomy technician

WHAT WOULD YOU DO?

You've been hired by Central Hospital for your first job as a phlebotomist. You start next Monday, but first you need to read the employee handbook, which includes a description of personal characteristics for the successful phlebotomist. Dependability? Check—you've been holding down a steady job for more than 2 years. Positive attitude? Check—your nickname at the warehouse is "Can do." Professional appearance? Uh-oh—no piercings, no visible tattoos, no artificial nails. You've got them all. When Monday rolls around, what should you do? Forget about the job? Tell your supervisor, "This is me—deal with it"? What would you do?

WHAT IS PHLEBOTOMY?

Phlebotomy is the practice of drawing blood. The word *phlebotomy* is derived from the Greek *phlebo-*, which means "vein," and *-tomy*, which means "to make an incision." Phlebotomy is an ancient profession, dating back at least 3500 years to the time of the ancient Egyptians. The earliest phlebotomists drew blood in an attempt to cure disease and maintain the body in a state of wellness. In Europe during the Middle Ages, barber-surgeons performed bloodletting to balance the four humors, or bodily fluids, because an imbalance of the humors was thought to underlie disease. The familiar stripes on the barber's pole date from this period, with red symbolizing blood and white symbolizing bandages. Early phlebotomists' tools included lancets (called fleams) and suction cups (Figure 1-1), and they used ornate ceramic bowls to collect the blood. Phlebotomists also applied leeches to patients' skin for hours at a time to remove blood. Today, removal of a prescribed volume of blood ("therapeutic phlebotomy") is used to treat a small number of blood disorders.

MODERN PHLEBOTOMY

Modern phlebotomy shares little more than a name with these ancient practices. Today, phlebotomy is performed primarily for diagnosis and monitoring of a patient's disease condition. It involves highly developed and rigorously tested procedures and equipment, all meant to ensure the safety and comfort of the patient and the integrity of the sample collected.

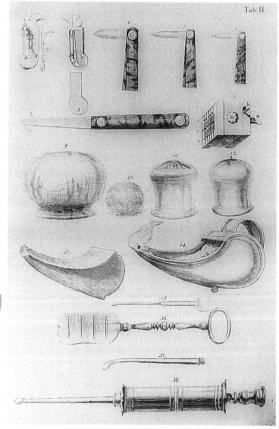

FIGURE 1-1 Tools of the earliest phlebotomists. (From Brambilla GA: *Instrumentarium chirurgicum.* Vienna, Matthias Andreas Schmidt, 1781. Courtesy U.S. National Library of Medicine, History of Medicine Division, Bethesda, Md.)

Job Skills

Today's phlebotomist is highly trained and uses a variety of skills in the workplace. Technical skills are required to collect specimens for analysis, and developing these skills will constitute a large part of your training. A phlebotomist also needs to be highly organized and detail-oriented in order to deal with the large number of samples that may be collected in a short time, while ensuring that each sample is properly labeled and correctly handled. The successful phlebotomist is able to prioritize multiple tasks and match his or her pace to the volume of work. Equally important are interpersonal skills. As a phlebotomist, you will spend a large part of your working day interacting with people, including patients, their families, and medical personnel. Another important job skill is being able to handle stress. A phlebotomist must occasionally deal with difficult patients, fainting patients, malfunctioning equipment, or demands for immediate action. As your technical skills increase, these situations will become less stressful, but the job will always carry some stress. Being able to cope with this in a calm, professional manner is vital to being a successful phlebotomist.

Job Duties

The principal purpose of phlebotomy is to obtain blood samples, at the request of a physician or a qualified health care professional such as a nurse practitioner, for analysis in the laboratory. Performing these duties correctly ensures that patients receive prompt and complete medical care. Failure to perform these duties correctly can lead to significant adverse consequences for the patient, including improper care and even death. Later chapters cover the details of how to perform each step of each procedure you will be required to perform. In brief, the steps in a routine collection are as follows:

1. Obtain a requisition from a licensed practitioner.
2. Correctly and positively identify the patient by asking the patient to state his or her name.
3. Choose the appropriate equipment for obtaining the sample.
4. Select and prepare the site for collection.
5. Collect the sample, ensuring patient comfort and safety.
6. Correctly label the sample with patient's name, date, and time of collection.
7. Transport the sample to the laboratory in a timely manner, using appropriate handling procedures.

8. Adhere to all safety and infection control regulations throughout the process.

In addition to collecting patient blood samples, phlebotomists must also:

1. Effectively interact with both patients and health care professionals.
2. Keep accurate records and be knowledgeable about the computer operations of the laboratory.
3. Develop other health care skills, such as performing blood pressure determinations, collecting nonblood specimens, processing specimens, instructing patients on collecting nonblood specimens (such as urine), performing point-of-care testing and quality-control procedures, maintaining point-of-care instruments, and performing some basic laboratory tests.

A trained phlebotomist can also be employed as a medical assistant, a laboratory assistant, or an accessioner, after receiving specialized training. A medical assistant works in a clinic or hospital to assist other staff in patient care and facility preparation. A medical assistant requires training in medical billing and coding with a specific certification process. A laboratory assistant assists in performing routine laboratory testing. An accessioner performs a variety of tasks related to specimen preparation in the clinical laboratory. A phlebotomist may be cross-trained to perform clerical duties such as patient registration.

Personal Characteristics

As a phlebotomist, you will often be the first medical professional a patient meets. You therefore represent not only yourself or the laboratory but the entire health care facility. This public relations aspect of your work is important because it sets the tone for the patient's stay in the health care facility and the patient's satisfaction with the service the facility provides. How you present yourself has an effect on everyone with whom you interact. The quality of care you provide has a direct effect on the patient's health and satisfaction, as well as on the health care facility's reputation in the health care setting. In addition, your interaction with a patient also affects scoring on patient satisfaction surveys. These survey results are monitored by The Joint Commission and influence the quality rating of the health care system.

The phlebotomist is a member of the health care profession and must display professional behavior at all times (Figure 1-2). Professionalism is both an attitude toward your work and a set of specific characteristics. A professional displays the following characteristics.

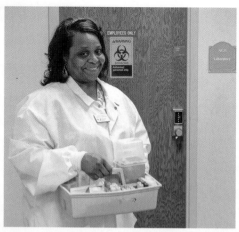

FIGURE 1-2 Phlebotomists spend much of the day interacting with people, and interpersonal skills are a vital part of the job.

Dependability

The phlebotomist plays a crucial role in the health care institution and is depended on to perform that role skillfully, efficiently, and without constant supervision. The phlebotomist must report to work on time and avoid all unnecessary absences or tardiness. Failure to do so can affect patient care. A late or absent phlebotomist decreases the overall function of the laboratory and may even prevent a patient from having a sample collected in a timely manner for monitoring of medication, for example.

Honesty and Integrity

Because the phlebotomist often works without supervision, unquestioned integrity is crucial. Everyone makes errors, and you will be no exception. It is vital for the health and safety of your patients that you admit to errors when they are made. Unreported errors can result in patient injury and death.

Positive Attitude

Your attitude affects everyone you interact with, and having a positive attitude toward your job makes others around you more positive as well. This is especially important in your interactions with patients and their families as well as other health care professionals.

Empathy and Compassion

The phlebotomist is often called on to interact with patients experiencing health crises or undergoing painful or unpleasant treatments. Patients may be worried about the procedure being performed, the condition for which they are being treated, or the

cost of their care. By being sensitive to patients' concerns and taking the time to reassure anxious patients, you can help make their stay less stressful (Figure 1-3).

Professional Detachment

Conversely, it is important to remain emotionally detached from patients. You will encounter many distressing situations in your career. Becoming emotionally involved on a personal level does not help your patients and can lead to stress and burnout. Your approach to patients in distress must be sympathetic and understanding, but you must retain enough professional distance to allow you to do your job efficiently. Developing this balanced approach is a significant step in your professional growth.

Professional Appearance

Appearance has a significant effect on how the phlebotomist is thought of by patients and treated by coworkers, including superiors. First impressions are often lasting ones. Cleanliness and scrupulous grooming is critical, with conservative clothing, hair, and makeup the general rule. Avoid long, dangling jewelry and earrings; exposed piercings other than in ears; strong perfume; and gaudy makeup. Employers usually set specific standards. In addition, keep your fingernails short, avoid artificial nails, and if you use nail polish, use neutral shades and avoid chips. Long nails and chipped polish breed bacteria and fungi, which may affect patients' health.

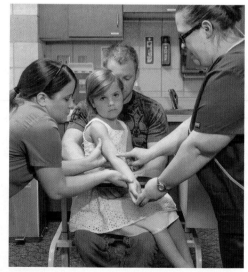

FIGURE 1-3 The phlebotomist is a member of the health care profession and must display professional behavior at all times.

Interpersonal Skills

The phlebotomist must be able to communicate effectively with patients and coworkers. Patients may be fearful, uncooperative, or excessively talkative. In all cases, the phlebotomist must be able to communicate clearly to patients what is to be done and to obtain consent for the procedure. Speaking slowly, clearly, and in a courteous tone will help you gain the patient's trust, which is necessary to perform the procedure effectively. Nonverbal communication is important as well. By making eye contact, smiling, and appearing relaxed, calm, and prepared, you communicate confidence and professionalism to patients. Reading patients' nonverbal communication, or body language, will let you know when you need to take extra steps to put them at ease. For example, anxious patients often fidget, tap their fingers, or bounce their legs. Fearful patients may have their eyes "glazed over," unable to focus. Take the time to reassure anxious patients by listening to their needs. Take the time to answer questions. Patients need empathetic attention—they are people, not just names on requisition forms. Treat all patients as if they are a family member.

Telephone Skills

The phlebotomist is often required to answer calls and take messages in the laboratory. The information that comes in over the phone may be critical for patient care or for the operation of the laboratory. It is essential that you display the same high level of professionalism in answering the phone as in dealing directly with patients and coworkers. If you are staffing the desk, do the following:

- Answer the phone promptly.
- Smile when speaking, even though you can't be seen; it will positively affect your voice tone.
- Identify the department and yourself, and ask how you can help.
- Write everything down, including the name of the person calling, their phone number, and the date and time of the call. Be prepared to take a message by having writing materials at hand.
- Speak slowly and clearly.
- Do not put the caller on hold until you determine it is not an emergency call.
- Make every attempt to help, but give only accurate information. If you do not know the answer to a question, find out and call back, if necessary.

An example of these telephone skills steps is illustrated in Box 1-1.

BOX 1-1   Answering the Phone

Here is an example of the correct way to answer the phone in the clinical laboratory:

[Phone rings]

Phlebotomist: Good afternoon, this is the clinical laboratory at Mercy Hospital. Sandy speaking. How may I help you?

Caller: This is Dr. Tom Watson from Fairview Clinic. Can you tell me if the results from the fecal test on a patient on Three West are ready yet?

Phlebotomist: I will try to find out. Can you tell me the patient identification number on the test request and the date that the specimen was sent?

Caller: The number is 243576-1. The date for the specimen was 8/12.

Phlebotomist: Thank you. Can you hold while I check?

Caller: Yes.

Phlebotomist: Thank you. Please hold.

[Phlebotomist places call on hold, checks for the results, and returns to the phone.]

Phlebotomist: Dr. Watson? What is your patient's name?

Caller: The patient is Harry Blum.

Phlebotomist: I'm sorry. The results are not back yet—we've had a slight delay here. May I take your number and call you when they are ready? It should be about 2 hours.

Caller: Yes. I'm at 555-5555.

Phlebotomist: [Writes down number.] I will call you as soon as the results are ready.

Caller: Thank you.

Phlebotomist: Thank you. Good-bye.

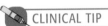 CLINICAL TIP

Always write down *all* pertinent information when answering the phone.

PROFESSIONAL ORGANIZATIONS AND STANDARDS

The high standards necessary for the proper practice of modern phlebotomy have led to the creation of several organizations that develop standards and monitor training in the field. There are three aspects of this type of professional monitoring: accreditation, certification, and continuing medical education. Accreditation is for institutions that train phlebotomists, whereas the other two are for phlebotomists themselves. The program in which you are training to become a phlebotomist should be accredited. Once you receive your training, you can become certified. After you become certified, you may need to participate in continuing medical education to remain certified.

Some of the organizations and the services they provide are shown in Table 1-1.

Membership in a professional organization for phlebotomists offers an additional way to follow changes in the field and to learn important new information. Some of the organizations listed in Table 1-1 publish journals with useful articles or sponsor workshops or seminars.

Accreditation

Programs that train phlebotomists receive **accreditation** or **approval** from a professional organization by meeting and documenting established requirements, called **standards**. An accredited education program exposes students to both classroom and clinical experiences and fully prepares them to become professional phlebotomists. As shown in Table 1-1, the organizations that provide accreditation or approval are the American Medical Technologists (AMT), the American Society of Phlebotomy Technicians (ASPT), the National Accrediting Agency for Clinical Laboratory Sciences (NAACLS), and the National Phlebotomy Association (NPA). The program you are enrolled in may be accredited by one or more of these organizations. As discussed later, California accredits training programs within that state.

Certification

After completing an accredited or approved program, you are eligible to take a certifying examination. **Certification** is evidence that an individual has demonstrated proficiency in a particular area of practice. As shown in Table 1-1, the organizations and companies that offer certification are American Allied Health, the American Certification Agency for Healthcare Professionals (ACA), the AMT, the American Society for Clinical Pathology (ASCP), the ASPT, the National Healthcareer Association (NHA), and the NPA. Once you pass the examination, you may use the title shown in Table 1-1 as part of your professional name.

State Licensure

Several states require that phlebotomists obtain a license directly from the state to perform phlebotomy within the state. These states include California, Louisiana, Nevada, and Washington. The requirements for each state as of late 2013 are discussed below.

California

Phlebotomists in California fall under a set of state regulations governing their education, training, and certification. Those who wish to become phlebotomists must show proof of having met several educational requirements, including the following:
- High school diploma or equivalent
- Forty hours of classroom instruction in phlebotomy (20 hours basic, 20 hours advanced) in a state-accredited program
- Forty hours of practical training in phlebotomy in a state-accredited program, including at least 50 venipunctures and 10 skin punctures
- Certification from a national phlebotomy organization that is approved by the state to administer examinations and issue certification

Once you have met all these requirements, you are eligible to apply to the state for certification to practice phlebotomy. (A high school diploma or equivalent plus 20 hours of training will allow you to qualify as a limited phlebotomy technician and perform skin punctures only; this does not require certification.) State certification is for 2 years, with renewal based on meeting continuing education requirements.

The initial certification granted is as a certified phlebotomy technician level I (CPT-I), which enables phlebotomists to perform dermal punctures and venipunctures without supervision and arterial punctures with the supervision of a physician, registered nurse, medical laboratory scientist, medical laboratory technician, or certified respiratory therapist. After performing 20 successful supervised arterial punctures, the CPT-I can apply to become a CPT-II, with the ability to perform unsupervised arterial punctures.

Practicing phlebotomists may need to show proof of classroom instruction to obtain state certification, even if they are already certified by a national organization.

Regardless of whether you plan to practice in California, it is wise to get the maximum amount of training before you start your career as a phlebotomist.

Louisiana

The state of Louisiana requires phlebotomists to apply for licensure through the State Board of Medical Examiners after receiving certification from one of the private national organizations. There are multiple exemptions from this requirement, however. If you fall into one of the categories for exemption in the board's rules, you do not need a state license to practice phlebotomy. Those exempted include phlebotomists supervised by a licensed physician, or a licensed clinic, hospital, nursing home, or other licensed health care facility authorized by licensure to perform clinical laboratory testing.

TABLE 1-1	Organizations That Provide Accreditation, Certification, or Continuing Education		
Name	Accredits or Approves Training Programs	Certifies Phlebotomists (Title Awarded)	Offers Continuing Education Units
American Allied Health, Inc. Testing and Certification PO Box 1487 Lowell, AR 72745 (479) 553-7614 www.americanalliedhealth.com	No	Yes	No
American Certification Agency for Healthcare Professionals (ACA) PO Box 58 Osceola, IN 46561 (574) 277-4538 www.acacert.com	No	Yes	Yes
American Medical Technologists (AMT) 10700 W. Higgins Rd., Suite 150 Rosemont, IL 60018 (847) 823-5169 www.americanmedtech.org	Yes	Yes (registered phlebotomy technician[RPT])	Yes
American Society for Clinical Laboratory Science (ASCLS) 1861 International Drive, Suite 200 McLean, VA 22102 (571) 748-3770 www.ascls.org	No	No	Yes
American Society for Clinical Pathology (ASCP) Board of Certification (BOC) 33 W. Monroe St., Suite 1600 Chicago, IL 60603 (312) 541-4999 www.ascp.org	No	Yes (phlebotomy technician [PBT])	Yes
American Society of Phlebotomy Technicians (ASPT) PO Box 1831 Hickory, NC 28603 (828) 294-0078 www.aspt.org	No	Yes (certified phlebotomy technician [CPT])	Yes
National Accrediting Agency for Clinical Laboratory Sciences (NAACLS) 5600 N. River Rd., Suite 720 Rosemont, IL 60018-5119 (773) 714-8880 www.naacls.org	Yes	No	No
National Center for Competency Testing (NCCT) 7007 College Blvd, Suite 385 Overland Park, KS 66211 (800) 875-4404 www.ncctinc.com	No	Yes	No
National Healthcareer Association (NHA) 11161 Overbrook Rd. Leawood, KS 66211 (800) 499-9092 www.nhanow.com	No	Yes (CPT)	Yes

Continued

TABLE 1-1	Organizations That Provide Accreditation, Certification, or Continuing Education—cont'd		
Name	Accredits or Approves Training Programs	Certifies Phlebotomists (Title Awarded)	Offers Continuing Education Units
National Phlebotomy Association (NPA) 1901 Brightseat Rd. Landover, MD 20785 (301) 386-4200 *www.nationalphlebotomy.org*	No	Yes	No

Nevada

In Nevada, you must present a high school diploma or equivalency degree. You must also be certified by one of two national certification agencies (either the ASCP or the AMT) or complete at least 6 months of training under the supervision of a state-approved practitioner. For the purposes of the application, phlebotomists are classified as either Office Lab Assistants (if you work in a physician's private practice) or Lab Assistants (if you work in an independent licensed laboratory, a hospital, or other facility serving more than a single physician's patients).

Washington

As of July 2013, phlebotomists in the state of Washington must obtain certification from the state as a "Medical Assistant–Phlebotomist." This is not to be confused with a medical assistant who has completed a training program specific to medical assistants. A Medical Assistant–Phlebotomist is trained specifically in the field of phlebotomy. Requirements for licensure as a Medical Assistant–Phlebotomist include a high school diploma or equivalency degree; the ability to read, write, and converse in English; 7 hours of acquired immunodeficiency syndrome (AIDS) education; and proof of appropriate training in phlebotomy. Acceptable proof includes one of the following: a transcript indicating successful completion of a phlebotomy program through an accredited postsecondary school, a statement from a health care practitioner that he or she supervised your training, or a transcript indicating you received phlebotomy education and training in the military.

Continuing Education

Certification programs usually require phlebotomists to participate in continuing education programs and

earn a certain number of **continuing education units (CEUs)** to remain certified. These programs provide updates on new information, regulations, and techniques and help phlebotomists refresh skills that are used less frequently. Larger health care institutions often sponsor such programs on site. As shown in Table 1-1, the organizations that provide continuing education are the AMT, the American Society for Clinical Laboratory Science (ASCLS), the ASCP, the ASPT, and the NPA.

LEGAL ISSUES IN PHLEBOTOMY

As in every other profession, phlebotomy is bound by laws and regulations governing the workplace, relations with customers (patients), and the privacy of privileged information, such as medical records. Failure to observe these laws and regulations may be cause for dismissal and may lead to a lawsuit against you or your institution. These issues are covered in more detail in Chapter 19. Here, we stress the two most important legal aspects of the phlebotomist's profession: informed consent and confidentiality.

> FLASH FORWARD

Legal issues are discussed in more detail in Chapter 19.

Informed Consent

Informed consent means that a patient must be informed of intended treatments and their risks before they are performed. For the phlebotomist, this means that the patient must understand that blood is to be drawn and must consent to that procedure before the phlebotomist may proceed. The patient has the right to refuse any medical treatment, including phlebotomy procedures requested by the physician. When a patient refuses, follow your institution's policy to ensure that the patient's physician is notified promptly. This usually involves notifying the patient's nurse, who will then notify the physician.

Confidentiality

All information regarding a patient's condition, including the types of tests ordered or the results of those tests, is confidential medical information. For the phlebotomist, this means that information regarding a patient should never be discussed with a coworker who is not involved in that patient's treatment. Discussions should never occur in common rooms or public areas, such as elevators, hallways, waiting rooms, or cafeterias. Furthermore, a phlebotomist should never discuss patients with their own friends and family.

Health Insurance Portability and Accountability Act

The privacy of medical information is covered by the Health Insurance Portability and Accountability Act (HIPAA), a law that went into effect in 1996. Under HIPAA, medical institutions must have procedures in place to actively protect the confidentiality of a patient's **protected health information (PHI)**. PHI includes any information about the patient's name, address, contact information, race, health status, treatment, or payment for health care. It may be in written, oral, or electronic forms. PHI is present on requisitions, labels, and other patient-specific materials.

As a phlebotomist, you will have access to some elements of a patient's PHI, and you are responsible for helping to protect the confidentiality of that information. That means, among other things, you must not discuss PHI with anyone who is not authorized to have access to it. For instance, you must not discuss a patient's health condition or treatment with a coworker who is not part of the patient's treatment team. Similarly, you must not have such discussions with family members or friends outside of work. If you are working at a computer screen displaying PHI, you must take care to prevent members of the public from viewing it. If you are carrying a stack of requisitions during your hospital rounds, as you enter a patient's room, you must ensure that the PHI of another patient is not visible.

REVIEW FOR CERTIFICATION

The modern professional phlebotomist must display technical, organizational, and interpersonal skills. The ability to communicate effectively with patients, the public, and coworkers is critical. Phlebotomy can be a stressful profession, and it is important to remain professionally detached even while showing compassion and care for all patients.

Phlebotomy training occurs at institutions that have received accreditation from one or more national agencies. After completing course work and practical training, the phlebotomist is eligible to take a national examination and receive certification from a national phlebotomy organization. Continuing education is often required to maintain certification. California, Louisiana, Nevada, and Washington have state licensure requirements.

Significant legal issues in phlebotomy include confidentiality and informed consent. The phlebotomist should never disclose information about a patient to third parties who are not involved in the patient's care. Every patient has the right to refuse treatment, including the withdrawal of blood. HIPAA regulates protected health information. The phlebotomist must ensure the confidentiality of PHI under his or her control.

BIBLIOGRAPHY

Clutterbuck H: *On the proper administration of bloodletting, for the prevention and cure of disease*, London, 1840. Excerpts retrieved from www.iupui.edu/~histwhs/h364.dir/Clutterbuck.html.

Ernst DJ: States fail to follow California's lead in certifying phlebotomists. *Medical Laboratory Observer,* 2009. Retrieved from www.entrepreneur.com/tradejournals/article/182040780.html.

Laboratory Field Services/DHS: *Phlebotomy certification* [in California], 2014. Retrieved from www.cdph.ca.gov/programs/lfs/Pages/Phlebotomist.aspx.

Louisiana Licensure Regulations: Retrieved from http://louisiana.gov/Services/POLicenses.

McPherson RA, Pincus MR: *Henry's clinical diagnosis and management by laboratory methods,* ed. 22, Philadelphia, 2012, Saunders.

Mitchell J, Haroun L: *Introduction to healthcare,* ed. 3, Clifton Park, N.Y., 2012, Delmar Cengage Learning.

Murdock SS, Murdock JR: From leeches to luers: The history of phlebotomy, *Journal of Medical Technology* 4(5), 1987.

Nevada Licensure Regulations: Retrieved from www.leg.state.nv.us/NRS/NRS-652.html#NRS652Sec127.

WHAT WOULD YOU DO?

Maintaining a professional appearance is part of what it means to be a professional phlebotomist. Dress codes may vary, but most institutions will not look kindly on any flamboyant aspect of personal appearance, including piercings, tattoos, revealing dress, or unusual hair colors. Artificial nails can interfere with your performance of your job, and broken nails can harbor infection. So if you want this job, you will need to do your best from the first day to meet the expectations of your employer, including for your appearance. You can remove the nails, take the piercings out while you are work, and cover up the tattoos so they are not visible. Do not wait to be told by your new employer—show up on the first day ready to be a part of the medical profession in every respect.

STUDY QUESTIONS

See answers in Appendix F.

1. Define phlebotomy.
2. List the six steps of routine blood collection.
3. Besides drawing blood samples, what other skills may a phlebotomist be trained to perform?
4. Define certification.
5. Explain the purpose of CEUs.
6. List three organizations that provide accreditation for phlebotomy programs.
7. List three organizations that provide certification for phlebotomists.
8. Why would a phlebotomist wish to become a member of a professional organization?
9. What is informed consent?
10. Describe two actions that would violate HIPAA's regulation of protected health information.
11. Describe some of the ancient phlebotomy practices and their uses.
12. Describe modern-day phlebotomy practices, their use in modern health care, and their similarities to ancient phlebotomy practices.
13. List and explain at least four responsibilities in the phlebotomist's job-related duties.
14. List at least four of the required personal characteristics of the phlebotomist.
15. Explain which one of the preceding four personal characteristics you feel is the most important to possess.
16. List the two most important legal aspects of the phlebotomist's profession.

CERTIFICATION EXAMINATION PREPARATION

See answers in Appendix F.

1. Phlebotomy skills would not include
   a. organization.
   b. handling patient correspondence.
   c. interpersonal skills.
   d. being able to handle stress.

2. The monitoring system for institutions that train phlebotomists is known as
   a. certification.
   b. accreditation.
   c. licensure.
   d. CEUs.

3. Once certified, what must a phlebotomist earn to ensure continued certification?
   a. CEUs
   b. Licensing points
   c. Accreditation
   d. A degree

4. Informed consent means
   a. patients must ask their physicians if they can have blood drawn.
   b. patients waive their rights.
   c. patients must be informed of intended treatments and their risks before they are performed.
   d. the phlebotomist may draw a patient's blood without the patient's permission.

5. Which characteristic is not a required personal characteristic of a professional phlebotomist?
   a. Dependability
   b. Honesty
   c. Compassion
   d. Sense of humor

6. When a patient in the hospital refuses to have blood drawn, the phlebotomist should
   a. persuade the patient to comply.
   b. perform the phlebotomy.
   c. notify a family member.
   d. notify the patient's nurse to ensure that the physician or other ordering practitioner is notified promptly.

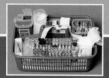

Phlebotomists may be employed in a variety of health care settings, including health maintenance organizations, clinics, urgent care centers, nursing homes, hospital laboratories, and physician office laboratories. Many phlebotomists, however, work in the clinical laboratory of a hospital. The various departments within the clinical laboratory are all involved in the analysis of patient samples, whether blood, urine, or other body fluids or tissues. To be accredited, all clinical laboratories must meet standards set by a variety of national organizations. In this chapter, you will learn about the organizational structures found in hospitals, how the phlebotomist fits into the larger health care environment, and how each department in the laboratory works with others to provide the many services offered.

OUTLINE

Hospital Organization
Fiscal and Information Services
Support Services
Nursing Services
Professional Services
Introduction to the Clinical Laboratory
Personnel
Anatomical and Surgical Pathology Area

Clinical Pathology Area
Functions of the Clinical Pathology Laboratory Departments
Blood Bank or Immunohematology
Chemistry
Specimen Processing
Coagulation and Hemostasis
Hematology
Microbiology

Molecular Diagnostics
Serology or Immunology
Urinalysis and Clinical Microscopy
Phlebotomy
Referrals
Standards and Accreditation for the Clinical Laboratory
Other Health Care Settings
Review for Certification

OBJECTIVES

After completing this chapter, you should be able to:

1. Describe the overall structure of a typical hospital.
2. Explain the roles of each of the following hospital branches, and list the kinds of jobs included:
   a. Fiscal and information services
   b. Support services
   c. Nursing services
   d. Professional services
3. Describe the departments and functions of the professional services branch of the hospital.
4. List the personnel who may work in the laboratory.
5. Describe the functions of the anatomic and surgical pathology laboratory.
6. List the major departments of the clinical laboratory.
7. Describe the kinds of samples typically analyzed and the kinds of tests that may be performed in each of the following clinical laboratory sections:
   a. Hematology
   b. Coagulation and hemostasis

   c. Chemistry
   d. Specimen
   e. Microbiology
   f. Urinalysis and clinical microscopy
   g. Serology or immunology
   h. Blood bank or immunohematology
   i. Molecular diagnostics
   j. Referrals
8. Explain the role of molecular diagnostics and flow cytometry in laboratory testing.
9. Explain how laboratory quality is monitored, and list at least four organizations that are involved in ensuring quality laboratory testing.
10. Describe other health care settings where a phlebotomist may work.

KEY TERMS

anatomical and surgical
  pathology area
autologous donation
blood bank
blood type
centrifuge
chemistry panel
Clinical and Laboratory
  Standards Institute (CLSI)
Clinical Lab Improvement
  Act of 1988 (CLIA '88)
clinical laboratory

clinical pathology area
coagulation
College of American
  Pathologists (CAP)
complete blood count
  (CBC)
culture and sensitivity
  (C&S) test
flow cytometry
forensic
health maintenance
  organization (HMO)

hemolyzed
hemostasis
icteric
immunochemistry
immunohematology
The Joint Commission
lipemic
molecular diagnostics
nursing home
physician office
  laboratory (POL)

preferred provider organization (PPO)
professional services
reagent
reference laboratory
serum separator tube
stat
urgent care center

ABBREVIATIONS

2-hr PPBS 2-hour postprandial blood sugar
AIDS acquired immunodeficiency syndrome
ALP alkaline phosphatase
ALT alanine aminotransferase
ANA antinuclear antibodies
aPTT activated partial thromboplastin time
AST aspartate aminotransferase
BMP basic metabolic panel
BUN blood urea nitrogen
C&S culture and sensitivity
CAP College of American Pathologists
CBC complete blood count
CCU cardiac care unit
CK creatine kinase
CK-MB creatine kinase-MB
CLIA '88 Clinical Laboratory Improvement Act of 1988
CLSI Clinical and Laboratory Standards Institute
CMP comprehensive metabolic panel
CNA certified nursing assistant
CT computed tomography
diff differential
DNA deoxyribonucleic acid
EDTA ethylenediaminetetraacetic acid
ER, ED emergency room, emergency department
ESR erythrocyte sedimentation rate
FBS fasting blood sugar
FDP fibrin degradation product
GTT glucose tolerance test
hCG human chorionic gonadotropin
Hct hematocrit
HDL high-density lipoprotein
Hb hemoglobin
Hb A$_{1c}$ glycated hemoglobin/glycosylated hemoglobin
HIV human immunodeficiency virus

HMO health maintenance organization
ICU intensive care unit
INR international normalized ratio
IV intravenous
LDL low-density lipoprotein
LIS laboratory information services
LPN licensed practical nurse
MCH mean corpuscular hemoglobin
MCHC mean corpuscular hemoglobin concentration
MCV mean corpuscular volume
MIS manager of information services
MLS medical laboratory scientist
MLTs medical laboratory technicians
MPV mean platelet volume
MRI magnetic resonance imaging
MTs medical technologists
NICU neonatal intensive care unit
NSY nursery
OR operating room
PCA patient care assistant
PCT patient care technician
PET positron emission tomography
Plt platelets
POLs physician office laboratories
PPOs preferred provider organizations
PT prothrombin time
RBCs red blood cells
RDW red blood cell distribution width
RN registered nurse
RPR rapid plasma reagin
SST serum separator tube
STAT short turnaround time
TDM therapeutic drug monitoring
WBCs white blood cells

WHAT WOULD YOU DO?

It's your third week on your new job as a phlebotomist at Green Hills Hospital. Your supervisor has been showing you the rounds, observing your technique, and helping you learn the routine, but today you are on your own. Your first three blood draws go just fine, but they took longer than you expected. You are now on your fourth patient, and there is a problem. Your instructions were to draw the sample by 7:30 AM, but it's now 7:45 AM and you are just getting started. If the blood sample isn't drawn, the patient may not be ready for his treatment later that morning. Should you take the sample even though it is after the specified time and just label it 7:30 AM?

HOSPITAL ORGANIZATION

The hospital laboratory in which a phlebotomist works is one part of a large organization. Organization of the hospital may vary, with larger hospitals having more complex and varied structures than smaller hospitals (Figure 2-1). The chief of staff oversees the medical staff. The hospital administrator oversees the central administration of the hospital. The hospital administrator also oversees the various branches of support personnel. These are divided into several branches, typically fiscal and information services, support services, nursing services, and professional services. Professional services include

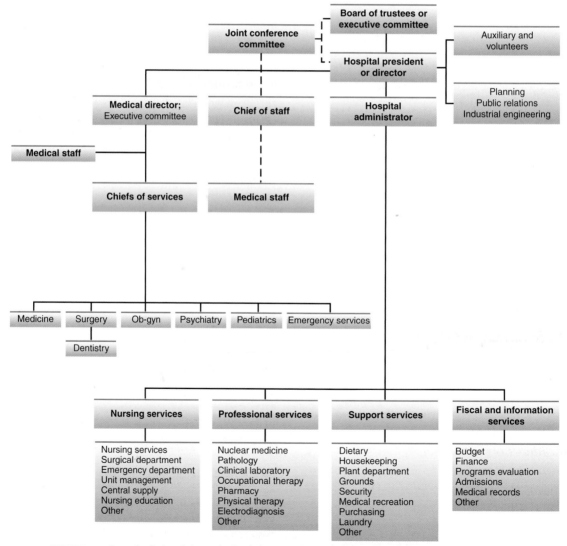

FIGURE 2-1 Example of a hospital organizational chart. (Modified from Hupp J, Tucker M, Ellis: *Contemporary oral and maxillofacial surgery,* ed. 6, St. Louis, 2014, Mosby.)

the clinical laboratory in which the phlebotomist works and are discussed in detail later.

Fiscal and Information Services

This branch is responsible for admissions and medical records, as well as for billing, accounting, and other financial aspects of the hospital. Human resources may be a part of this branch as well.

Support Services

This branch includes all aspects of the physical plant of the hospital, such as cleaning, maintenance, and security, as well as food service and purchasing.

Nursing Services

Nursing services personnel provide direct care to patients. Phlebotomists have a great deal of direct contact with nursing personnel. Some nursing services departments have their own phlebotomy team. Nursing services include a range of people with various levels of education and training, including the registered nurse (RN), licensed practical nurse (LPN), certified nursing assistant (CNA), patient care technician (PCT) or patient care assistant (PCA), and ward clerk or unit secretary. Nursing staff are divided among a number of units within the hospital, depending on the size of the institution. The most common divisions are the emergency room (ER) or emergency department (ED), operating room (OR), intensive care unit (ICU), cardiac care unit (CCU), nursery (NSY), maternity, pediatrics, and labor and delivery, as well as inpatient floors for medical, surgical, and psychiatric patients. Larger hospitals have specialty units such as neonatal intensive care unit (NICU), neurology, and pulmonology units. Nurses can also hold positions such as case managers, discharge planners, and other specialized service providers within the hospital.

Professional Services

Professional services personnel provide services at the request of licensed practitioners (including physicians and nurse practitioners) who aid in the diagnosis and treatment of patients. Each department provides specialized services.

Cardiac Catheterization

This department evaluates and treats patients with cardiovascular disease by inserting devices into the bloodstream that are threaded up to the heart.

FLASH FORWARD

You will learn more about these devices in Chapter 12.

Clinical Laboratory

The clinical laboratory analyzes samples from patients at the request of physicians or other licensed health care personnel. The samples may be blood, urine, or other body fluids, or they may be cells from aspiration procedures or pieces of tissue from biopsies. Results of these tests are used for making a diagnosis, monitoring treatment, or determining a patient's prognosis. A more detailed discussion of the clinical laboratory is presented later in this chapter.

Nuclear Medicine

This department uses radioisotopes to perform tests and treat diseases. Radioisotopes are unstable forms of certain elements that can be detected as they break down. They are often used as tracers; when injected into a patient's bloodstream, they can be tracked to reveal the structure and function of internal organs. In large doses, radioisotopes can be used to destroy cancerous tissue.

Occupational Therapy

Occupational therapists assess patients and design adaptive aids or compensatory strategies to help people with physical or mental impairments perform tasks of daily living and reach their maximum potential.

Pharmacy

The pharmacy prepares and dispenses drugs that have been prescribed by physicians.

Physical Therapy

Physical therapists assess patients both before and after treatment and devise plans of physical treatment. Physical therapists design exercises, stretching programs, and other physical treatments to aid in a patient's rehabilitation after injury or illness.

Radiation Therapy

The radiation therapy department also treats cancer, using x-rays or other high-energy radiation sources to destroy tumors.

Radiology or Medical Imaging

The radiologist interprets a range of diagnostic and therapeutic procedures using various forms of radiant energy. The radiologic technologist obtains radiographs, computed tomography (CT) scans, magnetic resonance imaging (MRI) scans, positron emission tomography (PET) scans, and fluoroscopy images.

Respiratory Therapy

Respiratory therapists provide treatment for respiratory disorders. They often perform arterial punctures for the determination of arterial blood gas measurements.

> **FLASH FORWARD**
> You will learn about arterial blood collection in Chapter 13.

INTRODUCTION TO THE CLINICAL LABORATORY

The clinical laboratory is divided into two main areas: the **anatomical and surgical pathology area**, which analyzes the characteristics of cells and tissues, and the **clinical pathology area**, which analyzes blood and other body fluids. The phlebotomist works in the clinical pathology area of the clinical laboratory.

Personnel

The clinical laboratory is usually under the supervision of a pathologist, who is a physician with special training in laboratory analysis of tissues and fluids or a physician who has a minimum of 2 years' experience directing or supervising high complexity testing or a one who holds an earned doctorate in chemical, physical, biological, or clinical laboratory science from an accredited institution. A laboratory manager directs the administrative functions of the laboratory, including hiring personnel. Management staff may include a manager of information services (MIS) and a laboratory information services (LIS) coordinator. Section supervisors supervise personnel, monitor equipment maintenance, and monitor test results. Medical laboratory scientists (MLSs) or medical laboratory technicians (MLTs) run routine tests, perform equipment maintenance, and collect specimens. MLSs have bachelor of science degrees in clinical laboratory science–medical technology, whereas MLTs have associate's degrees. The American Society for Clinical Pathology now assigns the title Medical Laboratory Scientist (MLS) to both MT and clinical laboratory technician positions. Phlebotomists collect blood specimens for analysis in the laboratory. Phlebotomists obtain certification from a nationally recognized certifying agency.

Anatomic and Surgical Pathology Area

This area is usually divided into three sections, or departments.

Cytogenetics

The cytogenetics department examines chromosomes for evidence of genetic disease, such as Down syndrome.

Cytopathology

The cytology department processes and stains cells that are shed into body fluids or removed from tissue with a needle (aspiration) and examines them for the presence of cancer or other diseases. The cytotechnologist assists in this work. One of the most common tests performed in cytology is the Pap smear.

Histology

The histology department prepares tissues from autopsy, surgery, or biopsy for microscopic examination by a pathologist. Special stains are used to highlight particular cell morphology. The histotechnologist helps prepare samples for the pathologist to examine.

Clinical Pathology Area

Blood and other body fluids can be analyzed in a number of ways, and the divisions within the clinical pathology area reflect these differences. The number of sections in this area depends on the size of the hospital. In some laboratories, some functions may be combined. The clinical departments in a typical laboratory are as follows:

- Blood banking or immunohematology
- Chemistry
- Specimen processing
- Coagulation and hemostasis
- Hematology
- Flow cytometry
- Microbiology
- Molecular diagnostics
- Serology or immunology
- Urinalysis and clinical microscopy
- Phlebotomy
- Referrals

FUNCTIONS OF THE CLINICAL PATHOLOGY LABORATORY DEPARTMENTS

Blood Bank or Immunohematology

The **blood bank** or **immunohematology** department deals with blood used for transfusions. Blood is tested there to identify the blood type of both patient and donor blood to determine their compatibility. Compatibility testing is performed to ensure that the patient's immune system does not reject the donor blood.

Specimens for this department are drawn in a plain red-top tube or a special pink-top tube containing a chemical called ethylenediaminetetraacetic acid (EDTA). The strictest attention must be paid to patient identification and sample labeling. A fatal transfusion reaction may occur if either patient identification or labeling are incorrect.

Blood type is determined by the presence and type of particular antigens on the surface of red blood cells (RBCs). In routine blood typing, two major antigen groups are tested for: the ABO group and the Rh group. In addition, dozens of other antigens can be determined to improve the match and prevent adverse transfusion reactions. This is important for patients receiving multiple transfusions over a lifetime, such as for leukemia or anemia.

In compatibility testing, patient serum is mixed with donor RBCs to look for clumping of cells, caused by a reaction between the patient's antibodies and the antigens on the donor cells. If clumping is seen, the donor blood cannot be used. Patients can also donate their own blood for use later, called **autologous donation**. This is often done several weeks before a patient is scheduled for surgery.

The blood bank department may also process donated blood to obtain blood components. Blood is donated and handled by the unit, which is equivalent to a pint. With use of a centrifuge, blood can be separated in several ways to obtain the following components:

- Packed cells, consisting of RBCs, white blood cells (WBCs), and platelets, without plasma
- Fresh frozen plasma, collected from a unit of blood and immediately frozen
- Platelets, harvested from several units of blood and combined in a single packet
- Cryoprecipitate, the component of fresh plasma that has clotting factors

Each of these has specific uses. For instance, cryoprecipitate may be used for patients with clotting disorders.

FLASH FORWARD

You will learn about blood bank collections in Chapter 14.

Chemistry

The chemistry department performs a range of tests on the chemical components of blood. Chemistry tests may be performed as either single tests or as groups, called **chemistry panels**. The most common tests and panels are shown in Table 2-1. The

TABLE 2-1	Common Chemistry Tests and Panels
Test or Panel	**Purpose**
Basic Metabolic Panel (BMP) • Blood urea nitrogen (BUN) • Calcium • Creatinine • Electrolytes • Glucose	Is used as a general metabolic screen
Coronary Risk or Lipid Panel • Cholesterol • High-density lipoprotein (HDL) • Low-density lipoprotein (LDL) • Triglycerides	Assesses risk for heart disease
Electrolytes • Bicarbonate • Chloride (Cl^-) • Potassium (K^+) • Sodium (Na^+)	Evaluates levels of ions in the blood
General Health or Comprehensive Metabolic Panel (CMP) • Alkaline phosphatase (ALP) • Aspartate aminotransferase (AST) • Bilirubin • BMP • Total protein or albumin	Assesses the overall health standard of the patient
Glucose • 2-Hour postprandial blood sugar (2-hr PPBS) • Fasting blood sugar (FBS) • Glucose tolerance test (GTT) • Glycolated hemoglobin (Hb A_{lc})	Assesses risk for diabetes mellitus (elevated levels indicate diabetes mellitus)
Liver Function Panel • Alanine aminotransferase (ALT) • Albumin • ALP • AST • Bilirubin—conjugated • Bilirubin—total • Globulin • Total protein	Assesses liver function
Myocardial Infarction • Creatine kinase (CK) • Creatine kinase-MB (CK-MB) • Troponin I	Determines the occurrence and timing of a myocardial infarction
Renal Disease • Albumin • Creatinine clearance • Phosphorus	Assesses kidney function

panels are used to screen for a variety of diseases or assess general wellness in patients.

General types of tests performed include toxicology, immunochemistry, and electrophoresis. Toxicology tests analyze plasma for levels of drugs and poisons. These tests are used for therapeutic drug monitoring (TDM), identification of illegal drugs, and detection of lead and other toxic substances. Immunochemistry tests use antibodies to detect a range of substances in the blood. Electrophoresis separates chemical components of blood based on differences in electrical charge. Electrophoresis is most often used to analyze hemoglobin, enzymes, and other proteins.

Most tests are automated, and advances in the instruments used to perform these tests allow them to be run using very small samples. In many cases, this means that less blood is needed from the patient, which can decrease patient discomfort significantly. For patients who require frequent blood monitoring, it can also reduce the chance of developing anemia. The clinical pathology laboratory must keep records of the amount of blood drawn from each patient.

> ### CLINICAL TIP
>
> Always determine the specimen volume requirements of tests requested by the physician.

> ### FLASH FORWARD
>
> You will learn how to determine collection volumes for newborns and infants in Chapter 12.

Specimen Processing

Chemistry tests are performed on either serum or plasma. Serum is collected in a tube without anticoagulants (a plain red-top tube) or in a **serum separator tube (SST)**. Plain red-top tubes need 45 to 60 minutes for full clot activation, and an SST needs a minimum of 30 minutes. When results are needed quickly (a **stat,** or short turnaround time requisition), blood can be collected in a tube with clot activators. After clotting, serum is separated out by centrifugation. A **centrifuge** spins the sample at high speeds to separate components based on density (Figure 2-2). Plasma, which is also used for stat results, is collected with the anticoagulants heparin sodium or sodium fluoride in the tube. These anticoagulants prevent blood from clotting, allowing for

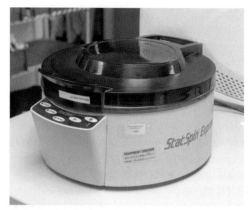

FIGURE 2-2 A centrifuge spins samples at high speeds.

immediate centrifugation, which shortens the TAT (turnaround time) for reporting the test results.

> ### FLASH FORWARD
>
> You will learn more about serum and plasma in Chapter 7.

Serum is normally a clear, pale yellow fluid. The color and appearance of the serum sample can be altered by both the patient's condition and the collection technique. Liver disease can increase the amount of bilirubin in the serum, making it appear a darker yellow (called **icteric** serum). Recent ingestion of fats or other lipids can make the sample cloudy (**lipemic** serum). Hemolysis, or breakage of RBCs, can give the serum a pink tinge (**hemolyzed** serum). Hemolysis may occur as a result of a poorly performed draw. Many laboratory tests measure the substance of interest by photometry, in which the substance is reacted with other chemicals to form a colored solution whose intensity is detected by passing light through the sample. If the original sample is degraded by hemolysis or other contamination, however, the results of photometry tests can be erroneous.

Serum quality can also be affected by post-collection handling procedures. Some samples must be chilled during transport, whereas others must be protected from light. Some tests must be performed within 1 hour of collection.

> ### FLASH FORWARD
>
> You will learn more about special specimen handling procedures in Chapters 14 and 16.

Chemistry tests are also performed on other body fluids, such as urine, cerebrospinal fluid, and synovial fluid (from joints).

Coagulation and Hemostasis

This department is usually part of the hematology department, but it may be separate in larger hospitals.

Hemostasis refers to the process by which the body stops blood from leaking out of a wound. Hemostasis involves coagulation and other processes. Coagulation depends on the presence of clotting factors and platelets.

Coagulation tests are performed on plasma (Box 2-1). Coagulation studies (samples) are collected in a tube containing the anticoagulant citrate, which preserves the coagulation factors better than other anticoagulants do. Coagulation tests are most often performed to monitor anticoagulant therapy, for instance, in a patient who has had a thrombotic stroke, heart attack, or thrombophlebitis. Drugs to prevent the formation of clots help avoid the recurrence of stroke, but the dosage must be adjusted to allow a minimal level of clotting and uncontrolled bleeding. The activated partial thromboplastin time (aPTT) is used to monitor intravenous (IV) heparin therapy, and the prothrombin time/protime (PT) and international normalized ratio (INR) are used to monitor oral warfarin (Coumadin) therapy. These tests aid in the diagnosis of a variety of clotting disorders, including hemophilia (Figure 2-3). The assays for specific clotting factors determine deficiencies and abnormalities.

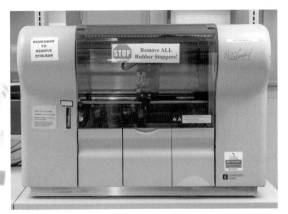

FIGURE 2-3 Automated coagulation instrument.

Hematology

The hematology department analyzes blood for evidence of diseases affecting the blood-forming tissues and the cells produced by those tissues— namely, RBCs, WBCs, and thrombocytes/platelets (Plt). This department also analyzes the clotting ability of the blood.

> **FLASH FORWARD**
>
> You will learn about the composition and function of blood in Chapter 7.

Hematology tests are most often performed on whole blood, which is blood that has not coagulated (clotted). To prevent the blood from clotting after it is collected from the patient, the blood is drawn into a tube containing an anticoagulant (usually EDTA). Thus the blood cells remain freely suspended in the liquid component of the blood, just as they are inside the body.

> **FLASH FORWARD**
>
> You will learn about hemostasis in Chapter 7.

> **FLASH FORWARD**
>
> You will learn about anticoagulants and other tube additives in Chapter 8.

In the hematology laboratory, blood is analyzed in a computer-controlled instrument that counts and identifies the various types of cells (Figure 2-4). The most common hematology test is the complete blood count (CBC). This automated test includes a hemoglobin (Hb) determination, hematocrit (Hct), WBC count, RBC count, and platelet count. It may also include a WBC differential (diff), which determines

---

BOX 2-1	**Coagulation Tests**

- *Activated partial thromboplastin time (aPTT):* Monitor heparin therapy, coagulation factor deficiency
- *D-Dimer:* Disseminated intravascular coagulation
- *Factor activity assays:* Coagulation factor deficiency
- *Fibrin degradation product (FDP):* Disseminated intravascular coagulation
- *Fibrinogen:* Risk of cardiovascular disease
- *International normalized ratio (INR):* Monitor coumadin therapy
- *Prothrombin time/protime (PT):* Coagulation factor deficiency
- *Thrombin time:* Heparin-like anticoagulants, antibody inhibitors of thrombin

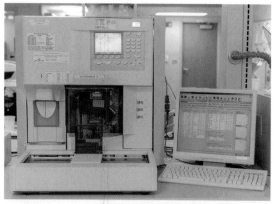

FIGURE 2-4 In the hematology laboratory, blood is analyzed by a computer-controlled instrument.

the kinds of WBCs present. Among other applications, the CBC is used to diagnose and classify types of anemia, leukemia, infectious diseases, and other conditions that affect the number and types of blood cells. The complete list of tests included in the CBC is given in Table 2-2. Other common hematology tests are listed in Table 2-3.

FLASH FORWARD

You will learn about the types of blood cells in Chapter 7.

Flow cytometry is a special analytic technique that is used in hematology, immunology, and anatomic pathology. Flow cytometry identifies cellular markers on the surface of WBCs. This is done to determine lymphocyte subclasses in patients with acquired immunodeficiency syndrome (AIDS), as a measure of the disease process, and to determine CD4/CD8 ratios of helper to suppressor cells, as a means of tracking the health of patients infected with human immunodeficiency virus (HIV). It is also used to diagnose and classify malignancies, aiding in the development of treatment plans. Either whole blood or bone marrow specimens are used to perform this testing.

FLASH FORWARD

You will learn about special patient populations, including patients with HIV, in Chapter 12.

TABLE 2-2   Complete Blood Count

Test	Purpose
White blood cell (WBC) count	Counts the number of WBCs in a sample of known volume
Red blood cell (RBC) count	Counts the number of RBCs in a sample of known volume
Hemoglobin (Hb)	Measures the level of Hb in the blood as a whole; this determines the oxygen-carrying capacity
Hematocrit (Hct)	Measures the percentage of blood volume attributable to RBCs
Mean platelet volume (MPV)	Assesses platelet volume and size
Mean corpuscular volume (MCV)	Determines the size of the average RBC
Mean corpuscular hemoglobin (MCH)	Measures the average amount of Hb in an RBC
Mean corpuscular hemoglobin concentration (MCHC)	Assesses the ratio of Hb to the size of the RBC
Red cell distribution width (RDW)	Determines the range of sizes of RBCs
Platelet count (Plt)	Counts the number of platelets in a sample of known volume
Differential (diff)	Classifies and counts the types of WBCs; morphologic (shape) abnormalities of RBCs or platelets detected by the analyzer can be checked by manual examination of a blood smear under a microscope

TABLE 2-3   Other Hematology Tests

Test	Purpose
Body fluid analysis	Determines the number and types of cells in body fluids
Bone marrow	Determines the number and types of cells in bone marrow
Erythrocyte sedimentation rate (ESR)	Determines sedimentation rate of red blood cells (RBCs) as a test for inflammation
Reticulocyte count	Evaluates bone marrow delivery of RBCs into the peripheral circulation
Sickle cell (solubility test)	Determines whether RBCs containing hemoglobin S are present; used to diagnose sickle cell anemia

Microbiology

The microbiology department isolates and identifies pathogenic microorganisms in patient samples and is responsible for infection control in the health care institution. The department also determines a pathogenic organism's susceptibility to specific antibiotic treatments. Microbiology comprises bacteriology (the study of bacteria), mycology (the study of fungi), parasitology (the study of parasites), and virology (the study of viruses). Specimens to be tested include blood, urine, throat swabs, sputum, feces, pus, and other body fluids.

FLASH FORWARD
Collection of blood cultures is discussed in Chapter 14, and nonblood samples are covered in Chapter 15.

The most common microbiology tests are **culture and sensitivity (C&S) tests**, which detect and identify microorganisms and determine the most effective antibiotic therapy. Bacteria are identified by their nutritional requirements and by the staining characteristics (shape and color) detected with Gram stain. Results are usually available in 24 to 48 hours. Identification of fungi usually takes much longer, because they take longer to grow in culture.

Molecular Diagnostics

Molecular diagnostics testing is used to diagnose genetic disorders, analyze forensic evidence, track disease, and identify microbiologic pathogens. At the heart of these techniques is the analysis of the deoxyribonucleic acid (DNA) in the sample. In the clinical laboratory, molecular diagnostic techniques are used most commonly to identify infectious agents, such as HIV, and genetic diseases, such as cystic fibrosis; to test for parentage; and to perform **forensic** studies on criminal evidence. Specimens analyzed include blood, body fluids, skin cells, hair, and other body tissues that contain DNA. Special tubes and handling procedures are required for these specimens. The most important aspect of this type of test is to keep the sample free from contamination with DNA from other sources. Keeping the laboratory clean is important, and usually only authorized personnel are allowed entrance.

FLASH FORWARD
You will learn about specimen handling and processing in Chapter 16.

Serology or Immunology

The serology or immunology department evaluates the patient's immune response through the detection of antibodies. Antibodies are proteins that help fight infection by binding to surface molecules of the infective agent, called antigens (Table 2-4).

Antibodies are found in the serum; thus samples for serology testing are serum samples, collected in either a plain red-top tube or an SST. Antibodies may be formed in response to infection by microorganisms such as bacteria, fungi, parasites, or viruses. For example, the presence of antibodies against HIV is a sign of exposure to that virus. Similarly, antibodies are used to diagnose syphilis, hepatitis, infectious mononucleosis, and other communicable diseases. Antibodies may also form against antigens in the body's own tissues in a process called autoimmunity. Detection of such autoantibodies is part of the diagnostic process for systemic lupus erythematosus, for instance.

FLASH FORWARD
The immune system is discussed in Chapter 7.

Urinalysis and Clinical Microscopy

Urine is examined to assess kidney disease and metabolic disorders that alter the levels of substances in the urine. Diabetes, for instance, causes elevated glucose, and damage to the kidneys themselves may lead to protein in the urine. Many urinalysis tests are performed with plastic dipsticks with pads embedded with reagents that are dipped

TABLE 2-4 A Sample of Common Immunology Tests

Test	Purpose
Anti-*Haemophilus influenzae* B antibody	Detects exposure to *Haemophilus influenzae* B
Antinuclear antibodies (ANA)	Detects autoimmune disease
C-reactive protein	Detects inflammatory disease
Hepatitis B surface antigen	Detects hepatitis B infection
Human chorionic gonadotropin (hCG)	Detects pregnancy
Rapid plasma reagin (RPR)	Detects syphilis infection
Rheumatoid factor	Detects rheumatoid arthritis
T- and B-cell markers	Are used to quantify types of white blood cells (WBCs)

into the sample. The reagents (test chemicals) embedded in the pads change color, indicating the results of the test. The tests commonly performed on urine are shown in Table 2-5.

Feces may be examined for blood—called occult blood—as a screen for colorectal cancer. They are also examined for parasites and their ova (eggs). Other body fluids (e.g., spinal fluid and joint fluid) may also be analyzed in this section.

Phlebotomy

The phlebotomy department is responsible for collection of blood samples from inpatients and outpatients. The phlebotomist is also responsible for proper handling and timely delivery of samples to the laboratory for analysis. You will learn much more about all of these responsibilities in the coming chapters.

Referrals

The referrals department handles and ships specimens for any tests not done by the laboratory. These are usually newer tests that may require special equipment or training not available in the laboratory. Some of these tests are approved diagnostic tests, whereas others are used for research only. Physicians often call the referral department requesting information about a new and uncommon test. Referral personnel will do research to find a laboratory that performs the test so that the specimen can be sent to that laboratory. Frequently, a hospital laboratory will contract with a single, large, national, commercial laboratory to handle all of the tests not done in-house.

STANDARDS AND ACCREDITATION FOR THE CLINICAL LABORATORY

The clinical laboratory must meet rigorous performance standards to ensure the quality of its procedures and results. Congress passed the Clinical Laboratory Improvement Act of 1988 (CLIA '88), which mandated the regulation of all facilities that perform patient testing. Standards and guidelines are set by the Clinical and Laboratory Standards Institute (CLSI), a nonprofit organization formerly known as the National Committee for Clinical Laboratory Standards (NCCLS). Laboratories that meet these standards are eligible to receive accreditation from one or more agencies. Accreditation is required for the health care facility to receive Medicare or Medicaid reimbursement. The following agencies are involved in the accreditation of clinical laboratories:

- The Joint Commission: Laboratories must be inspected and accredited every 2 years. This organization was previously known as the Joint Commission on Accreditation of Healthcare Organizations, and you may still hear it referred to by its acronym JCAHO (pronounced "Jayco").
- College of American Pathologists (CAP): Inspection and accreditation occur every 2 years.

TABLE 2-5	Complete Urinalysis
Test	Purpose
Clarity	Detects crystalline and cellular elements
Color	Detects blood, bilirubin, and other pigments
Specific gravity	Measures urine concentration
Chemical Examination	
Bilirubin	Indicates liver disease when level is elevated
Blood	Detects red blood cells (RBCs) or hemoglobin
Glucose	Indicates diabetes mellitus when level is elevated
Ketones	Indicates diabetes mellitus or starvation when level is elevated
Leukocyte esterase	Detects white blood cells (WBCs)
Nitrite	Detects bacterial infection
pH	Determines the acidity of the urine
Protein	Indicates kidney disease when level is elevated
Urobilinogen	Indicates liver disease or hemolytic disorder when level is elevated
Microscopic Examination	
Cells and other structures	Detects WBCs, RBCs, epithelial cells, bacteria, yeast, and parasites; also detects crystals and casts (structures sloughed off renal tubules)

As of 2006, unannounced inspections occur within 6 months of the accreditation renewal date.
- State agencies: In states with their own licensure requirements, these agencies require laboratories to participate in proficiency testing and inspections.

OTHER HEALTH CARE SETTINGS

In addition to working in hospitals, phlebotomists may be employed in other health care settings, including the following:
- **Health maintenance organizations (HMOs):** HMOs have become major providers of health care in the past two decades. HMOs typically function as full-service outpatient clinics, providing most medical specialties under one roof.
- **Preferred provider organizations (PPOs):** A PPO is a group of doctors and hospitals that offer their services to large employers to provide health care to employees.
- **Urgent care center:** An urgent care center is an outpatient clinic that provides walk-in services to patients who cannot wait for scheduled appointments with their primary health care providers or who do not have a primary health care provider.
- **Physician office laboratories (POLs):** Physicians in a group practice may employ a phlebotomist to collect patient samples, which are then usually analyzed by a separate reference laboratory or, if the facility is large enough, in an on-site laboratory.
- **Reference laboratories and private testing laboratories:** These are independent laboratories that analyze samples from other health care facilities or from outpatients sent to the laboratory by their health care providers. The phlebotomist may travel to other facilities to obtain samples (mobile phlebotomy) or may collect samples on site.
- **Nursing homes:** Phlebotomists may be employed by a nursing home to obtain samples from clients for analysis by a reference laboratory.
- Blood donor services or health fairs: Phlebotomists may be hired to draw blood donations,

either in a stationary setting such as a clinic, or a mobile setting such as a Bloodmobile. Health fairs are mobile health services that move within a community to reach those who may not otherwise have access to them.

In any of these settings, you may be required to perform clerical tasks, such as patient registration or telephone follow-up. As always, you will be most successful in your career if you bring a high level of professionalism to your work, whatever the task you are performing. Exhibiting skill and care in performing these tasks shows you are able to handle multiple kinds of responsibilities, an ability that is highly valued by most employers.

REVIEW FOR CERTIFICATION

Most phlebotomists work in hospitals, in the clinical laboratory. The clinical laboratory is divided into two major sections: the anatomic and surgical pathology area and the clinical pathology area. Clinical pathology is further divided into a number of departments, each responsible for the analysis of one or more types of samples. Blood bank or immunohematology focuses on compatibility testing and blood storage. Chemistry measures the chemical composition of the fluid portion, coagulation and hemostasis is concerned with the coagulation process, and hematology analyzes the cells of the blood. Microbiology tests for bacterial and other infections. Molecular diagnostics analyzes DNA in a variety of tissues. Serology or immunology is concerned with elements of the immune response. Urinalysis and clinical microscopy is responsible for performing urine and feces analysis. Phlebotomy is responsible for collection and delivery of blood samples. Finally, the referrals department handles and ships specimens for any tests not done by the laboratory.

All clinical laboratories are monitored and accredited by one or more national organizations. Other health care settings in which the phlebotomist may work include HMOs, reference laboratories, urgent care centers, and nursing homes.

BIBLIOGRAPHY

Berger D: A brief history of medical diagnosis and the birth of the clinical laboratory, Parts 1 & 2, July 1999, *Medical Laboratory Observer*.

Butch S: Professional organizations: Part of the package, *Advance for Medical Laboratory Professionals,* 14(3): 173–182, February 28, 2000.

Doig K, Beck SJ, Kolenc K: CLT and CLS job responsibilities: Current distinctions and updates, *Clinical Laboratory Science,* 2001, Summer.

McPherson RA, Pincus MR: *Henry's clinical diagnosis and management by laboratory methods,* ed. 22, Philadelphia, 2012, Saunders.

Turgeon ML: *Linné & Ringsrud's clinical laboratory science: The basics and routine techniques,* ed. 7, St. Louis, 2016, Mosby.

WHAT WOULD YOU DO?

You should not take the sample. Instead, immediately inform the patient's nurse and your supervisor to determine what to do. It is possible that the physician ordering the sample will not want the sample if it is not drawn by the time specified, and taking an unnecessary sample increases the patient's discomfort and puts him at unnecessary risk. Most important, you should never alter the information on a sample to match what it "should" be—that puts the patient at even greater risk, because medical decisions may be made based on incorrect information. Honesty and integrity are vital to the practice of phlebotomy. You may be admonished for not taking the sample on time, but you will have done the right thing—making sure the patient has received the best possible care.

STUDY QUESTIONS

See answers in Appendix F.

1. Name the branches of support personnel in the hospital organizational system.

2. Name the two main areas of the laboratory, and identify which area the phlebotomist works in.

3. Name the specialty of the physician who oversees the laboratory.

4. Name two common laboratory tests performed in the coagulation department, and explain which therapy each test monitors.

5. Describe the tests the immunology department performs.

6. Define molecular diagnostics.

7. Name five liver function tests.

8. C&S testing is performed in which department?

9. Describe the significance of CLIA '88.

10. Name two organizations that accredit clinical laboratories.

11. What organization sets laboratory standards and guidelines?

12. Name four health care settings, besides the hospital, in which a phlebotomist may be employed.

13. Name the laboratory department that has a special specimen or patient identification system. What might be the outcome of mislabeling or mishandling specimens within this laboratory?

14. Describe the details the blood bank technologist looks for in compatibility testing to determine test results.

15. Define professional services, and give at least two examples of them.

CERTIFICATION EXAMINATION PREPARATION

See answers in Appendix F.

1. Fiscal services is responsible for
   a. cleaning and maintenance.
   b. performing tests.
   c. diagnosis and treatment of the patient.
   d. admitting, medical records, and billing.

2. In addition to the laboratory, the following department may draw arterial blood gases:
   a. physical therapy
   b. occupational therapy
   c. respiratory therapy
   d. radiology

3. The following department uses radioisotopes to perform tests:
   - a. respiratory therapy
   - b. cytogenetics
   - c. nuclear medicine
   - d. hematology

4. The clinical laboratory is typically under the direction of a
   - a. pathologist.
   - b. phlebotomist.
   - c. pharmacist.
   - d. medical assistant.

5. The analytic tool used to identify cell markers in HIV patients is
   - a. a syringe.
   - b. a flow cytometer.
   - c. an electrolyte.
   - d. a C&S test.

6. A CBC is performed in the _____ department.
   - a. chemistry
   - b. urinalysis
   - c. serology
   - d. hematology

7. aPTT testing monitors
   - a. chemotherapy.
   - b. physical therapy.
   - c. heparin therapy.
   - d. warfarin/coumadin therapy.

8. The type of chemistry test associated with drug analysis is known as
   - a. immunology.
   - b. cardiology.
   - c. toxicology.
   - d. electrophoresis.

9. The _____ department identifies pathogenic microorganisms in patient samples.
   - a. virology
   - b. microbiology
   - c. mycology
   - d. parasitology

10. A C&S test is analyzed in the _____ department.
    - a. microbiology
    - b. chemistry
    - c. hematology
    - d. urinalysis

11. Occult blood testing is performed on
    - a. plasma.
    - b. feces.
    - c. serum.
    - d. cerebrospinal fluid.

12. When patients donate their blood for use during their own surgery, this is known as
    - a. autologous donation.
    - b. platelet donation.
    - c. cryoprecipitate donation.
    - d. fresh frozen plasma donation.

13. Independent laboratories that analyze samples from other health care facilities are known as
    - a. physician office laboratories.
    - b. urgent care centers.
    - c. reference laboratories.
    - d. waived laboratories.

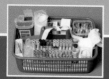

CHAPTER 3   Safety

Like any workplace, a hospital or other health care facility contains certain hazards that must be treated with caution and respect to prevent injury. These hazards include biological, physical, chemical, radioactive, electrical, and fire factors, as well as the most significant hazard involved in phlebotomy—sharps in the form of needles, lancets, and glass. Latex sensitivity is also a growing concern in the workplace. Here, we discuss the variety of potential hazards you may encounter and outline the proper precautions to take to prevent accidents or injuries. The Occupational Safety and Health Administration (OSHA) is the governmental agency responsible for workplace safety.

OUTLINE

Occupational Safety and Health
  Administration
Types of Safety Hazards
  Physical Hazards
  Sharps Hazards
  Chemical Hazards
  Radioactive Hazards

Electrical Hazards
Fire and Explosive Hazards
Magnetic Resonance Imaging
  Hazards
Emergency First-Aid Procedures
  Cardiopulmonary Resuscitation
  Bleeding Aid

First Aid for Shock
Disaster Emergency Plan
Sensitivity to Latex and Other
  Materials
  Preventing Latex Reactions
Review for Certification

OBJECTIVES

After completing this chapter, you should be able to:

1. Explain the role of the Occupational Safety and Health Administration (OSHA) in workplace safety.
2. List eight types of safety hazards.
3. Describe six precautions that can reduce the risk of injury.
4. Explain steps to be taken to lessen the risk of physical or sharps hazards.
5. List the items that must be included on a chemical label according to the Globally Harmonized System.
6. List two other kinds of labels used to identify hazardous materials.
7. Explain the purpose of the safety data sheet (SDS).
8. Describe the components of a chemical hygiene plan.

9. Discuss safety precautions to be used when handling hazardous chemicals.
10. Identify the radioactive hazard symbol.
11. Describe precautions to be taken to reduce the risk of electrical hazards.
12. Describe the four classes of fire, and identify the type or types of fire extinguisher used to combat each.
13. Explain what to do in case of the following:
    a. bleeding wound
    b. no sign of breathing
    c. shock
    d. latex sensitivity

KEY TERMS

allergic contact dermatitis
anaphylaxis
cardiopulmonary
  resuscitation (CPR)
chemical hygiene plan
Department of
  Transportation (DOT)
  label

Globally Harmonized
  System (GHS) of
  Classification and
  Labeling of Chemicals
irritant contact dermatitis
latex sensitivity

National Fire Protection
  Association (NFPA) label
Occupational Safety and
  Health Administration
  (OSHA)

radioactive hazard symbol
safety data sheet (SDS)
sharps

ABBREVIATIONS

AED automated external defibrillator
CHP chemical hygiene plan
CPR cardiopulmonary resuscitation
DOT Department of Transportation
FDA Food and Drug Administration
GHS Globally Harmonized System
HBV hepatitis B virus
HCl hydrochloric acid

HCV hepatitis C virus
HIV human immunodeficiency virus
MRI magnetic resonance imaging
NFPA National Fire Protection Association
OSHA Occupational Safety and Health Administration
PPE personal protective equipment
SDS safety data sheet

WHAT WOULD YOU DO?

It's 9 AM, and you are heading to your first draw on the chronic care wing of Mercy Hospital. As you pass the nurse's station, a nurse offers you one of the doughnuts from the box on the desk. You have a tight schedule and cannot stop to eat one now, so the nurse suggests you take it along with you. "It should fit right there in your tray next to your tubes. I'll wrap it up good and tight for you," she offers. Is it appropriate to take the snack for later?

FLASH FORWARD

You will learn about infection control and the special precautions needed to collect and handle biological specimens in Chapter 4.

OCCUPATIONAL SAFETY AND HEALTH ADMINISTRATION

Workplace safety is regulated by OSHA. The regulations are designed both to inform workers about hazards in the workplace (e.g., by requiring that workers know the health effects of the chemicals they use) and to protect workers from harm (e.g., by requiring an emergency shower nearby in case of chemical spills). Your employer is required by OSHA to maintain a safe workplace, provide a comprehensive safety training program, and report accidents that occur on the job. OSHA regulations are revised as needed to increase workplace safety in light of new information or new hazards. Therefore you should keep up to date on all relevant information as it changes throughout your career.

TYPES OF SAFETY HAZARDS

Despite their goal of promoting health, health care facilities can be dangerous places for people who are not aware of the potential risks. Types of hazards include the following:

- *Biological:* Infectious agents, including airborne or bloodborne organisms such as bacteria and viruses

- *Physical:* Wet floors, heavy lifting (e.g., boxes and patient transfers)
- *Sharps:* Needles, lancets, and broken glass
- *Chemical:* Preservatives and reagents (laboratory-grade chemicals)
- *Radioactive reagents*
- *X-ray equipment*
- *Electrical:* Dangerous high-voltage equipment
- *Fire or explosive:* Open flames, oxygen, and chemicals (e.g., nitrous oxide)
- *Gases under pressure*
- *Latex sensitivity:* Allergic reaction to latex in gloves or other equipment

In addition to specific safety precautions for phlebotomy procedures, a number of general precautions can reduce your risk of injury:

- Practice hand hygiene, as discussed in Chapter 4.
- Always wear the appropriate personal protective equipment (PPE) when handling specimens.
- Avoid touching your face, nose, or mouth in the work area. Do not rub your eyes, handle contact lenses, or apply cosmetics, especially when wearing gloves.
- Never store food or beverages in the laboratory refrigerator with reagents or specimens.
- Do not let anything hang loose that might get contaminated or caught in equipment. Tie back shoulder-length hair, and never wear long chains, large or dangling earrings, or loose bracelets.
- Protect your feet from spills, slips, and falling objects. Never wear open-toe or open-back shoes. Shoes should be sturdy, made of nonabsorbent material, and have nonskid soles.

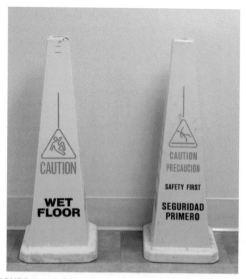

FIGURE 3-1 Safety cones; note English and Spanish warnings.

- Avoid putting anything in your mouth in the work area. This means no eating, drinking, smoking, or chewing gum while in the laboratory area. Never put pens or pencils in your mouth.

Physical Hazards

Avoiding physical hazards in the workplace is mostly a matter of common sense, plus learning some important habits:

- Avoid running. This is not only a safety rule but also a consideration for patients, who may become concerned or agitated.
- Watch for wet floors. Your facility should use cones or other types of signs to warn when a floor is wet and should have cleanup equipment for spills (Figure 3-1).

- Bend your knees when lifting heavy objects or transferring a patient (Figure 3-2).
- Maintain a clean, organized work area.

Sharps Hazards

Sharps, especially needles and lancets, are the most common hazards you will encounter as a phlebotomist. Sharps are dangerous both because of the physical injury they may cause and because they may carry bloodborne pathogens such as human immunodeficiency virus (HIV), hepatitis B virus (HBV), or hepatitis C virus (HCV). To prevent contact, always use the safety engineering features as specified for the device you are using. Safety engineering features for sharps include shielded or self-blunting needles for both vacuum tube systems and butterflies, as well cylindrical sheaths for syringe needles, used when transferring blood into vacuum tubes.

> **FLASH FORWARD** ⟶ »»
>
> Bloodborne pathogens are discussed in Chapter 4.

The safety feature must be activated as soon as the needle is removed from the vein, unless it is an in-vein safety activation device. Never detach the needle from the plastic tube holder, because this will expose the rubber-covered needle that punctures the tube. The needle-vacutainer unit is disposed of in its entirety in a sharps container. A used needle should never be removed from a syringe by hand, and you should never bend or break a needle. Dispose of sharps in a puncture-resistant container immediately after activating the safety feature (Figure 3-3). It is best to keep the needle disposal device within arm's reach during the procedure.

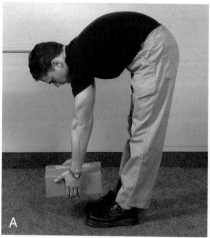
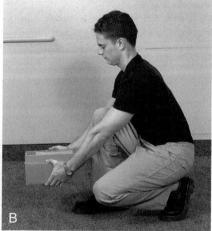

FIGURE 3-2 A, Improper lifting technique. **B,** Proper lifting technique. The knees should be bent while lifting; this allows the legs to bear the weight, instead of the back.

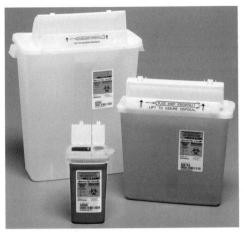

FIGURE 3-3 Sharps containers.

The Needle Stick Safety and Prevention Act of 2001 required all employers to switch to safety needle devices to minimize the risk of accidental sticks and solicited employee input in choosing safer devices. Failure to comply with the 2001 regulation can result in high fines for the institution and the individual who violates the act.

If you are stuck by a used needle or other sharp object that has been in contact with blood, or if you get blood in your eyes, nose, mouth, or broken skin, you should perform the following steps:

1. *Immediately* flood the exposed area with water and clean any wound with soap and water or a skin disinfectant.
2. Report this immediately to your employer. Your employer is required to keep a log of such incidents. Follow your facility's exposure control plan for reporting and medical treatment for an accidental needle exposure.
3. Seek immediate medical attention, including counseling for exposure to HIV, HBV, and HCV.

FLASH FORWARD ⤳⟫

You will learn more about exposure control plans in Chapter 4.

Some phlebotomists may be tempted to cut some safety corners, especially as they gain more confidence in their handling of needles and other sharps. However, there is never a good enough reason to take such risks. The risk of infection is always present, and there can be months of psychological trauma while waiting to learn the results of serologic testing after an accidental needle stick. In many institutions, not following safety procedures is grounds for dismissal.

Chemical Hazards

You will encounter many different chemicals in your work as a phlebotomist, including several that can be quite harmful if handled improperly. For example, hydrochloric acid (HCl), which burns mucosal tissue and skin, is used as a preservative for urine. Bleach, which causes irritation of mucosal tissue and skin, is used as a disinfectant in the laboratory.

Identification of Chemicals

The safe handling of chemicals begins with proper labeling. All chemicals should have labels that identify the chemical by name, and you should read the label carefully before using any chemical. Do not use a chemical that is not labeled.

In 2012, OSHA adopted the **Globally Harmonized System (GHS) of Classification and Labeling of Chemicals**. The new GHS label contains information on the identity of the chemical, the chemical manufacturer or other responsible party, appropriate hazard warnings communicated through the visual symbols called pictograms, explanations of the hazards involved in exposure to the chemical, and first-aid measures to take in the event of exposure (Figure 3-4).

OSHA also requires that each chemical come with a **safety data sheet (SDS**; also called a materials safety data sheet), which provides information about the chemical, its hazards, and the procedures for cleanup and first aid. The SDS has 16 sections, with each section providing specific information on that chemical (Table 3-1). These data sheets must

TABLE 3-1	SDS Sections
1	Identification
2	Hazard identification
3	Composition/information on ingredients
4	First-aid measures
5	Fire-fighting measures
6	Accidental release measures
7	Handling and storage
8	Exposure controls/personal protection
9	Physical and chemical properties
10	Stability and reactivity
11	Toxicological information
12	Ecological information
13	Disposal considerations
14	Transport information
15	Regulatory information
16	Other information

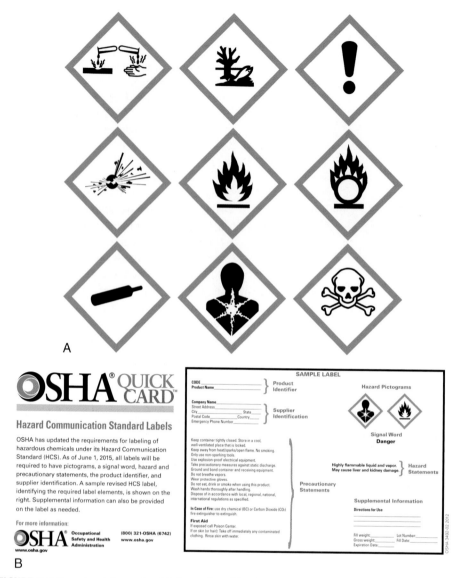

A

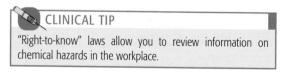

B

FIGURE 3-4 Example of Occupational Safety and Health Administration (OSHA)-mandated labeling; Globally Harmonized System label. (From OSHA: Hazard communication, 2013. Retrieved from *www.osha.gov/dsg/hazcom/index.html.*)

be kept on file in the workplace, and you have a right to review them. It may also be possible to access these sheets through your facility's intranet. By June 2015 all chemicals will be required to include the GHS label and the SDS information.

> ### CLINICAL TIP
> "Right-to-know" laws allow you to review information on chemical hazards in the workplace.

Two other types of secondary labels are still in use to identify hazardous materials. The **Department of Transportation (DOT) label** (Figure 3-5)

displays the type of hazard, the United Nations hazard class number, and an identifying number. The **National Fire Protection Association (NFPA) label** (Figure 3-6) is a design recognized by firefighters that warns of the location of hazardous materials in the event of a fire. It uses a diamond-shaped symbol whose four quadrants contain numbers indicating the relative danger level in four areas: health, fire, chemical stability, and specific hazard types. Higher numbers indicate higher risk. Primarily designed for fixed installations, this symbol has been widely used to indicate hazards at the entrances to laboratory facilities within buildings. How the DOT

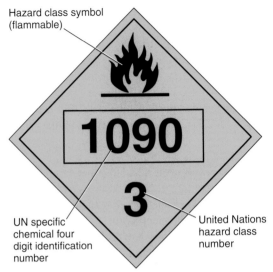

FIGURE 3-5 Department of Transportation label displaying the type of hazard, the United Nations hazard class number, and an identifying number.

Hazard class symbol (flammable)

UN specific chemical four digit identification number

United Nations hazard class number

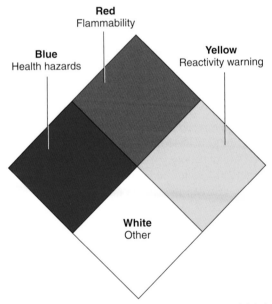

FIGURE 3-6 National Fire Protection Association (NFPA) label.

Red
Flammability

Blue
Health hazards

Yellow
Reactivity warning

White
Other

and NFPA labels will be used in conjunction with the GHS will be determined as time goes on.

Reducing Risk

OSHA further requires that every workplace develop and train its employees in a **chemical hygiene plan (CHP)**. The plan describes all safety procedures, special precautions, and emergency procedures used when working with chemicals.

Each employee must receive training in the details of the plan.

Although some chemicals are more dangerous than others, you should treat every chemical as if it were hazardous. This means that you should always use PPE when working with chemicals, including eye protection, a laboratory coat, and gloves.

Follow protocols and instructions carefully. For instance, if a protocol says to add an acid to water, do not add the water to the acid instead. Combining acid and water releases heat. By adding acid to water, you allow the large amount of water to heat up slowly. By adding water to concentrated acid, the small amount of water may boil on contact (Figure 3-7). This can cause the acid to splash out of the container onto the skin or mucous membranes, causing burns.

CLINICAL TIP

Never add water to acid. Always add acid to water.
Other important precautions include the following:
- Follow the written chemical hygiene plan of your facility.
- Never mix chemicals together unless you are following an approved protocol.
- Never store chemicals above eye level.
- Always store a chemical in its original container
- Know the location of safety showers and eyewash stations in the laboratory.

When Accidents Happen

Despite precautions, chemical accidents occasionally occur. In such cases, you must be prepared to act quickly to prevent or minimize a serious injury.

If a chemical spills on you, proceed immediately to the safety shower or eyewash station. Flush the affected area with water for a minimum

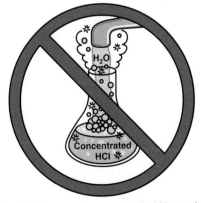

FIGURE 3-7 Adding water to concentrated acid is very dangerous.

of 15 minutes. Report your accident to the appropriate supervisor in your department, and then proceed to the emergency room to be evaluated for further treatment.

If a chemical spills on the floor or a work surface, alert nearby personnel of the danger, and then follow laboratory protocol for cleanup. Cleanup kits should be available, with different types of equipment and neutralizing chemicals used for different types of spills. You must take the time to learn how to use the clean-up kit in your facility.

Radioactive Hazards

Radioactive materials are used in health care facilities to perform diagnostic tests and deliver treatment. In areas in which radioactivity is used, the **radioactive hazard symbol** is displayed (Figure 3-8). Although the duties of a phlebotomist do not involve direct handling of radioactive materials, you may be exposed to small amounts of such materials when drawing blood from a patient in the radiology department, for instance, or when drawing blood from a patient receiving radioactive treatments or undergoing imagery with a radioactive substance. X-rays are used for diagnosis. Precautions taken by the staff of the radiology department should prevent you from ever being exposed to x-rays. You should not be drawing blood while a patient is receiving an x-ray.

The effects of radiation exposure increase with the length of exposure, the distance to the radiation source, the dose of radiation, and the shielding in place. Appropriate shielding devices are required to protect employees from unnecessary exposure to radiation. Pregnant women need to be especially careful to minimize their exposure because of the risk to the fetus. There are several important guidelines to follow to minimize your risk:

• Recognize the radioactive hazard symbol.

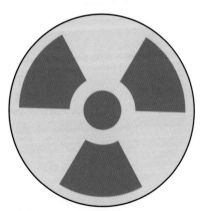

FIGURE 3-8 Radioactive hazard symbol.

• Exercise extra caution in areas where radioactive materials are in use.
• Learn your institution's procedures for minimizing exposure and responding to accidents.

Pregnant women in the first trimester should not enter a patient's room or a laboratory facility if there is a radiation alert posted at the door; this precaution can prevent a possible adverse effect on the fetus.

Electrical Hazards

Electrical hazards in the laboratory may result in shock or fire. General rules of electrical safety apply in health care institutions as well, including the following:

• Avoid using extension cords.
• Report frayed cords, overloaded circuits, and ungrounded equipment.
• Unplug a piece of equipment before servicing it.
• If a piece of equipment is marked with an electrical caution warning, do not attempt to open it, even for inspection. It may contain batteries or electrical capacitors that store electricity even when unplugged.
• Know the location of the circuit breaker box for the equipment you are using.
• Avoid contact with any electrical equipment while drawing blood. Electricity may pass through you and the needle and shock the patient.

Emergency Response to Electric Shock

If someone receives an electric shock in the workplace, turn off the equipment, either by unplugging it or by switching off the circuit breaker. In the event you cannot turn off the electricity, break contact between the source and the victim using a nonconductive material, such as a wooden broom handle. Do not touch the victim until the risk of further shock is removed. Call for medical assistance (call 911), start **cardiopulmonary resuscitation (CPR)** if indicated, and keep the victim warm (CPR is discussed later in this chapter).

Fire and Explosive Hazards

Fires or explosions in the laboratory may occur as a result of chemical or electrical accidents or carelessness with flames or other fire sources. In addition to preventive measures, the most important steps to take to minimize the risk of injury are summarized in the acronym **RACE:**

Rescue. Remove any patients from the immediate area where fire risk is present (Figure 3-9).
Alarm. Call 911 or the appropriate number for fire emergency in your facility.
Confine. Close all windows and doors.

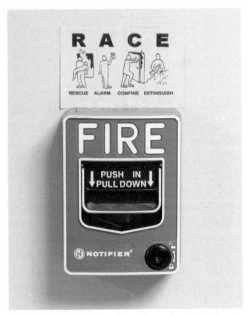

FIGURE 3-9 Fire extinguisher. Fire pull and RACE card.

TABLE 3-2	Classes of Fire	
Class	Fuel	Extinguisher
A	Wood, paper, and cloth	A, ABC
B	Grease, oil, and flammable liquids	ABC, BC, and halogenated agents
C	Energized electrical equipment	C
D	Flammable metals	D, special equipment
K	Cooking oils and grease	K, special equipment

Also know the location of all fire extinguishers and emergency exits in your facility. Exit signs should be plainly marked with written escape routes posted around the office or facility.

Classes of Fire

There are five classes of fire, as identified by the NFPA, based on the fire's fuel source. These correspond to the type of extinguisher that should be used to combat the fire, as shown in Table 3-2. Type A fire extinguishers may contain water or dry chemicals. Type B extinguishers may contain dry chemicals, carbon dioxide, or environmentally safe fluorocarbons. Type C extinguishers are safe for electrical fires. Type D extinguishing agents are dry powders that may be contained in a pressurized extinguisher or in sealed cans for careful application. The newest class of extinguisher is the type K unit, which is used for kitchens or grease fires.

Magnetic Resonance Imaging Hazards

A magnetic resonance imaging (MRI) machine uses an extremely powerful magnet to create images of the body. The strength of the magnet poses significant safety risks when proper precautions are not taken. The magnet is strong enough to pull metal objects toward it from across the room at great speed. Warning signs are posted outside the MRI examination room. Anyone entering the MRI examination room must remove all metallic objects, including jewelry, belt buckles, and even zippers. People with implanted metallic devices may be barred from entering. The instructions of the MRI staff must be followed to prevent serious injury or death.

Extinguish. If the fire is small and contained, use a fire extinguisher (Figure 3-10) or fire blanket to put it out.

Know how to use a fire extinguisher. The proper technique is summarized in the acronym **PASS:**

Pull the pin.
Aim at the base of fire.
Squeeze the handle.
Sweep.

EMERGENCY FIRST-AID PROCEDURES

A full review of first-aid techniques is beyond the scope of this chapter. Here we review the most common types of emergencies and the major steps that

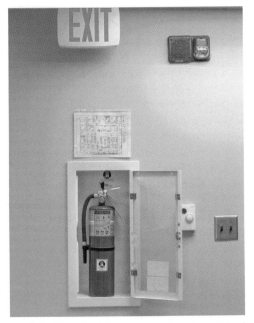

FIGURE 3-10 Fire extinguisher with evacuation plan and fire alarm.

should be taken to deal with them. Health care workers should be trained in the techniques of CPR and should refresh their skills biannually.

Cardiopulmonary Resuscitation

A victim of cardiac arrest will be unresponsive and will not be breathing normally. Quick intervention may save the person's life. Guidelines issued by the American Heart Association in 2010 emphasize that continual chest compressions should be the initial CPR action for all victims, regardless of their age, and that breathing aid is less important than continual compression, especially in adults. If you are not trained in rescue breathing or cannot provide rescue breathing, you should perform compression only ("hands-only CPR") after determining the victim is not responsive and not breathing normally.

1. Determine whether the victim is conscious by asking loudly, "Are you okay?" If there is no response, alert emergency medical personnel (either within the hospital or by calling 911).
2. Determine whether the victim is breathing normally. If the victim is unresponsive and is not breathing or is only gasping, begin chest compressions immediately. (If there is an automated external defibrillator [AED] device nearby, use that instead.)
3. To perform chest compressions, push down on the chest, right between the nipples, compressing the chest between 1½ and 2 inches. Compressions should be at the rate of 100 per minute, so each compression should take less than 1 second. Continue compressions until professional help arrives.

Bleeding Aid

1. Apply direct pressure to a bleeding wound; first place a clean cloth, if available, against the wound.
2. Elevate the limb unless you suspect a fracture.
3. Maintain pressure until medical assistance is available.

First Aid for Shock

Recognize the early signs of shock: pale, cold, or clammy skin; rapid pulse; shallow breathing; weakness; and possible nausea or vomiting. In the event of possible shock, perform the following actions:

- Call for professional assistance.
- Keep the victim lying down.
- Elevate the injured person's legs, unless you suspect a fracture.

- In case of vomiting, keep the individual's airway open by turning the person's head to the side and sweeping out his or her mouth with your finger.
- Keep the person warm.

DISASTER EMERGENCY PLAN

Most institutions have disaster emergency plans that describe procedures in the event of a large-scale disaster, such as a flood, hurricane, fire, or earthquake. Learn your institution's procedures so that you are prepared to respond in an emergency. Pay special attention to your responsibilities. These may range from reporting to a specific place or person outside your facility in case of a fire in your building to helping remove patients from danger. If you are assigned to multiple institutions, be sure to check procedures and your responsibilities at each one.

You may also have responsibilities as a responder in the event of a health-related emergency, for instance, when a surge of injured patients arrives at your hospital, as they might in the event of a multicar accident or building collapse. In such an event, you may be called on to take on responsibilities outside of your normal duties, whether in processing patients as they arrive, taking samples in the emergency room, or working longer shifts. Again, know your institution's plan and your responsibilities, and be prepared to respond quickly.

SENSITIVITY TO LATEX AND OTHER MATERIALS

Latex sensitivity is an important problem in the health care field. Today, many health care facilities have stopped using latex gloves, replacing them with stretch nitrile or vinyl. The reaction to latex products can take a variety of forms.

Irritant contact dermatitis occurs as a result of direct skin contact with materials left on the latex surface during manufacturing, such as processing chemicals. Redness, swelling, and itching may occur within minutes to hours of exposure. Removing the glove and washing the exposed area are enough to reduce the reaction within several hours. The skin may become highly sensitized with repeat exposure.

Allergic contact dermatitis is a true allergic response in which the body's immune system reacts to the proteins or other components of the latex that are absorbed through the skin. Perspiration increases absorption. Absorption may also occur through inhalation of glove powder. Symptoms may not be localized to the exposed area.

Anaphylaxis is a rapid, severe immune reaction that can be life threatening if not treated. During anaphylaxis, the airway may swell shut, the heart rate may increase, and the blood pressure drops. Epinephrine injection and emergency room management are needed for anaphylaxis.

Regulations by the Food and Drug Administration (FDA) require the labeling of medical gloves that contain natural rubber latex or powder. Glove boxes are required to bear caution statements whose wording depends on the actual content of the gloves.

Nitrile and vinyl are much less allergenic but may nonetheless cause a reaction in some individuals. In addition, they may react with chemicals in some hand lotions, causing irritant or allergic dermatitis. Only approved lotions or hand creams should be used to prevent these reactions.

FLASH FORWARD

You will learn about latex tourniquets in Chapter 8.

Preventing Latex Reactions

Individuals with known sensitivity to latex should wear a medical alert bracelet. Patients should be asked about allergies or other reactions to previous latex exposure. The substances causing latex allergy are similar to ones found in chestnuts and some tropical fruits, such as kiwi, avocado, and banana. Patients should be asked about allergies or reactions to any of these fruits.

REVIEW FOR CERTIFICATION

Safety is a paramount concern in the health care workplace. OSHA is responsible for workplace safety and has created rules and regulations to improve safety. These regulations govern the handling of sharps, chemicals, and other occupational hazards. The phlebotomist must pay close attention to workplace safety and learn the most effective ways to avoid hazards such as biologic, physical, sharps, chemical, radioactive, electrical, and fire dangers. Most important of all is the danger of accidental contamination with blood or other body fluids.

BIBLIOGRAPHY

Francis AL: Glove me tender, *The Scientist,* May 15, 2000. Retrieved from www.the-scientist.com/?articles.view/articleNo/12845/title/Glove-Me-Tender/.

McPherson RA, Pincus MR: *Henry's Clinical Diagnosis and Management by Laboratory Methods,* ed. 22, Philadelphia, 2012, Saunders.

Muller BA: Minimizing latex exposure and allergy, *Postgraduate Medicine,* 113(4):91–97, 2003.

Travers AH, Rea TD, Bobrow BJ, et al: Part 4: CPR Overview: 2010 American Heart Association Guidelines for Cardiopulmonary Resuscitation and Emergency Cardiovascular Care, *Circulation* 122:S676–S684, 2010. Retrieved from http://circ.ahajournals.org/cgi/content/full/122/18_suppl_3/S676.

WHAT WOULD YOU DO?

Unfortunately, you must pass on the snack. Food and beverages should never be stored or transported along with specimens because of the risk that one or the other will become contaminated. It is also a violation of OSHA regulations, and your employer could be fined. If you eat contaminated food, you could become ill or even die. If the sample becomes contaminated, the patient may suffer from incorrect results or may need another sample drawn.

STUDY QUESTIONS

See answers in Appendix F.

1. Name six types of safety hazards in the workplace and give an example of each.

2. List five safety precautions that can reduce the risk of injury in the workplace.

3. Because needle sticks are a major concern, what should you never do after performing a venipuncture?

4. List the five identifying features that all hazardous material labels must display.

5. Describe the purpose of an SDS.

6. Explain the purpose of a chemical hygiene plan.

7. In the event a chemical spills on your arm, what steps should be taken?

8. Describe the steps in the emergency response to electric shock.

9. List the types of fire extinguishers and what each contains.

10. Describe the protocol for hands-only CPR.

11. Describe three types of reaction associated with latex usage.

12. Name the organization that regulates workplace safety, and define its purpose.

13. Explain the process that should be followed in controlling a bleeding emergency.

14. List the signs of shock and the steps to take to prevent further complications.

15. What is the best way for a phlebotomist to prepare for a disaster that occurs in the community?

16. Choose a local health care institution. Research its disaster emergency plan, and find out what responsibilities phlebotomists have in the plan.

CERTIFICATION EXAMINATION PREPARATION

See answers in Appendix F.

1. OSHA stands for
   a. Occupational Standards in Health Associations.
   b. Outline of Safety Hazards and Accidents.
   c. Occupational Safety and Health Administration.
   d. Occupational Standards and Health Administration.

2. When mixing acids and water, you should
   a. add acid to water.
   b. add water to acid.
   c. never mix acids and water together.
   d. add equal amounts in an empty container.

3. Chemicals should be
   a. stored above eye level.
   b. labeled properly.
   c. cleaned up using soap and water.
   d. disposed of in the sink.

4. The first action to take in the event of fire is to
   a. call the fire department.
   b. close the windows and doors.
   c. remove patients from danger.
   d. pull the fire alarm.

5. In the event of electric shock, the first thing you should do is
   a. call 911.
   b. attempt to turn off the electrical equipment.
   c. break contact between the source and the victim.
   d. start CPR.

6. Class C fires involve
   a. wood.
   b. grease or oil.
   c. flammable materials.
   d. electrical equipment.

7. Which of the following does the NFPA symbol not warn about?
   a. Protective equipment
   b. Fire
   c. Chemical stability
   d. Health

8. The first thing to do when giving CPR to a victim is
   a. clear the airway.
   b. place the victim on a firm, flat surface.
   c. begin mouth-to-mouth ventilation.
   d. determine whether the victim is conscious.

9. Safety equipment in the laboratory may include
    a. personal protective equipment.
    b. an emergency shower.
    c. an eyewash station.
    d. all of these.

10. An SDS provides information on
    a. sharps.
    b. patients.
    c. chemicals.
    d. office procedures.

11. Reaction to latex products may include
    a. irritant contact dermatitis.
    b. allergic contact dermatitis.
    c. anaphylaxis.
    d. all of these.

12. The yellow diamond in the NFPA label indicates
    a. health hazards.
    b. flammability.
    c. reactivity warning.
    d. other.

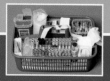

The goal of infection control is to develop and maintain an environment that minimizes the risk of acquiring or transmitting infectious agents to hospital personnel, patients, and visitors. It is not always possible for you to know if a patient is infectious or is incubating an infection. Therefore it is important that you understand how infections occur and follow infection control practices and policies to protect yourself and your patients from infectious agents. Infection control requires recognizing potential sources of transmission and breaking the chain of infection. Techniques for preventing transmission include hand hygiene, use of personal protective equipment (PPE), and use of both Standard and Expanded Precautions. In Chapter 3, you learned how to recognize and prevent physical safety hazards on the job. In this chapter, we examine in detail the biologic hazards with which you may come in contact. By taking appropriate precautions against potentially infectious organisms, you can make the workplace safe for you, your patients, and your coworkers.

OUTLINE

Infection
Bloodborne Pathogens
  Contact with Bloodborne
    Pathogens
  Viral Survival
Chain of Infection
  Means of Transmission

Breaking the Chain of Infection
  Hand Hygiene
  Personal Protective Equipment
  Standard Precautions
Occupational Safety and Health
  Administration's Bloodborne
  Pathogens Standard

Isolation Control Measures
  Airborne Precautions
  Droplet Precautions
  Contact Precautions
Cleaning Up a Spill
Review for Certification

OBJECTIVES

After completing this chapter, you should be able to:

1. Define infection, and differentiate between community-acquired and health care–associated infections.
2. Explain how organisms found in a hospital differ from those found in the community.
3. Describe four ways that infectious agents may be transmitted, and give examples of each.
4. Discuss the importance of proper hand hygiene in breaking the chain of infection.
5. Describe the proper handwashing technique, including the sequence of steps.
6. Define personal protective equipment (PPE) and describe at least four types.
7. Describe the order and procedure for putting on and removing PPE.
8. Define Occupational Safety and Health Administration (OSHA) and explain its role in infection control.
9. Define bloodborne pathogen and give examples.
10. Explain how bloodborne pathogens may be transmitted.
11. Explain the components of Standard Precautions.
12. Define Expanded Precautions and describe the types.
13. Explain general procedures for cleaning up a blood spill.

KEY TERMS

Airborne Infection Isolation
  Precautions
airborne transmission
bloodborne pathogens
  (BBPs)
chain of infection
common vehicle
  transmission
Contact Precautions

contact transmission
droplet nuclei
Droplet Precautions
droplet transmission
Expanded Precautions (EPs)
exposure control plan
fomite
health care–associated
  infection

hepatitis B virus (HBV)
high-efficiency particulate
  air (HEPA)
human immunodeficiency
  virus (HIV)
infection
isolation
micrometer
nosocomial infection

pathogen
personal protective
  equipment (PPE)
protective environment (PE)
reservoir
sepsis
Standard Precautions
vectors

ABBREVIATIONS

AIDS acquired immunodeficiency syndrome
BBP bloodborne pathogen
CDC Centers for Disease Control and Prevention
ECP exposure control plan
EPs Expanded Precautions
HAI health care–associated infection
HBV hepatitis B virus
HEPA high-efficiency particulate air
HIV human immunodeficiency virus

HTLV human T-cell lymphotropic virus
MRSA methicillin-resistant *Staphylococcus aureus*
NIOSH National Institute for Occupational Safety and Health
OSHA Occupational Safety and Health Administration
PE protective environment
PPE personal protective equipment
SARS severe acute respiratory syndrome
VRE vancomycin-resistant *Enterococcus*

WHAT WOULD YOU DO?

You have just finished up with your fifth patient of the morning on your rounds at Mercy Hospital, and before you leave the room, you use an alcohol-based rub to sanitize your hands. You stop at the nurses' station to sort your requisitions. You borrowed a pen from the desk, and because you recognize the potential that it may be contaminated, you sanitize your hands again as you leave the station. Your next draw is just around the corner, and after entering the room and greeting the patient, you begin to prepare your materials. The patient, who looks upset, says to you, "You haven't yet washed your hands. Please do so immediately." What would you do?

INFECTION

The human body is host to a variety of microorganisms that normally do not cause illness. Such organisms are said to colonize the body. For example, the skin has several common types of bacteria that live harmlessly on its surface. Although these microorganisms can live and multiply on and within the body without causing disease, the correct conditions, such as a break in the skin, can allow these organisms to enter the body and cause an infection. An infection is an invasion and growth of a microorganism in the human body that causes disease. Infectious organisms, also called pathogens, can be viruses, bacteria, fungi, protists (single-celled organisms), helminthes (wormlike animals), or prions (molecules of infectious proteins). Some common infectious organisms from different classes are listed in Table 4-1. The number of potential pathogens is large, however, and the list is not comprehensive. New pathogens will likely continue to emerge in the future.

The infectious agents found in a hospital are often more virulent and more resistant to treatment than are most organisms found at large in the community. This is true for three reasons.

1. A more virulent organism is more likely to cause a more serious disease, meaning that an infected person is more likely to be admitted for treatment.
2. Hospitalized patients usually have a lowered resistance to infection by potential pathogens and opportunistic organisms.

3. Treatment with antibiotics may leave the most resistant organisms alive through the process of natural selection. These organisms then cause even more serious disease, requiring more aggressive treatment, usually in a hospital.

Infections contracted by patients during a hospital stay are termed health care–associated infections (also called nosocomial infections). Health care–associated infections (HAIs) may be caused by direct contact with other patients, but they are most often caused by failure of hospital personnel to follow infection control practices, such as hand hygiene.

BLOODBORNE PATHOGENS

Bloodborne pathogens (BBPs) are infectious agents carried in the blood, certain body fluids, and unfixed (unpreserved) tissues as defined in the Occupational Safety and Health (OSHA) Bloodborne Pathogens Standard. Contracting a BBP infection from an accidental needle stick is the principal occupational risk for a phlebotomist. The most common BBPs are listed in Box 4-1.

Contact With Bloodborne Pathogens

The phlebotomist may be exposed to BBPs in a number of ways. Exposures to blood or body fluids can occur through the following:

- Percutaneous injury via needle stick or puncture. Percutaneous contact occurs through the surface

TABLE 4-1	Common Infectious Organisms and Diseases They Cause
Organism	**Disease**
Viruses	
Adenovirus	Upper respiratory infections
Hepatitis virus (A to E and G)	Hepatitis
Herpes simplex	Oral and genital herpes
Human immunodeficiency virus (HIV)	Acquired immunodeficiency syndrome (AIDS)
Influenza virus	Influenza, or "flu"
Poliovirus	Polio
Varicella-zoster virus	Chickenpox and shingles
Bacteria	
Bordetella pertussis	Pertussis or whooping cough
Corynebacterium diphtheria	Diphtheria
Escherichia coli	Food poisoning; some types are normal residents of the colon
Haemophilus influenza	Meningitis, pink eye, and upper respiratory infections
Mycobacterium tuberculosis	Tuberculosis
Neisseria gonorrhoeae	Gonorrhea
Neisseria meningitides	Meningococcal meningitis
Salmonella	Food poisoning
Staphylococcus aureus	Skin and wound infections and food poisoning
Streptococcus	"Strep throat," rheumatic fever, and other types of infections
Treponema pallidum	Syphilis
Fungi	
Candida albicans	Candidiasis
Cryptococcus neoformans	Cryptococcosis
Protists	
Entamoeba histolytica	Amebiasis and dysentery
Giardia lamblia	Giardiasis
Plasmodium	Malaria
Trichomonas vaginalis	Trichomoniasis

BOX 4-1   Bloodborne Pathogens (BBPs)

- Babesiosis
- Colorado tick fever
- Hepatitis B, C, and D
- Human immunodeficiency virus (HIV)
- Human T-cell lymphotropic virus (HTLV) types I and II
- Malaria
- Syphilis

From Centers for Disease Control and Prevention, Atlanta, Ga.

---

of the skin, such as by scalpel cuts, transfusions, sharps injuries, or other means that penetrate the skin. Inoculation by accidental needle stick can occur any time a needle is unsheathed. In Chapters 8 and 9 you will learn important safety techniques to minimize the chances of a needle stick.

- Contact of mucous membranes (eyes, nose, and mouth) via splashes or touching eyes, nose, or mouth with contaminated glove or hands.
- Contact of nonintact skin via splashes or contact with contaminated gloves or hands. Nonintact skin contact occurs through preexisting wounds, scratches, abrasions, burns, or hangnails.
- Human bite.
- Contact with equipment or laboratory instruments contaminated with body fluid, as well as contact through nail biting, smoking, eating, or manipulating contact lenses.
- Droplet transmission. Such transmission can occur by removal of rubber stoppers; centrifuge accidents; splashing or spattering, especially during transfer of blood or other body fluids between containers; or failure to wear a proper face shield.

CLINICAL TIP

As you remove a stopper or lid from a blood tube, always tilt the top away from you and the bottom toward you, to direct any droplets away from you. Place the stopper bottom side up on a paper towel to prevent contamination of laboratory surfaces.

Viral Survival

Bloodborne viruses have been reported to survive outside the body for much longer than was once believed possible. For example, hepatitis B virus (HBV) can survive in dried blood for up to 1 week. This prolonged survival means that, as a phlebotomist, you must be even more aware of potential sources of infection in your environment. HBV is very infectious—there are about 1 million infectious viral particles per milliliter of a body fluid. Laboratory equipment such as centrifuges or quality-control products that use human blood or body fluids should be handled with appropriate precautions. Always use PPE when handling samples. Learn the procedures in your laboratory for minimizing risk, including equipment-related precautions, work practice controls, and spill cleanup procedures. Routinely disinfect your phlebotomy tray with a 10% bleach solution. The 10% solution is made fresh once a week by mixing one part household bleach with nine parts water. All contaminated surfaces should be cleaned with 10% bleach.

CHAIN OF INFECTION

The **chain of infection** requires a continuous link through three primary elements: the reservoir, the means of transmission, and the susceptible host (Figure 4-1). In addition, other links in this chain include a portal of exit (the means by which the infectious agent leaves the source) and a portal of entry (the means by which the infectious agent enters the host, resulting in infection or colonization). The **reservoir**, the source of the infection, can be an infected person, who may be either symptomatic or asymptomatic. The source may also be a contaminated object (called a **fomite**), such as equipment or supplies, or it may be food or water contaminated with the infectious agent. The susceptible host may be a patient, a health care professional, or a visitor. Microorganisms can be transmitted by contact (either direct or indirect), droplet, or airborne routes. The means of transmission of infectious agents can be as obvious as a puncture with a contaminated needle or as inconspicuous as exposure to airborne droplets from a person with tuberculosis. In some cases, a person may carry and transmit the agent without being sick; this person is considered a reservoir. Breaking the chain of infection requires understanding the continuous links in

the chain and applying appropriate interventions to interrupt a link.

Means of Transmission

Infectious agents can spread by five means:
1. Contact, both direct and indirect
2. Droplet
3. Airborne
4. Common vehicle
5. Vector

Contact Transmission

Contact transmission is the most frequent and important transmission route for health care–associated infections. Direct contact involves the transfer of microorganisms from an infected or colonized person directly to a susceptible host by physical contact between the source and the susceptible host. Indirect contact involves contact between a susceptible host and a fomite, such as a medical instrument, needle, dressing, or bed rail. Phones, pencils, computer keyboards, gloves, and other objects can also act as sources of indirect contact transmission.

Droplet Transmission

Droplets are particles that are generated from the source by coughing, sneezing, or talking. Transmission of infectious agents by this route can also occur from liquid splashes or aerosols formed by uncapping a blood collection tube or transferring blood from a syringe to a tube. Because droplet particles

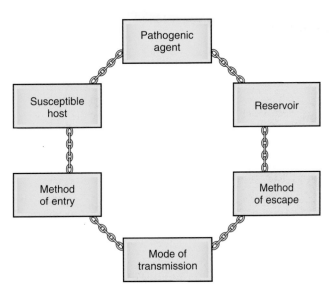

FIGURE 4-1 The chain of infection. The disease cycle continues to repeat unless measures are taken to stop the cycle, such as practicing meticulous hand hygiene and isolating the patient. (From Gerdin J: *Health Careers Today*, ed. 5, St. Louis, 2012, Mosby.)

are bigger than 5 μm, they are propelled only a short distance before falling and coming to rest. Therefore **droplet transmission** is likely for only a brief time and within a short distance (approximately 3 feet) of the source, meaning that specialized ventilation or air-filtering equipment is not needed to prevent the transmission of infectious agents via droplets.

Airborne Transmission

Airborne transmission involves either airborne **droplet nuclei** or dust particles that contain the infectious microorganism. Droplet nuclei are particles smaller than 5 μm that can remain suspended in the air for long periods. These droplet nuclei can be transported long distances by air currents and can cause disease when inhaled. Droplet nuclei can be formed by sneezing or coughing or simply by singing or talking. They may also form during aerosol-producing procedures, such as suctioning or bronchoscopy. Examples of microbes spread in this manner are *Mycobacterium tuberculosis,* rubeola virus (measles), and varicella-zoster virus (chickenpox). Special ventilation and air-handling equipment designed to prevent airborne transmission include **high-efficiency particulate air (HEPA)** filters (Figure 4-2).

Infectious agents found in the environment that can cause disease via the airborne route include *Aspergillus* (a fungus) and anthrax (a bacterium). *Aspergillus* species can be aerosolized from construction dust. Patients who are immunocompromised or immunosuppressed are at risk for *Aspergillus* infection. Anthrax in a finely milled powder can also be transmitted via the airborne route. These agents are not generally thought to be transmitted from person to person.

Common Vehicle Transmission

Common vehicle transmission involves a common source that causes multiple cases of disease. This type of transmission is caused by contaminated items such as food, water, medications, devices, and equipment. An example of this is foodborne illness, such as salmonellosis or listeriosis, which can occur by ingesting food (e.g., chicken or hot dogs) contaminated with the bacteria *Salmonella* or *Listeria.* Although some infectious agents are inactivated in the gastrointestinal tract, many others are not.

Vector Transmission

Some infectious agents are carried by agents such as arthropods (e.g., insects and ticks) that are not harmed by their presence. Such organisms are called **vectors.** Mosquitoes, for instance, may carry malaria and yellow fever, and ticks may carry Lyme disease and Rocky Mountain spotted fever.

BREAKING THE CHAIN OF INFECTION

The chain of infection is broken by disrupting the continuous chain from source to host, thus preventing transmission of infectious microorganisms. Transmission is prevented by practicing appropriate hand hygiene, using PPE, and using the set of practices known as Standard Precautions. In addition, patients at risk for spreading or contracting infections may be isolated. OSHA requires all facilities to have an **exposure control plan** (ECP) that describes all these elements for preventing spread of infection. ECPs include the following elements to ensure compliance with OSHA standards:

- Determination of employee exposure
- Implementation of various exposure controls such as Universal Precautions; engineering and work practice controls (i.e., handwashing, PPE, use of safety needles); and housekeeping
- Hepatitis B vaccine
- Postexposure evaluation and follow-up
- Communication of hazards to employees and training
- Record keeping
- Procedures for evaluating circumstances surrounding an exposure incident

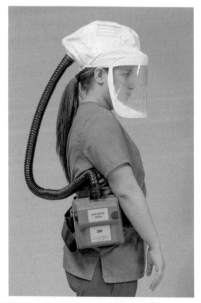

FIGURE 4-2 A health care worker wearing a respirator.

Hand Hygiene

Hand hygiene is the most important and effective means of preventing the spread of infection and antibiotic-resistant microorganisms. Hand hygiene includes (1) washing your hands with plain or antimicrobial soap and water and (2) rubbing your hands with an alcohol-based hand agent. In some institutions, an alcohol-based agent may be preferred, but CLSI guidelines indicate that it should not be used as a substitute for hand washing.

While performing your duties, your hands continually come in contact with patients and with potentially contaminated material and microorganisms. Wearing gloves reduces but does not eliminate the chance of your hands carrying infectious agents. Performing appropriate hand hygiene significantly reduces the likelihood of passing potentially infectious agents on to yourself or other people.

You should perform hand hygiene at the following times:

- Before and after patient contact
- Before donning and after removing gloves
- Before performing procedures
- After removing PPE
- After touching contaminated equipment
- Before going to break and after returning from break
- Before leaving the laboratory at the end of your shift

You should clean your hands when you enter a patient's room, even if you just cleaned them in the last patient's room, because it gives the patient confidence that you are doing all you can to prevent health care–associated infection. Always wash your hands when entering the patient's room in front of the patient even though you have washed them or sanitized several times between patients.

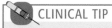

> **CLINICAL TIP**
>
> Perform hand hygiene upon entering and before exiting a patient's room and before donning and after removing gloves.

Hand hygiene sanitizes your hands by removing or killing most of the organisms present. In this way, the sanitizer acts as an antiseptic. An antiseptic is an agent used to clean living tissue, preventing sepsis, or infection.

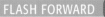 **FLASH FORWARD**
You will learn more about antiseptics and disinfectants in Chapter 8.

Procedure 4-1 illustrates proper handwashing technique. To sanitize your hands with waterless alcohol-based antiseptic hand rub, apply the product to the palm of one hand, making sure to pump enough of the product to cover all the surfaces of your hands and fingers. Rub your hands together, covering all surfaces of your hands and fingers, until your hands are dry.

Personal Protective Equipment

Personal protective equipment (PPE) consists of barriers and respirators used alone or in combination to protect skin, mucous membranes, and clothing from contact with infectious agents. PPE includes fluid-resistant gowns, aprons, masks and respirators, face shields, goggles, shoe covers, and gloves. The types of PPE you use depend on the tasks or procedures being performed, the amount of fluids you are working with, and the potential for exposure to these fluids.

Fluid-resistant gowns provide full-body coverage and prevent body fluids or spills from passing through and contacting the skin or clothing. The cuffs are designed to close tightly around the wrists and are covered by the gloves for further protection. Alternatively, a cloth gown may be worn to prevent contamination of skin and clothing with transmissible infectious microorganisms when protection from fluid penetration is not necessary.

Face protection is worn to protect mucous membranes of the eyes, mouth, and nose from splashes or sprays of blood and body fluids (including excretions and secretions). Face protection includes goggles and a mask or chin-length face shield.

Face shields can prevent droplets or spatters from contacting nonintact skin of the face. In some models, the shield can be flipped up out of the way, if necessary. Masks cover the mouth and nose to protect mucous membranes from large droplets of respiratory secretions from a coughing patient and from splashes of blood or body fluids generated during certain procedures (Figure 4-3).

Goggles and a mask or face shield must be worn during procedures that may generate splashes of blood or body fluid excretions or secretions. Masks can also worn by health care workers to prevent transmission of infectious microorganisms to patients (e.g., lung transplant or bone marrow transplant patients). Masks are secured to the head either with elastic loops or with two cloth straps for tying behind the head. They also have a metal band at the nose to seal the mask over the bridge of the nose.

PROCEDURE 4-1

Hand-Washing Technique

1. Wet your hands.
   Remove any rings you are wearing, and wet
      your hands with warm water.

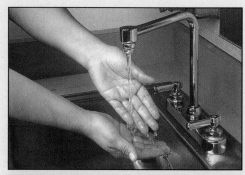

2. Apply soap.
   Soap should be applied from an easily
      accessible container.

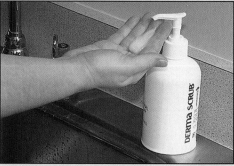

3. Scrub vigorously.
   The friction of rubbing hands together loosens
      debris and creates a lather to wash away
      surface material. Rub palms, backs of hands,
      between fingers, and under nails for at least
      15 seconds.

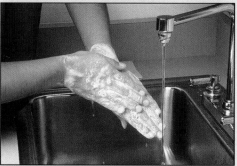

4. Rinse your hands.
   While rinsing your hands, be sure to hold them
      in a downward position. This allows water
      and lather to run into the sink instead of
      back on clean hands.

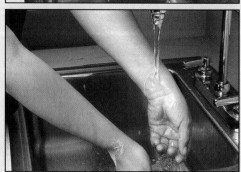

PROCEDURE 4-1—cont'd

Hand-Washing Technique

5. Dry your hands.
   Use a paper towel, being careful not to touch the paper towel dispenser as you are obtaining the towel. Dry your hands thoroughly. Hands should be dried by blotting with the towel, not by rubbing.

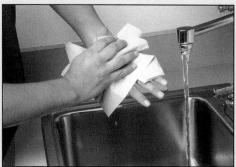

6. Turn off the faucet.
   Use a new, dry paper towel to turn off the faucet. (The faucet is considered contaminated, whereas your hands are now considered clean.) When finished, throw the paper towel in the waste container.

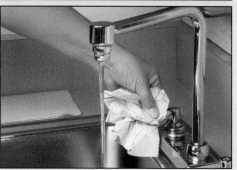

Respirators are designed to prevent inhalation of airborne microorganisms. These masks fit tightly and have filters whose efficiency capability is set by OSHA and must be certified by the National Institute for Occupational Safety and Health (NIOSH). Such masks are known as N95 masks or N95 respirators, meaning they filter out a minimum of 95% of airborne particles if they are worn correctly. Before you wear a respirator, you must receive medical clearance and be fit-checked to the specific respirator. You must check the fit each time you wear the respirator by checking for leaks on both inhalation and exhalation.

Gloves are made of a variety of materials (e.g., vinyl, nitrile, latex) and come in a variety of sizes. Latex used to be the most common material for gloves, but because of the increase in latex allergies, most health care facilities are phasing out their use of latex gloves and replacing them with gloves made of either vinyl or nitrile. Gloves provide a protective barrier against blood and other body fluids and from contamination of hands with microorganisms. They are designed to fit tightly over the hand and fingers to allow precision work. Gloves are not meant to be washed. If they become soiled or come in contact with potentially infectious material, dispose of them and put on a new pair. Never cut the finger tip off a glove to allow for a better feel on a patient's vein. Also, you must not use an oil-based hand lotion, as this may break down the glove material. Instead, use a nonprotein-based hand lotion.

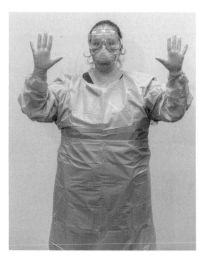

FIGURE 4-3 Health care worker wearing gown, goggles, and gloves.

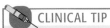

> **CLINICAL TIP**
>
> If your gloves become soiled or come in contact with a potentially infectious material, remove them, perform hand hygiene, and put on a new pair.

> **FLASH FORWARD**
>
> You learned about latex allergy in Chapter 3.

Shoe covers can protect your shoes and feet from spills of biohazardous materials or chemicals. Shoes that are not protected by shoe covers and that cannot be appropriately disinfected may need to be disposed of after a spill.

Putting on and Removing Personal Protective Equipment

The order in which you don and remove your PPE is chosen to ensure that you do not contaminate your skin or clothing with infectious agents. Procedures for putting on and removing PPE are illustrated in Procedures 4-2 and 4-3.

Standard Precautions

Standard Precautions refer to infection control measures that use barrier protection and work practice controls to prevent contact between skin or mucous membranes and blood, other body fluids, and tissues from all people. Standard Precautions are based on the difficulty of identifying all individuals who are infected or harboring infectious agents with whom the health care worker may come in contact. Standard Precautions should be the minimum level of precautions applied when coming in contact with all patients. Guidelines for Standard Precautions were published by the Centers for Disease Control and Prevention (CDC) in 1996 and include the following:

- *Hand hygiene.* Disinfect hands whether or not gloves are worn. Use an alcohol-based hand agent unless hands are visibly contaminated, in which case, use soap and water.
- *Gloves.* Wear gloves when collecting or handling blood, body fluids, tissue samples, secretions, excretions, and items contaminated with blood or body fluids. Remove gloves promptly after use and disinfect your hands.
- *Gowns.* Wear fluid-resistant gowns when there is a likelihood of contamination of your clothing or skin with blood or body fluids.
- *Face protection.* Wear appropriate protection (mask and goggles or chin-length face shield) when there is a danger of spray, spatter, or aerosol formation.
- *Sharps disposal.* Dispose of all needles and other sharps in a puncture-proof container after engaging the safety device. Do not recap the needle.
- *Respiratory hygiene and cough etiquette.* This component of Standard Precautions was added in 2003 in response to the severe acute respiratory syndrome (SARS) outbreak. These infection control measures are aimed at preventing transmission of respiratory infections. These measures apply to patients, their families and friends, and any person with signs of a cold and respiratory infection. The precautions include posting signs to instruct people who are coughing to cover mouth and nose with tissues, dispose of used tissues in the trash, and perform hand hygiene after contact with respiratory secretions. There should also be a supply of tissues and alcohol-based hand agents available for these patients, and people who are coughing should be asked to wear a surgical mask and separate themselves from other patients in the waiting room if possible.

> **CLINICAL TIP**
>
> Activate the safety device before disposing of the sharp in the needle box. Never recap a used needle.

OCCUPATIONAL SAFETY AND HEALTH ADMINISTRATION'S BLOODBORNE PATHOGENS STANDARD

OSHA is a regulatory enforcement agency for employee health and safety that has authority over all industries, including hospitals and health care facilities. In 1992 OSHA gave the Standard Precautions the force of law by making them part of a larger set of standards designed to protect health care workers from infection. The bloodborne pathogen rule was revised in 2001 to clarify issues related to sharps safety. The Bloodborne Pathogens Standard set by OSHA includes the following:

- Employers must have a written bloodborne pathogen exposure control plan in the workplace, and it must be readily accessible to employees.
- Employers must provide the proper PPE to employees at no charge, train employees in the use of PPE, and require employees to wear PPE.
- Employers must mandate that all blood and body fluids and other potentially infectious materials

PROCEDURE 4-2

Putting on Personal Protective Equipment

Perform hand hygiene before donning PPE.

1. Put on the gown.
   Tie the gown behind your back.

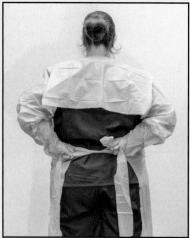

2. Put on the mask, respirator, and goggles or face shield.
   Secure the mask straps. Crimp the metal band down across the bridge of your nose. If you are donning a respirator, secure the elastic band at the middle of your head and neck. Crimp the metal band down across the bridge of your nose. Perform a fit check. Don goggles or a face shield. Adjust the face shield headband for a firm, comfortable fit.

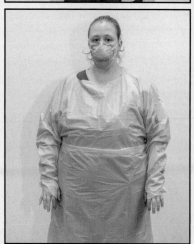

3. Put on the gloves.
   Pull the gloves on tightly, and stretch the ends of the gloves over the cuffs of the gown. The gloves should fit snugly over the cuffs.

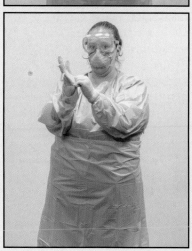

PROCEDURE 4-3

Removing Personal Protective Equipment*

The order of removal is important to prevent contamination of your skin and clothing. Except for the respirator, your PPE should be removed at the doorway, before leaving the patient's room, or in the anteroom. Remove the respirator outside the room, after the door has been closed, to avoid airborne transmission.

1. Remove the gown and gloves.
   These are likely to be the most heavily contaminated items, so they are removed first. If the gown has ties, be sure to untie before removal. Begin removing it by peeling it off over your arms, turning the sleeves inside out as you go. Before you complete removal of the gown, you will begin removing your gloves. Grasp the cuff of one glove with the opposite hand. Peel it off your hand, turning it inside out as you go. Repeat for the other glove, grasping it not with your bare hand but with the fabric of the gown. (In this way, your hands do not touch the contaminated outside surfaces of either the glove or the gown.) Complete removal by rolling the gloves and gown together and disposing of them according to hospital policy.

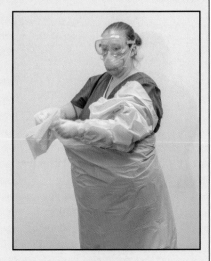

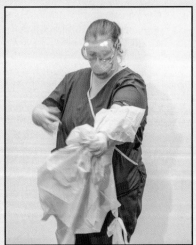

PROCEDURE 4-3–cont'd

Removing Personal Protective Equipment

2. Perform hand hygiene.
3. Remove the goggles or face shield.
   The outside of the goggles or face shield is contaminated. To remove, handle by the clean headband or earpieces. Follow hospital infection control policy for proper disposal.

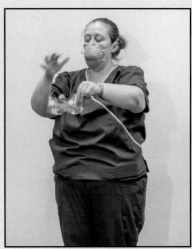

4. Remove the mask or respirator.
   The front of the mask or respirator is contaminated. Grasp the bottom ties or elastics and then the top ones, and remove. Follow hospital infection control policy for proper disposal.

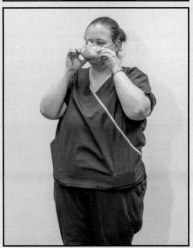

5. Perform hand hygiene again after removing all PPE.

*These steps follow the World Health Organization guidelines. Each facility has its own procedures that may differ slightly; check with your facility for its procedure.

be treated as if they are infectious and must implement work practice and engineering controls to minimize or prevent occupational exposure.

- Employers must provide immunization against HBV to employees free of charge. If the employee declines the vaccine, the employer must document that the vaccine was offered by having the employee sign a declination statement, which must be kept in the employee's personnel file.
- Employers must provide free medical follow-ups to employees in the event of accidental exposure.
- Employers must provide education and safety

training for employees at the time of hire and annually thereafter.

- Employers must provide additional training, education, and containment policies for human immunodeficiency virus (HIV) and HBV research laboratories.
- All biohazardous materials must be appropriately identified with a biohazard label (Figure 4-4) or a color-coded system and contained to prevent leakage. Regulated medical waste must be disposed of into appropriate containers (e.g., sharps and needles into puncture-resistant, leak-proof containers).

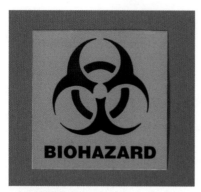

FIGURE 4-4 The biohazard symbol.

- Employers must provide a written schedule for cleaning, including a procedure for how to clean blood and other potentially infectious materials and the type of disinfectant to use. Employees must carry out daily and as-needed disinfection protocols on countertops and workspaces (e.g., bleach disinfection).
- Employers must maintain records on occupational exposure and employee training sessions.

Following these mandated standards significantly reduces the likelihood of infection.

All specimens should be handled as if they contain bloodborne pathogens. This is the best way to ensure your safety and that of others in the workplace. All tubes should be placed in a biohazard bag after filling, and the bag should be sealed before transport.

ISOLATION CONTROL MEASURES

Isolation means the separation of an infection source from susceptible hosts, thereby breaking the chain of infection. Isolation control measures can be used to protect the patient from infectious agents in the environment or carried by staff or visitors, or they can be used to protect staff, visitors, and other patients from patients with certain infectious diseases and conditions. Such patients may be in private rooms with specific isolation precautions (e.g., droplet, contact, and airborne) posted outside the door. In some cases, a separate floor of a hospital may be reserved for patients with infections that are transmitted via the airborne route and therefore require special ventilation and air handling. An example of this is tuberculosis, which requires negative-pressure air (so that air flows in, not out, of the unit). Air is exhausted directly to the outside or recirculated through HEPA filtration.

Immunocompromised patients may have their own isolation unit. This is termed a **protective environment (PE)**. These units are designed to minimize risk of acquiring environmental fungal infections (e.g., *Aspergillosis*). Such patients may include patients receiving chemotherapy and those who have had transplants. PE rooms have HEPA-filtered air and positive air pressure (air flows out, not in) with respect to adjacent areas. In addition, there may be special requirements for wearing gloves, mask, and gowns when providing care for these patients. Be sure to check with the infection control practice policies at your facility.

Isolation Precautions are based on a two-tiered system.

Tier 1 includes precautions used for all patients in the hospital without regard to their diagnosis or infection status. Standard Precautions are used for tier 1 isolation. Standard Precautions are meant to protect against transmission of infectious agents by means of blood, body fluids, secretions, and excretions; through exposure to mucous membranes and nonintact skin surfaces; and through punctures. The purpose of these precautions is to prevent transmission of pathogens regardless of a patient's diagnosis or infection status.

Tier 2 isolation uses **Expanded Precautions (EPs)**. This tier is targeted at patients known to be or suspected of being infected with a highly transmissible pathogen. It also applies to pathogens that are considered epidemiologically important, such as methicillin-resistant *Staphylococcus aureus* (MRSA) and vancomycin-resistant *Enterococcus* (VRE). EPs begin with Standard Precautions and add additional precautions based on the potential means of transmission of the suspected or identified disease or condition. There are three types of EPs: airborne, droplet, and contact. Some diseases may require a combination of precautions. An example of this is varicella (chickenpox), which requires that a nonimmunized person use both Airborne and Contact Precautions. Immunized people need to use only Contact Precautions when caring for a patient with varicella.

Airborne Precautions

In addition to Standard Precautions, **Airborne Infection Isolation Precautions** are used for patients known to have or suspected of having a disease transmitted by airborne droplet nuclei. Examples of such illnesses are measles, varicella (including disseminated zoster), and tuberculosis. Airborne Precautions include having the patient in a room with special air handling and ventilation. People entering the room must perform hand hygiene and wear an N95 respirator. A fit check must be done each time the respirator is put on.

Droplet Precautions

In addition to Standard Precautions, **Droplet Precautions** are used for patients known to have or suspected of having a disease transmitted by large infectious droplets that can be deposited on the conjunctivae or mucous membranes of a susceptible host. Examples of such diseases are listed in Box 4-2. Droplet Precautions include performing hand hygiene and wearing a mask when within 3 feet of a patient. The mask is usually donned when entering the room.

Contact Precautions

In addition to Standard Precautions, **Contact Precautions** are used for patients known to have or suspected of having diseases or conditions transmitted by direct patient contact or by contact with items in the patient's environment. Examples are listed in Box 4-3. Contact Precautions include performing hand hygiene, donning gloves, and wearing a gown for all interactions with the patient or if you will be exposed to materials in the patient's room. PPE should be donned when entering the patient's room

---

BOX 4-3 Diseases for Which Contact Precautions Should Be Used

- Enteric infections with a low infectious dose or prolonged environmental survival, including *Clostridium difficile*
- Gastrointestinal, respiratory, skin, or wound infections or colonization with multidrug-resistant bacteria judged by the infection control program, based on current state, regional, or national recommendations, to be of special clinical and epidemiologic significance
- In diapered or incontinent patients, enterohemorrhagic *Escherichia coli* O157:H7, *Shigella* species, hepatitis A, or rotavirus
- In infants and young children, respiratory syncytial virus, parainfluenza virus, or enteroviral infections
- Skin infections that are highly contagious or that may occur on dry skin:
  - Diphtheria (cutaneous)
  - Herpes simplex virus (neonatal or mucocutaneous)
  - Impetigo
  - Major (noncontained) abscesses, cellulitis, or decubitus
  - Pediculosis
  - Scabies
  - Staphylococcal furunculosis in infants and young children
  - Viral hemorrhagic infections (Ebola, Lassa, or Marburg)
  - Viral or hemorrhagic conjunctivitis
  - Zoster (disseminated or in an immunocompromised host; also airborne)

BOX 4-2 Diseases for Which Droplet Precautions Should Be Used*

Bacterial Diseases
- Diphtheria (pharyngeal)
- Invasive *Haemophilus influenzae* type b disease, including meningitis, pneumonia, epiglottitis, and sepsis
- Invasive *Neisseria meningitidis* disease, including meningitis, pneumonia, and sepsis
- *Mycoplasma pneumoniae*
- Pertussis
- Pneumonic plague
- Streptococcal (group A) pharyngitis, pneumonia, or scarlet fever in infants and young children

Viral Diseases
- Adenovirus
- Influenza
- Mumps
- Parvovirus B19
- Rubella

*Certain infections require more than one type of precaution.
From Centers for Disease Control and Prevention, Atlanta, Ga.

and removed before exiting to prevent the spread of infectious agents.

In all cases the phlebotomist should not take anything into the room except the specific equipment needed, including the phlebotomy tray. Only the specimen should come back out, and it should be placed in a biohazard-labeled bag. Remove your gloves and gown, and perform hand hygiene before leaving the room. Contaminated items should be disposed of in the appropriate receptacle in the patient's room. For used needles, the safety device should be activated, and it should be disposed of into the needle box in the room. There should be a dedicated tourniquet in the patient's room, or the tourniquet should be discarded.

FLASH FORWARD

You will learn about needle safety devices and procedures in Chapter 8.

CLEANING UP A SPILL

Despite careful technique, spills do occur. Careful and thorough cleanup protects you and your co-workers from exposure to infectious agents and potential infection. Although each laboratory has its own detailed procedures, general guidelines include the following:

- Wear gloves.
- Use 10% bleach as a disinfectant. Bleach solutions must be made fresh once a week from concentrated bleach. When you make a fresh solution, label the container as "10% bleach" and indicate the date it was made.
- Clean up the visible blood first, then disinfect the entire area of potential contamination.
- Allow the bleach to remain in contact with the contaminated area for 20 to 30 minutes to ensure complete disinfection.

Kits that contain powder or gels for absorption are available in all laboratories and work well for large spills.

REVIEW FOR CERTIFICATION

Infection transmission can occur by contact (either direct or indirect), droplet, air, common vehicle, or vector. Hand hygiene is the most important means of preventing the spread of infection and should be done before and after coming in contact with patients, before donning and after removing gloves, before performing procedures, after removing PPE, after touching potentially contaminated equipment, before eating, after eating and before coming back to work, and whenever you enter or leave a patient's room, as well as at other times.

Breaking the chain of infection is accomplished through the use of Standard Precautions and EPs and by following practices outlined in your facility's exposure control plan. The goal of Standard Precautions is to protect both the health care worker and the patient from infectious agents through hand hygiene, use of PPE (gowns, gloves, and face protection), engineering controls, and respiratory etiquette. EPs are used to guard against the transmission of specific organisms or types of diseases or conditions that require more than Standard Precautions.

Phlebotomists are at a high risk for exposure to infection from BBPs, which can occur by an accidental needle stick or other routes of exposure to blood. Use of appropriate PPE, engineering controls, and safe work practices can reduce your exposure to BBPs and other infectious agents. Cleaning up spills properly and according to protocol reduces the risk of infection transmission should a spill occur.

BIBLIOGRAPHY

Association for Professionals in Infection Control and Epidemiology: *APIC text of infection control & epidemiology,* ed. 2, Washington, DC, 2005, The Association.

Centers for Disease Control and Prevention: *Guideline for disinfection and sterilization in healthcare facilities,* 2008. Retrieved from www.cdc.gov/hicpac/pdf/guidelines/Disinfection_Nov_2008.pdf.

Centers for Disease Control and Prevention: Workplace safety and health topics: Model Plans and Programs for the OSHA Bloodborne Pathogens and Hazard Communications Standards. OSHA 3186-06R 2003, 2010. Retrieved from www.cdc.gov/niosh/topics/correctionalhcw/plan.html.

CLSI: *Protection of laboratory workers from occupationally acquired infections; Approved guideline—fourth edition. CLSI document M29-A4.* Wayne, Pa., 2014, Clinical and Laboratory Standards Institute.

Siegel JD, Rhinehart E, Jackson M, Chiarello L: The Healthcare Infection Control Practices Advisory Committee, Guideline for isolation precautions: *Preventing transmission of infectious agents in healthcare settings,* 2010. Retrieved from www.cdc.gov/hicpac/2007ip/2007isolationprecautions.html.

World Health Organization: *How to put on and take off personal protective equipment (PPE),* 2010. Retrieved from www.who.int/csr/resources/publications/PPE_EN_A1sl.pdf.

WHAT WOULD YOU DO?

You should sanitize your hands in front of the patient and thank the patient for the reminder. It is possible that you touched an infectious agent on the way to the room. Regardless of whether or not you did, performing hand hygiene in front of the patient instills confidence that you are doing all you can to keep the patient free from a health care–associated infection. You may explain to the patient you cleaned your hands just before entering the room, but that is not a reason not to do so again once in the room. Hand hygiene is the most important step in breaking the chain of infection, and it should be practiced both after you enter the room and before you leave it.

STUDY QUESTIONS

See answers in Appendix F.

1. Define infection.

2. Name four classes of pathogens.

3. List the infectious organisms that cause each of the following diseases:

  a. Acquired immunodeficiency
     syndrome (AIDS)   _____
  b. Gonorrhea   _____
  c. Hepatitis   _____
  d. Malaria   _____
  e. Oral and genital herpes   _____
  f. Strep throat   _____
  g. Syphilis   _____
  h. Trichomoniasis   _____
  i. Tuberculosis   _____

4. What are health care–associated infections, and how are they typically caused?

5. What three main elements make up the chain of infection?

6. List three ways in which you can break the chain of infection.

7. Explain the difference between direct and indirect contact transmission.

8. What is the difference between a vector and a fomite?

9. What is the most important and effective way of preventing the spread of infection?

10. Name four items included among PPE.

11. Explain what Standard Precautions are and why they are used.

12. Name three BBPs.

13. HBV may be stable in dried blood for at least _____ days.

14. Bleach should be in contact with a contaminated area for _____ minutes for complete disinfection.

15. Explain the possible reasons behind the 1992 OSHA standards, and give the policies set within this standard.

CERTIFICATION EXAMINATION PREPARATION

See answers in Appendix F.

1. Which of the following would not be considered a pathogen?
  a. Bacteria
  b. Viruses
  c. Fungi
  d. Vectors

2. Varicella-zoster is the cause of
  a. syphilis.
  b. chickenpox.
  c. malaria.
  d. hepatitis.

3. HIV is the causative agent of
  a. gonorrhea.
  b. food poisoning.
  c. AIDS.
  d. hepatitis B.

4. Vectors include
  a. doorknobs.
  b. medical instruments.
  c. needles.
  d. insects.

5. Some types of E. coli are normal flora of the
   a. urinary tract.
   b. respiratory tract.
   c. colon.
   d. circulatory system.

6. The most important way to stop the spread of infection is through
   a. isolation procedures.
   b. Standard Precautions.
   c. hand hygiene.
   d. PPE.

7. In putting on PPE, the first article that is put on is the
   a. mask.
   b. face shield.
   c. gown.
   d. pair of gloves.

8. Which of the following is not an OSHA standard?
   a. All biohazard material must be labeled.
   b. Employees must practice Standard Precautions.
   c. Employers must have written airborne pathogen exposure control plans in the workplace.
   d. Employers must provide their employees with immunization against HBV free of charge.

9. Although Standard Precautions apply to all potentially infectious situations, EPs are chosen based on
   a. whether isolation is employed.
   b. the potential means of transmission of the disease or condition.
   c. airborne transmission.
   d. the risk to the health care worker from accidental needle sticks.

10. Ten percent bleach used as a cleaning agent should be made fresh every
    a. week.
    b. 3 hours.
    c. day.
    d. 6 hours.

11. The continuous links in the chain of infection are, in order,
    a. means of transmission, susceptible host, and source.
    b. source, means of transmission, and susceptible host.
    c. susceptible host, source, and means of transmission.
    d. none of these.

12. The purpose of a PE for highly immunosuppressed patients is to
    a. prevent transmission of infection to the patient.
    b. protect the public from disease.
    c. prevent transmission of infection from the patient.
    d. protect the patient from spores in the environment.

UNIT 2
Phlebotomy Basics

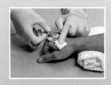

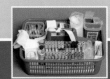

CHAPTER 5 Medical Terminology

The practice of medicine requires many specialized words whose meanings may at first seem impenetrably mysterious. However, most medical terms are formed from Latin or Greek and use prefixes, roots, combining vowels, and suffixes. Understanding the way in which words are constructed and memorizing the meanings of some of the most common word parts will allow you to decipher many terms encountered in the workplace. Abbreviations are also common and should become familiar to you.

OUTLINE

How to Use This Chapter
Parts of a Word

Abbreviations

Review for Certification

OBJECTIVES

After completing this chapter, you should be able to:

1. Define selected roots, suffixes, and prefixes.
2. Translate the English or common word for a condition or system into the appropriate medical form.
3. Use selected medical terms or expressions in their proper context.
4. Define and use correctly specific medical terms that apply to phlebotomy.
5. Define selected medical abbreviations, and use them correctly in accordance with The Joint Commission requirements.

KEY TERMS

combining form
combining vowel
prefix

root
suffix

HOW TO USE THIS CHAPTER

Medical terminology is a vital part of communicating in the health care environment. To do your job well, you will need to learn a significant number of terms you are probably unfamiliar with at the moment. Once you begin your job as a phlebotomist, many of these will become part of your daily practice, and they will quickly become a regular part of your vocabulary. Others you will likely encounter much less often. Therefore you should use this chapter in two ways. First, it provides an introduction to many of the most common terms you will encounter and with which you need to become familiar. Second, it can serve as a reference to you in the future, to remind you of the meaning of some

less common terms. But remember also that this chapter is not an exhaustive list of medical terminology. As you go on, you will likely learn more terms that you will find here. A good medical dictionary is invaluable as a complete reference.

PARTS OF A WORD

Most medical terms have several parts. For instance, *phlebotomy* is a combination of two parts, *phlebo-* and *-tomy*. *Phlebo-* means "vein," and *-tomy* means "cutting into," so *phlebotomy* literally means "to cut into a vein." Similarly, *phlebitis* is a combination of two parts, *phlebo-* and *-itis*. Once you know that *-itis* means "inflammation," you can deduce that *phlebitis* is inflammation of a vein.

The parts of a word include the **root**, or main part; a **prefix**, or part at the beginning; and a **suffix**, or part at the end (Figure 5-1). The reading of the word starts with first defining the suffix, moving to the prefix, and then to the root word. For instance, *antecubital* includes the suffix *-al,* meaning "pertaining to"; the prefix *ante-*, meaning "forward of" or "before"; and the root *cubit,* meaning "elbow." Therefore the word means "pertaining to the region forward of the elbow." Tables 5-1 through 5-3 list commonly used prefixes, suffixes, and roots.

Words may also contain a **combining vowel**, added to make pronunciation easier. For instance,

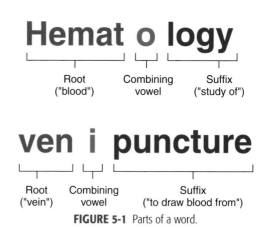

FIGURE 5-1 Parts of a word.

TABLE 5-1	Prefixes					
Prefix	**Meaning**	**Examples**	**Prefix**	**Meaning**	**Examples**
a-, an-	Without, lack of	Anemia (lack of blood)	*iso-*	Same	Isoagglutinin (protein that causes clumping when it encounters similar proteins)
ambi-, ampho-	Both	Ambidextrous (using both hands equally)			
ante-	Before, forward of	Antecubital (forward of the elbow)	*macro-*	Large	Macrophage
anti-	Against	Anticoagulant (coagulation preventer)	*mega-*	Large	Megakaryocyte
			micro-	Small	Microcyte
brady-	Slow	Bradycardia (slow heartbeat)	*neo-*	New	Neoplasm
			para-	Beside	Parathyroid gland
cryo-	Cold	Cryoagglutinins (proteins that clump in the cold)	*per-*	Throughout, through	Percutaneous (through the skin)
dys-	Bad, difficult	Dyspnea (difficulty breathing)	*peri-*	Around, surround	Pericardium (sac surrounding the heart)
ecto-, exo-	Outside	Exogenous (originating from outside)			
endo-	Inside	Endoscope (apparatus for looking inside the body)	*poly-*	Many	Polycythemia (elevated levels of blood cells)
epi-	On, over	Epicardium (outermost layer of the heart)	*post-*	After	Postprandial (after a meal)
			pre-	Before	Preexisting
			pro-	For, in front of	Prothrombin
hyper-	Above, more, increased	Hyperbilirubinemia (excess bilirubin in the blood)	*tachy-*	Fast	Tachycardia (fast heartbeat)
hypo-	Below, less, decreased	Hypodermic needle	**Prefixes for Numbers**		
			hemi-, semi-	Half	Hemiplegia (paralysis of half the body)
inter-	Between	Interstitial (relating to spaces between tissues)			
intra-	Within	Intramuscular injection	*mono-, uni-*	One	Mononuclear (having a round, or one-lobed, nucleus)

TABLE 5-1	Prefixes—cont'd				
Prefix	Meaning	Examples	Prefix	Meaning	Examples
bi-, di-	Two	Bilaterally (on both sides)	micro-	Millionth	microgram (one millionth of a gram)
tri-	Three	Tricuspid valve	nano-	Billionth	nanogram (one billionth of a gram)
tetra-, quad-	Four	Quadriceps (four-part muscle of the anterior thigh)			
Metric Prefixes			**Prefixes for Color**		
deca-	10	decaliter (10 L)	albi-	White	Albino
kilo-	1000	kilogram (1000 g)	cirrho-	Tawny yellow	Cirrhosis
deci-	10th	deciliter (1/10th of a liter)	cyan-	Blue	Cyanotic
			erythro-	Red	Erythrocyte
centi-	100th	centimeter (1/100th of a meter)	leuk-, leuko-	White	Leukocyte
			lute-	Yellow	Corpus luteum
milli-	1000th	milliliter (1/1000th of a liter)	melano-	Black	Melanoma
			nigr-	Black	Substantia nigra
			rube-	Red	Rubella

TABLE 5-2	Suffixes	
Suffix	Meaning	Examples
-ectomy	Surgical removal	Appendectomy
-emia	Blood condition	Anemia, bacteremia
-gen, -genic, -genous	Originating from, caused by	Iatrogenic (caused by medical treatment)
-itis	Inflammation	Arthritis
-oma	Tumor, growth	Hematoma
-osis	Condition	Tuberculosis
-pathy	Disease	Cardiopathy
-penia	Deficiency	Thrombocytopenia
-plasty	Shape, form	Angioplasty (surgical repair or reshaping of a blood vessel)
-plegia	Paralysis	Tetraplegia (paralysis of all four limbs)
-stasis	Stopping, control	Hemostasis
-stomy	Opening	Colostomy
-tomy	Cut	Phlebotomy

called the **combining form** of the root. Combining vowels usually are not used when the suffix begins with a vowel. For instance, no combining vowel is used to form *leukemia,* which combines the root *leuk* and the suffix *-emia,* meaning "blood condition."

The spelling of roots can also change slightly when they are combined with different suffixes. For instance, *erythema,* meaning "redness of the skin," uses a slightly modified form of the root *erythro.*

The plurals of some medical terms are formed by changing the end of the word rather than adding an *s.* For instance, words ending in *-us* typically change to *-i* for the plural, as in *nucleus* to *nuclei* and *thrombus* to *thrombi.* A list of such plurals is given in Table 5-4.

By memorizing some of the most common roots and remembering these simple guidelines, you should be able to deduce the meanings of many common medical terms. Keeping a medical dictionary handy allows you to learn terms you do not know. Medical dictionaries often have tables of word roots.

leuk is a root meaning "white," and *cyte* means "cell." An *o* is added to make *leukocyte,* a white blood cell. Similarly, *cyt* and *-logy,* meaning "study of," are joined with a combining vowel to form *cytology,* the study of cells. The combination of a word root and a combining vowel (usually an *o*) is

ABBREVIATIONS

Abbreviations are used widely in the health care field. In most cases, a particular abbreviation has only one widely used meaning within the medical

TABLE 5-3	Word Roots	
Root	Meaning	Examples
agglut	Clump together	Agglutinin
angio	Vessel	Angioplasty (reshaping a blood vessel)
arterio	Artery	Arteriosclerosis
arthro	Joint	Arthritis
bili	Bile	Bilirubin
cardio	Heart	Cardiologist (one who treats heart disease)
cephal	Head	Encephalitis
colo	Colon	Colostomy
cubit	Elbow	Antecubital fossa
cyst	Bladder	Cystitis, cystogram
derm	Skin	Dermal puncture
gastr	Stomach	Gastrostomy (opening into the stomach)
heme	Blood	Hematology, hemagglutinins
hepato	Liver	Hepatitis
necro	Death	Necrosis (cell or tissue death)
nephr	Kidney	Nephron
oste	Bone	Osteoma
phago, phage	Eat	Phagocyte, macrophage
phlebo	Vein	Phlebotomy
pneu, pnea	Breath	Pneumatic, apnea (lack of breathing)
pulmon	Lung	Pulmonary insufficiency
ren	Kidney	Renal artery
spleno	Spleen	Splenomegaly (enlarged spleen)
thromb	Clot	Thrombin, thrombosis
tox, toxico	Poison	Toxicology, detoxification
veno	Vein	Venopressor

TABLE 5-4	Plurals	
Singular Word Ending	Plural Form	Examples
-a	-ae	Axilla, axillae Fossa, fossae
-en	-ina	Lumen, lumina
-is	-es	Naris, nares
-ix	-ices	Fornix, fornices Cervix, cervices
-nx	-nges	Pharynx, pharynges
-on	-oa	Spermatozoon, spermatozoa
-um	-a	Ovum, ova
-us	-i	Articulus, articuli Nucleus, nuclei
-ux	-uces	Hallux, halluces

instance, AE may mean "above the elbow" to a phlebotomist reading a chart about a burn victim's scars, but it may mean "adverse effects" to a pharmacist comparing side effects of two drugs. Table 5-5 lists many of the abbreviations you will encounter. Because of the potential for confusion, The Joint Commission has recommended avoiding certain abbreviations, shown in Table 5-6. Abbreviations of medical tests are found in later chapters as they are covered.

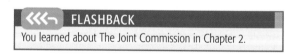

FLASHBACK

You learned about The Joint Commission in Chapter 2.

REVIEW FOR CERTIFICATION

Medical terms are most commonly formed from Greek or Latin. Each term contains a root and may contain a prefix, suffix, combining vowel, or other root. A combining vowel, usually an *o*, is used with a root to create a combining form for ease of pronunciation. A large number of abbreviations are used in the health care environment. Most abbreviations have unique meanings within a medical context.

field. For instance, MD, HIV, and Rx have unambiguous meanings in virtually any medical context (meaning "doctor of medicine," "human immunodeficiency virus," and "prescription," respectively). A few abbreviations are more context specific. For

TABLE 5-5	**Commonly Encountered Abbreviations**		
Abbreviation	Definition	Abbreviation	Definition
AC	Accommodation	DM	Diabetes mellitus
AC, ac	Before meals	DNA	Deoxyribonucleic acid
adeno-CA	Adenocarcinoma	DO	Doctor of osteopathy
ad lib	As desired	DOB	Date of birth
AE	Above the elbow, adverse effects	DPT	Diphtheria–pertussis–tetanus
AGN	Acute glomerulonephritis	DVT	Deep vein thrombosis
AIDS	Acquired immunodeficiency syndrome	Dx	Diagnosis
AK	Above the knee	ECG, EKG	Electrocardiogram
ALL	Acute lymphocytic leukemia	EEG	Electroencephalogram
AMA	American Medical Association, against medical advice	EENT	Eye, ear, nose, and throat
		ENT	Ear, nose, and throat
AMI	Acute myocardial infarction	ER, ED	Emergency room, emergency department
AML	Acute myelocytic leukemia	et	And
ARDS	Adult respiratory distress syndrome	F	Fahrenheit
ASAP	As soon as possible	FACP	Fellow of the American College of Physicians
BK	Below the knee		
BM	Bowel movement	FACS	Fellow of the American College of Surgeons
BP	Blood pressure		
Bx	Biopsy	FDA	Food and Drug Administration
C	Celsius, centigrade	Fe	Iron
c̄	With	FHR	Fetal heart rate
Ca	Calcium	FHT	Fetal heart tone
CA	Cancer	FS	Frozen section
CAD	Coronary artery disease	FTND	Full-term normal delivery
CAT	Computed axial tomography	FUO	Fever of undetermined origin
CC	Chief complaint	Fx	Fracture
CCU	Coronary care unit	g, gm	Gram
CDC	Centers for Disease Control and Prevention	GC	Gonorrhea
		GI	Gastrointestinal
CGN	Chronic glomerulonephritis	gr	Grain
CHF	Congestive heart failure	gt, Gtt, gtt	Drop, drops
Cl	Chloride	Gyn, gyn	Gynecology
CLL	Chronic lymphocytic leukemia	h, hr	Hour
cm	Centimeter	H	Hypodermic
CML	Chronic myelocytic leukemia	HCl	Hydrochloric acid
CNS	Central nervous system	HCO_3^-	Bicarbonate
CO_2	Carbon dioxide	Hg	Mercury
COLD	Chronic obstructive lung disease	HIV	Human immunodeficiency virus
contra	Against	hypo	Hypodermically
COPD	Chronic obstructive pulmonary disease	I&D	Incision and drainage
CPR	Cardiopulmonary resuscitation	ICU	Intensive care unit
CS, C-section	Cesarean section	ID	Intradermal
CT	Computed tomography	Ig	Immunoglobulin
CV	Cardiovascular	IM	Intramuscular
CVA	Cerebrovascular accident	IQ	Intelligence quotient
CVD	Cardiovascular disease	IS	Intercostal space
CXR	Chest x-ray, chest radiograph	IUD	Intrauterine device
d	Day, 24 hours	IV	Intravenous, intravenously
/d	Per day	IVC	Intravenous cholangiography
D&C	Dilation and curettage	IVP	Intravenous pyelogram
D&E	Dilation and evacuation	K	Potassium
dB	Decibel	KD	Knee disarticulation

Continued

TABLE 5-5 Commonly Encountered Abbreviations—cont'd

Abbreviation	Definition	Abbreviation	Definition
kg	Kilogram	PID	Pelvic inflammatory disease
KUB	Kidney, ureter, and bladder	PMP	Previous menstrual period
L	Liter	PO	Orally (per os; os = mouth)
LAT, lat	Lateral	postop, p/o	After operation
lb	Pound	pp	Postprandial
LE	Lupus erythematosus	preop	Before operation
LMP	Last menstrual period	prep	Prepare
LPN	Licensed practical nurse	prn	As required
M, m	Meter	pt	Patient
mcg	Microgram	PT	Physical therapy, physical therapist
MD	Doctor of medicine	PVC	Premature ventricular contraction
mets	Metastases	q	Every
Mg	Magnesium	qns	Quantity not sufficient
MH	Marital history	qs	Quantity sufficient
MI	Myocardial infarction	R	Respiration
MICU	Medical intensive care unit	RD	Respiratory disease
mL	Milliliter	REM	Rapid eye movement
mm	Millimeter	RN	Registered nurse
MRI	Magnetic resonance imaging	RNA	Ribonucleic acid
MS	Multiple sclerosis	ROM	Range of motion
MVP	Mitral valve prolapse	Rx	Prescription
NB	Newborn	s̄	Without
NICU	Neonatal intensive care unit	SICU	Surgical intensive care unit
NPO	Nothing by mouth (os = mouth)	SLE	Systemic lupus erythematosus
O_2	Oxygen	SOB	Short(ness) of breath
OA	Osteoarthritis	SOS	If necessary
OB	Obstetrics	Sp. gr.	Specific gravity
OC	Oral contraceptive	Staph	*Staphylococcus*
OHS	Open heart surgery	stat	Immediately
OR	Operating room	STI	Sexually transmitted infection
Ortho, ORTH	Orthopedics	Strep	*Streptococcus*
OT	Occupational therapy, occupational therapist	T	Temperature
Oto	Otology	T&A	Tonsillectomy and adenoidectomy
oz	Ounce	TB	Tuberculosis
P	Pulse, phosphorus	THR	Total hip replacement
Pap	Papanicolaou (smear)	TIA	Transient ischemic attack
paren	Parenterally	TPN	Total parenteral nutrition
Path	Pathology	TPR	Temperature, pulse, and respiration
PC, pc	After meals		
PD	Postprandial (after meals)	URI	Upper respiratory infection
PE	Physical examination	UTI	Urinary tract infection
Peds	Pediatrics	VA	Visual acuity
pH	Hydrogen ion concentration	VD	Venereal disease
PICU	Pulmonary intensive care unit, pediatric intensive care unit	wt	Weight
		X	Multiplied by

TABLE 5-6	Abbreviations That Should Not Be Used: Official "Do Not Use" List*	
Do Not Use	Potential Problem	Use Instead
U (unit)	Mistaken for 0, 4, or cc	unit
IU (International Unit)	Mistaken for IV (intravenous) or 10	International Unit
QD, Q.D., qd, q.d. (daily)	Mistaken for each other	daily
Q.O.D., QOD, q.o.d, qod (every other day)	Period after the Q mistaken for I, O mistaken for I	every other day
Trailing zero (X.0 mg)†	Decimal point missed	X mg
Lack of leading zero (.X mg)	Decimal point missed	0.X mg
MS	Can mean morphine sulfate or magnesium sulfate	morphine sulfate
MSO_4, $MgSO_4$	Confused for each other	magnesium sulfate

Copyright The Joint Commission, 2010. Reprinted with permission.
*Applies to all orders and all medication-related documentation that is handwritten (including free-text computer entry) or on preprinted forms.
†Exception: A "trailing zero" may be used only where required to demonstrate the level of precision of the value being reported, such as for laboratory results, imaging studies that report size of lesions, or catheter/tube sizes. It may not be used in medication orders or other medication-related documentation.

BIBLIOGRAPHY

Davis NM: *15,000 Medical abbreviations: Conveniences at the expense of communication and safety,* ed. 15, Philadelphia, 2011, Neil M Davis Associates: Temple University.

Dorland illustrated medical dictionary, ed. 32, Philadelphia, 2011, Saunders.

Joint Commission: *Official* "Do Not Use" *list.* Retrieved from www.jointcommission.org/patientsafety/donotuselist.

Leonard PC: *Quick & easy medical terminology,* ed. 7, St. Louis, 2013, Saunders.

STUDY QUESTIONS

See answers in Appendix F.

1. The parts of a word always include a _____ and may include a _____ or _____.

2. Give the meaning of the following prefixes:

ante-	before
anti-	against
brady-	slow
cirrho-	yellow
cyan-	blue
epi-	on, over
erythro-	red
hemi-	half
hyper-	above
hypo-	below
inter-	between
intra-	within
leuko-	white
lute-	yellow
micro-	small
nano-	billionth
neo-	new
peri-	around
poly-	many
post-	after
rube-	red

tachy-   Fast
tetra-   four

3. Give the meaning of the following roots:
   agglut   clump together
   angio   vessel
   arthro   joint
   bili   bile
   cardio   heart
   derm   skin
   heme   blood
   hepato   liver
   oste   bone
   nephro   kidney
   phago   eat
   phlebo   vein
   pnea   breath
   pulmon   lung
   ren   kidney
   thromb   clot
   tox   poison

4. Give the meaning of the following suffixes:
   -ectomy   surgical removal
   -emia   blood condition
   -genous   originating from
   -itis   inflammation
   -oma   tumor, growth
   -pathy   disease
   -penia   deficiency
   -plasty   shape
   -plegia   paralysis
   -stasis   stopping
   -tomy   cut

5. List what each of the following abbreviations stands for:
   AIDS   acquired immunodeficiency syndrome
   ASAP   as soon as possible
   BP   blood pressure
   CCU   cardiac care unit
   COLD   chronic obstructive pulmonary disease
   CPR   cardiopulmonary resuscitation
   CV   cardiovascular
   CVA   cerebrovascular accident
   DM   diabetes mellitus
   DOB   date of birth
   DVT   deep vein thrombosis
   Dx   diagnosis
   ECG/EKG   electrocardiogram
   FUO   fever of unknown origin
   GI   gastrointestinal
   hypo   hypodermically
   ICU   intensive care unit
   ID   identification
   IM   intramuscular

IV _intravenously_
LMP _last menstrual period_
MI _myocardial infarction_
NB _newborn_
NPO _nothing by mouth_
O₂ _oxygen_
OB _obstetrics_
OR _operating room_
P _____
PD _____
Pp _post-prandial_
prep _prepare_
pt _patient_
q _every_
qns _quantity not sufficient_
Rx _prescription_
SOB _shortness of breath_
stat _immediately_
STI _sexually transmitted infection_
TB _tuberculosis_
URI _upper respiratory infection_
UTI _urinary tract infection_

6. Write the plural form of each of the following words:

appendix _appendices_
larynx _larynges_
papilla _papillae_
scapula _scapulae_
testis _testes_
vertebra _vertebrae_

CERTIFICATION EXAMINATION PREPARATION

See answers in Appendix F.

1. _Hepato_ refers to the
   a. liver.
   b. kidney.
   c. heart.
   d. blood.

2. _Cyan-_ refers to
   a. red.
   b. yellow.
   c. black.
   d. blue.

3. _Hemi-_ means
   a. many.
   b. half.
   c. whole.
   d. two.

4. _-tomy_ means
   a. study of.
   b. to cut.
   c. shape or form.
   d. opening.

5. _Anti-_ means
   a. between.
   b. among.
   c. against.
   d. for.

6. _Leuko-_ refers to
   a. red.
   b. yellow.
   c. blue.
   d. white.

7. *-emia* means
   a. blood condition.
   b. tumor.
   c. opening.
   d. paralysis.

8. *Pulmon* refers to the
   a. liver.
   b. lung.
   c. colon.
   d. heart.

9. *Thromb* refers to
   a. hemolysis.
   b. clotting.
   c. lymphostasis.
   d. tumor.

10. *Derm* refers to
   a. death.
   b. bone.
   c. skin.
   d. blood.

11. Nephro refers to
   a. vein.
   b. kidney.
   c. brain.
   d. lung.

12. Cardio refers to
   a. heart.
   b. bone.
   c. liver.
   d. skin.

13. Heme refers to
   a. clot.
   b. vessel.
   c. blood.
   d. joint.

14. Erythro refers to
   a. black.
   b. cell.
   c. white.
   d. red.

15. Poly- refers to
   a. few.
   b. after.
   c. inside.
   d. many.

16. –logy refers to
   a. form.
   b. tumor.
   c. to cut.
   d. study of.

17. –ectomy refers to
   a. inflammation.
   b. surgical removal.
   c. cut.
   d. opening.

18. Inter- refers to
   a. between.
   b. above.
   c. within.
   d. below.

19. Intra- refers to
   a. same.
   b. many.
   c. after.
   d. within.

20. –oma refers to
   a. cut.
   b. tumor.
   c. disease.
   d. control.

21. –stomy refers to
   a. opening.
   b. cut.
   c. study.
   d. disease.

22. Phlebo refers to
   a. capillary.
   b. artery.
   c. vein.
   d. cut.

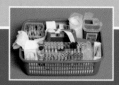

CHAPTER 6 Human Anatomy and Physiology

An understanding of human anatomy and physiology allows the phlebotomist to interact more knowledgeably with both patients and other health care professionals. The tissues, organs, and body systems work together to create and maintain homeostasis, the integrated control of body function that is characteristic of health. Each body system is prone to particular types of diseases and is subject to particular tests that aid in diagnosing those diseases. As a phlebotomist, many of the patients you collect samples from will be undergoing diagnosis or treatment for diseases or other disorders. Others may require blood collection for reasons not related to illness, such as pregnancy or blood donation. In this chapter, we discuss all aspects of human anatomy and physiology except the circulatory system and the related lymphatic and immune systems. Because of their special importance to phlebotomy, these systems are covered separately in the next chapter.

OUTLINE

OBJECTIVES

After completing this chapter, you should be able to:

1. Describe the three levels of organization of the human body.
2. Name four structures of the cell and describe the functions of each.
3. Name four kinds of tissue and explain the roles of each.
4. Define each anatomic term discussed and use it to locate various structures and position a patient.
5. Describe the eight major body cavities and list at least one organ contained in each.

6. For each of the following body systems describe major features, organs, and functions and list associated diseases and common laboratory tests:
   a. Skeletal
   b. Muscular
   c. Integumentary
   d. Nervous
   e. Digestive
   f. Urinary
   g. Respiratory
   h. Endocrine
   i. Reproductive

KEY TERMS

abdominal cavity
abduction
adduction
adrenal cortex
adrenal medulla
adrenocorticotropic
   hormone (ACTH)
afferents
agonist
aldosterone
alveoli
amino acid derivatives
amphiarthrosis
anatomic position
antagonist
anterior
antidiuretic hormone
   (ADH)
arachnoid
articular cartilage
autonomic motor system
bile
Bowman's capsule
brainstem
bronchi
bronchioles
bulbourethral glands
calcitonin
carbohydrases
cardiac muscle
central nervous system
   (CNS)
cerebellum
cerebral cortex
cerebrospinal fluid
   (CSF)
cerebrum
cervix
chyme
cilia
collecting duct
connective tissue
corticosterone
cortisol
cortisone
cranial cavity

cytoplasm
dermis
diarthrosis
distal
distal convoluted
   tubule
dorsal
dura mater
efferents
epidermis
epididymis
epinephrine
epithelial tissue
esophagus
estrogens
extension
external respiration
fallopian tube
feedback loops
flexion
follicle-stimulating
   hormone (FSH)
frontal plane
glomerulus
glucagon
glucocorticoids
gonads
ground substance
growth hormone (GH)
hematopoiesis
homeostasis
hormones
human chorionic
   gonadotropin (hCG)
hypothalamus
inferior
insulin
internal respiration
interneuron
larynx
lateral
ligaments
lipases
loop of Henle
luteinizing hormone
   (LH)

marrow
medial
melanocyte-stimulating
   hormone (MSH)
meninges
mineralocorticoids
mitochondria
motor neurons
myelin
nephron
nerves
neuromuscular junction
neurons
neurotransmitter
nonstriated involuntary
   muscle
norepinephrine
nucleus
osteoblasts
osteoclasts
ovaries
ovulation
oxyhemoglobin
oxytocin
parathormone
parathyroid hormone
   (PTH)
pelvic cavity
penis
peptides
pericardial cavity
peripheral nervous system
   (PNS)
peristalsis
peritoneal cavity
pharynx
pia mater
plasma membrane
pleural cavity
posterior
progesterone
prolactin
prone
prostate
proteases
proximal

proximal convoluted
   tubule
sagittal plane
scrotum
section
semen
seminal vesicles
skeletal muscle
smooth muscle
somatic motor system
sphincter
spinal cavity
steroid hormones
striated involuntary
   muscle
striated voluntary
   muscle
superior
supine
synapse
synaptic cleft
synarthrosis
synovial cavity
tendons
testosterone
thalamus
thermoregulation
thoracic cavity
thymosin
thyroid-stimulating
   hormone (TSH)
thyroxine (T_4)
tissues
trachea
tracts
transverse plane
triiodothyronine (T_3)
ureter
urethra
uterus
vagina
vas deferens
ventral
ventricles
villi

ABBREVIATIONS

ABGs arterial blood gases
ACE angiotensin-converting enzyme
ACTH adrenocorticotropic hormone
ADH antidiuretic hormone
ALP alkaline phosphatase
ALS amyotrophic lateral sclerosis
ALT alanine aminotransferase
ANA antinuclear antibody
AST aspartate aminotransferase
ATP adenosine triphosphate
BUN blood urea nitrogen
C&S culture and sensitivity
CBC complete blood count
CK creatine kinase
CK-BB creatine kinase-BB
CK-MB creatine kinase-MB
CK-MM creatine kinase-MM
CNS central nervous system
COPD chronic obstructive pulmonary disease
CSF cerebrospinal fluid
CT computed tomography
DNA deoxyribonucleic acid
ENT ear, nose, and throat
ESR erythrocyte sedimentation rate
FBS fasting blood sugar (glucose)
FSH follicle-stimulating hormone
FTA-ABS fluorescent treponemal antibody absorption test
GGT γ-glutamyltransferase
GH growth hormone

HBsAG hepatitis B surface antigen
hCG human chorionic gonadotropin
HCV hepatitis C virus
HIV human immunodeficiency virus
IRDS infant respiratory distress syndrome
KOH potassium hydroxide
LH luteinizing hormone
MRI magnetic resonance imaging
MSH melanocyte-stimulating hormone
O&P ova and parasites
PCR polymerase chain reaction
PID pelvic inflammatory disease
PMS premenstrual syndrome
PNS peripheral nervous system
PPD purified protein derivative
PSA prostate-specific antigen
PTH parathyroid hormone
RA rheumatoid arthritis
RF rheumatoid factor
RPR rapid plasma reagin
RSV respiratory syncytial virus
SLE systemic lupus erythematosus
STI sexually transmitted infection
T$_3$ triiodothyronine
T$_4$ thyroxine
TSH thyroid-stimulating hormone
TSS toxic shock syndrome
URI upper respiratory infection
UTI urinary tract infection

LEVELS OF ORGANIZATION

Just as a complex institution such as a hospital has different levels of organization, so does the human body. At the most basic level, the body is composed of cells. Cells of similar type join to form tissues, and tissues interact to form discrete units of function called organs. When different organs interact to carry out common tasks, they form an organ system. Organ systems themselves interact, making an integrated, functioning body.

At each level, the body acts to maintain homeostasis, or the dynamic steady state we think of when we refer to good health. Homeostasis requires many functions: nutrition, materials processing, and waste elimination; repair of injury, defense against infection, and regulation of growth; and communication and coordination among the parts of the body.

Cells

Cells are the smallest living units in the body. Cells are much like small factories, using raw materials to produce products for internal use or export. For cells, the raw materials include oxygen from the air and food molecules such as sugars and amino acids; the products are often more complex molecules, such as hormones or proteins. Muscle cells use up large amounts of sugar and oxygen to power their own movement, and neurons (nerve cells) use these same raw materials to create electrical and chemical signals.

The structures within cells that allow these functions to occur are complex (Figure 6-1). Among the most important are the following.

Nucleus

The **nucleus** contains deoxyribonucleic acid (DNA). DNA is arranged in functional units called genes,

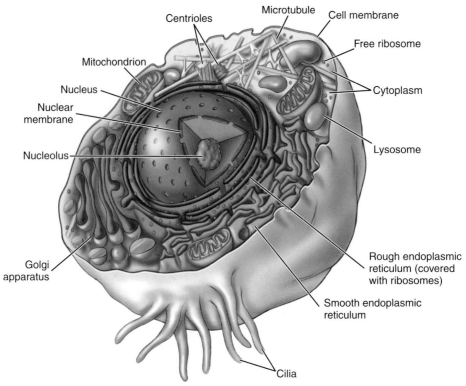

FIGURE 6-1 Cell structures include the plasma membrane, nucleus, mitochondria, and other organelles responsible for maintaining cellular homeostasis. (From Herlihy B: *The human body in health and illness,* ed. 5, St. Louis, 2015, Saunders.)

and genes are linked together in long strings called chromosomes. Genes perform two functions. During the normal life of the cell, they act as blueprints for making proteins. During cell reproduction, they act as the material of heredity, forming copies of themselves so that each new cell formed has a complete and identical set of blueprints. Defects in genes are responsible for hereditary diseases such as hemophilia and sickle cell disease. All cells in the body begin with a nucleus, but red blood cells push out theirs at maturity.

Mitochondria

Mitochondria are the cell's power plants, burning fuels such as sugar and fat with oxygen to supply energy for the cell in the form of adenosine triphosphate (ATP). Neurons and muscle cells contain very high numbers of mitochondria.

Cytoplasm

Cytoplasm refers to all the cellular material except the plasma membrane and the nucleus. Cytosol is the fluid portion of the cytoplasm.

Plasma Membrane

The **plasma membrane** encloses the cell and tightly regulates the flow of materials in and out of it. Membranes are flexible, allowing cells to change shape if necessary. For instance, the red blood cell must squeeze through tiny capillaries that are thinner than its normal diameter, a feat made possible by the flexibility of the membrane.

Tissues

Cells of similar structure and function combine to form **tissues**. The human body is composed of the following four basic types of tissues:
1. Epithelial
2. Muscle
3. Nerve
4. Connective

Epithelial Tissue

Epithelial tissue forms flat sheets and is most often found on surfaces where exchange with the environment takes place, such as the lining of the gut (Figure 6-2), or where rapid regeneration must

Stratified squamous

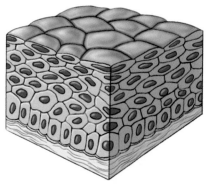

FIGURE 6-2 An example of epithelial tissue. (From Herlihy B: *The human body in health and illness,* ed. 5, St. Louis, 2015, Saunders.)

body just below the epithelial tissue, such as around the gut, lungs, bladder, and circulatory and reproductive systems. Smooth muscle contractions regulate the passage of materials through the vessel. For instance, contraction of intestinal smooth muscle propels food along the digestive system. Contraction of smooth muscle surrounding veins constricts the vessel, decreasing flow through the vein. Smooth muscle also is found in the skin, where it is responsible for hair erection.

FLASH FORWARD

As you will learn in Chapter 7, primary hemostasis (bleeding control) involves smooth muscle constriction.

occur to protect internal structures, such as the skin or the surface of the eye. Epithelium may contain glands, which produce and secrete substances such as saliva, sweat, or insulin.

Muscle Tissue

Muscle tissue is contractile, meaning that it can shorten its length. Muscle cells contain long fibers of the proteins actin and myosin, whose movements produce muscle contraction. Muscles receive the stimulus to contract when the axon terminals of motor neurons (neurons that stimulate muscle) make contact with the muscle. The neuron releases a chemical (called a neurotransmitter) onto the muscle cell surface at the **neuromuscular junction,** causing the chemical changes within the muscle that lead to contraction.

Muscle tissue occurs in three forms, which differ in both structure and function (Figure 6-3):

1. **Skeletal muscle,** or **striated voluntary muscle,** is the most widespread type, constituting all the muscles that move the skeleton. Under the microscope, striated muscle has a striped appearance.
2. **Cardiac muscle,** or **striated involuntary muscle,** is found in the heart. It looks similar to skeletal muscle but has features that are unique to it. Cardiac muscle cells do not need stimulation by the nervous systems to start a contraction. However, electrical stimulation is required to maintain the coordinated rhythm of the cells. This function is performed by the heart's physiologic pacemaker, found in the right atrium.
3. **Smooth muscle,** or **nonstriated involuntary muscle,** lines blood and lymph vessels within the

Nerve Tissue

Nerve tissue is specialized for intercellular communication by the conduction of electrical impulses and release of chemical messages. Nerve tissue is composed of neurons and neuroglial cells. **Neurons** are excitable cells, meaning that they can be stimulated to undergo electrical and chemical changes. Neurons are found in the brain and spinal cord and throughout the body. Neuroglial cells nourish and support neurons in the brain and spinal cord.

The three major portions of the neuron are the dendrite, cell body, and axon (Figure 6-4). Axons can be extremely long; each of the motor neurons controlling the toes, for instance, has an axon that stretches from the spinal cord, down the leg, through the ankle, and to the muscles of the foot. Axons are insulated by a fatty sheath of **myelin.**

One neuron conveys information to another by releasing a chemical, called a **neurotransmitter,** at the small gap where they meet, called the **synaptic cleft,** or **synapse.** The neurotransmitter leaves the axon of the first neuron, crosses the synaptic cleft, and lands on a receptor on the dendrite of the second neuron, beginning a cascade of chemical changes down the length of the neuron. This may ultimately cause the second neuron to release its own neurotransmitter, thereby conveying information farther along the neural chain.

Connective Tissue

The general function of **connective tissue** is to bind and support the other three types of tissue. Connective tissue is characterized by a relative scarcity of cells and a relative abundance of extracellular **ground substance** secreted by the cells. Bone is a

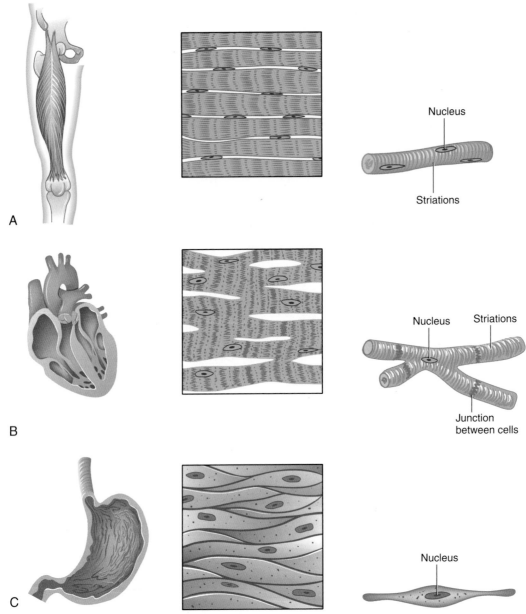

FIGURE 6-3 The three forms of muscle tissue. **A,** Skeletal. **B,** Cardiac. **C,** Smooth.

connective tissue—its ground substance is collagen, impregnated with mineral crystals. Blood is also a connective tissue, with plasma as its ground substance.

Organs

An organ is a distinct structural unit in the body, specialized for some complex function. Organs such as the heart, lungs, and kidneys incorporate all four tissue types. In the lungs, for instance, epithelial tissue lines the airways, cleaning and moistening them and providing a barrier to infection. Smooth muscle constricts or relaxes to regulate the size of the airway. Neurons in the bronchi detect the presence of excess mucus or other irritants and provoke a cough. Cartilage—a type of connective tissue—supports the larger airways to prevent collapse.

Body Systems

Body systems are groups of organs functioning together for a common purpose. The respiratory system, for instance, involves not only the lungs but

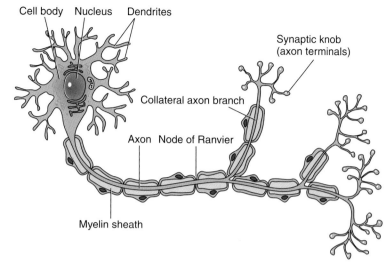

FIGURE 6-4 Neurons are specialized for communication. Signals travel from dendrite to cell body to axon, causing the release of neurotransmitters into the synaptic cleft separating the two neurons.

also the upper airway, including the nasal passages and throat. It also includes the muscles that inflate the lungs, such as the diaphragm, the rib muscles, and the muscles of the neck.

After a brief discussion of anatomic terminology, we review the structure and function of the body systems, discuss how they may be involved in disease, and indicate what tests can be ordered to monitor their function.

ANATOMIC TERMINOLOGY

Medical anatomists describe the location and direction of body structures with reference to the **anatomic position** (Figure 6-5). In this position, the body is erect and facing forward, and the arms are at the side with palms facing forward and thumbs pointed outward. When you look at a picture of a person in the anatomic position, their left hand is on the right-hand side of the picture. You can avoid becoming confused by remembering that "left" and "right" always refer to the person's left and right, not that of the picture. This is especially important to keep in mind when discussing internal structures, such as the heart.

Directional Terms

Directional terms are used to describe the relation of one body part to another or to describe a motion in relation to some part of the body. These terms remove any confusion or doubt that might ensue from such phrases as "insert the needle below the elbow," which could be interpreted to mean on the

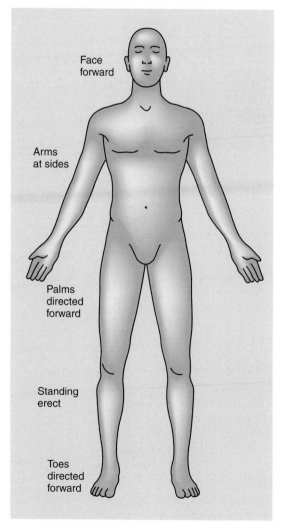

FIGURE 6-5 The body in the anatomic position.

underside of the elbow rather than on the forearm. Understanding and careful use of these terms will allow you to perform procedures correctly and improve your ability to communicate with other health care professionals. Refer to Figure 6-6 as you learn the following pairs of terms.

- Ventral and anterior refer to the front surface of the body. Routine venipuncture is performed on the ventral surface of the forearm. Dorsal and posterior refer to the back surface of the body. Hand venipuncture is usually performed on the dorsal surface of the hand.
- Lateral means more toward the side, away from the body's central axis. In the anatomic position (see Figure 6-5), the thumb is lateral to the other fingers. Medial means more toward the middle.
- Distal means farther from the point of origin of the structure in question. The elbow is distal to the shoulder, and the hand is distal to the wrist. Proximal means closer to the point of attachment.
- Inferior means below. The mouth is inferior to the nose. Superior means above. The eyebrows are superior to the eyes.
- Prone means lying on the abdomen with the face down. Supine means lying on the back with face up. Patients may be placed in the supine position during venipuncture if they are likely to faint.
- Flexion refers to a movement that bends a joint. Extension straightens the joint.
- Abduction is a movement that takes a body part farther from the central axis, and adduction brings it closer.

Body Planes

Depicting internal organs is often best done by slicing through them to make a section, or an imaginary flat surface. There are three sectional planes—two vertical and one horizontal (Figure 6-7):
1. Sagittal plane: A vertical plane dividing the body into left and right
2. Frontal plane: A vertical plane dividing the body into front and back
3. Transverse plane: A horizontal plane dividing the body into top and bottom

Body Cavities

Body cavities are spaces within the body that contain major organ systems. There are two large body cavities: the ventral cavity and the dorsal cavity. These are subdivided to form the eight major body cavities (Figure 6-8).

Ventral Cavity Subdivisions

The thoracic cavity contains the heart (within the pericardial cavity) and lungs (within the pleural cavity).

The abdominal cavity contains the stomach, small and large intestines, spleen, liver, gallbladder, pancreas, and kidneys (all but the kidneys are within the peritoneal cavity). The pelvic cavity contains the bladder, rectum, ovaries, and testes.

Dorsal Cavity Subdivisions

The cranial cavity contains the brain, and the spinal cavity contains the spinal cord.

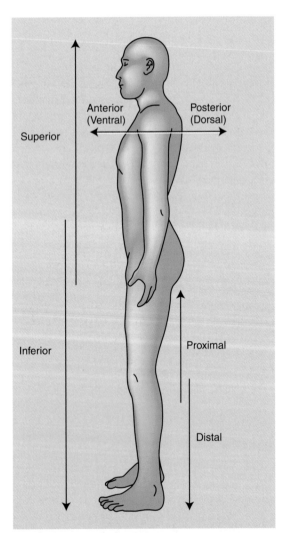

FIGURE 6-6 Directional terms are used to indicate relative positions and direction on the body.

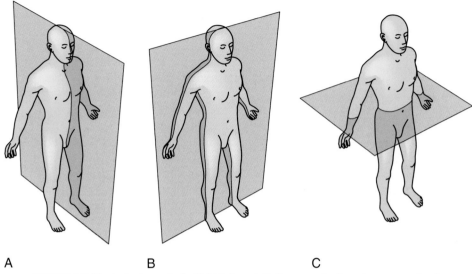

FIGURE 6-7 The body planes. **A,** Sagittal. **B,** Frontal. **C,** Transverse (horizontal or cross-sectional).

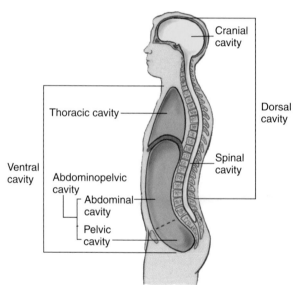

FIGURE 6-8 The body cavities. Note that some smaller cavities are within others and not shown. (From Applegate E: *The anatomy and physiology learning system,* ed. 4, St. Louis, 2011, Saunders.)

SKELETAL SYSTEM

The skeletal system includes all the bones, plus the connective tissue at the joints. It functions to support the body, provide movement, and protect the internal organs. Bones also store the minerals phosphorus and calcium, and the marrow of certain bones is the site of hematopoiesis, formation of blood cells.

Features of Bone

Bone is formed by osteoblasts. These cells produce collagen fibers and deposit calcium salts (principally calcium phosphate). This mixture of protein and mineral gives bone its unique combination of hardness and resiliency. Bone growth and development involve a complex balance between the action of osteoblasts and that of other cells, called osteoclasts, whose job is to break down bone and release stored minerals. This dynamic balance allows the growth of bone despite its rigidity and allows it to be remodeled to accommodate changing stresses.

There are 206 bones in the adult skeleton. Bones are classified by their shapes as long, short, flat, sesamoid, or irregular.
- Long bones include those in the arms and legs
- Short bones are found in the wrists and ankles
- Flat bones protect inner organs such as the heart and brain
- *Sesamoid* means "shaped like a sesame seed"; the patella (kneecap) is an example

Irregular bones are those that are not classified as one of the other types, for example, the vertebrae. The principal bones of the skeleton are illustrated in Figure 6-9.

Hematopoiesis takes place principally in spongy tissue within bone called marrow. In children, hematopoiesis takes place principally in the long bones, especially the tibia and femur. In adults, most hematopoiesis occurs in the vertebrae, rib cage, scapulae, and skull.

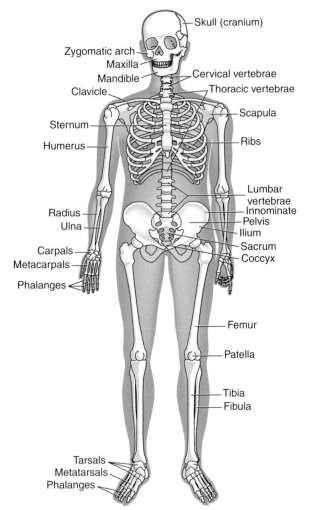

FIGURE 6-9 The major bones of the human skeleton.

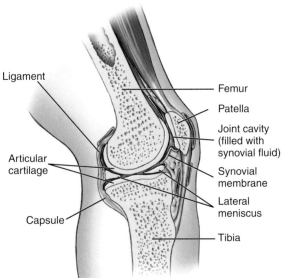

FIGURE 6-10 A typical joint in cross section. (Modified from Herlihy B: *The human body in health and illness,* ed. 5, St. Louis, 2015, Saunders.)

Features of Joints

Joints connect one bone to another. There are three types of joints:

1. **Synarthrosis** (immovable): Fixed or immovable joints include the sutures of the cranium and facial bones
2. **Amphiarthrosis** (partially movable): The vertebral joints are partially movable, restrained to protect the spinal cord from trauma.
3. **Diarthrosis** (free moving): The appendicular joints, such as the shoulder, elbow, and knee, are free moving

The structure of a typical free-moving joint is shown in Figure 6-10. The two bones are held together with **ligaments**, a type of tough, fibrous connective tissue. The fluid-filled **synovial cavity** is enclosed within the synovial membrane. The bearing surfaces of the bones are lined with smooth articular cartilage. The combination of synovial

fluid and **articular cartilage** allows the two bone surfaces to slide against each other without becoming damaged or irritated.

Bone and Joint Disorders

Bone disorders include fractures, metabolic diseases, neoplastic diseases, infections, and developmental abnormalities (Box 6-1). Joint disorders include trauma, inflammation caused by infections and autoimmune diseases, degenerative changes, and metabolic diseases. An orthopedist is a specialist who treats bone disorders. Joint disorders are treated by a rheumatologist. Common laboratory tests ordered for these disorders are listed in Table 6-1.

MUSCULAR SYSTEM

Skeletal muscles move the skeleton, allowing the vast range of activities that make up daily life. Cardiac muscle pumps the blood for the circulatory system. The primary function of smooth muscle is to regulate the passage of materials through vessels.

Features of Skeletal Muscle

Skeletal muscles are those attached to the skeleton. Skeletal muscles account for 45% of the weight of the body. Muscles attach to the skeleton by means of **tendons**, a type of fibrous connective tissue. A muscle's two points of attachment are on opposite sides of a joint, so contraction of the muscle bends

BOX 6-1 Disorders of Bones and Joints

Bones

Fracture

- Comminuted: Break that has splintered into many pieces
- Complicated: Broken bone plus injured soft tissue
- Compound: Bone protrudes through the skin
- Greenstick: Bone is bent or partially broken
- Impacted: Broken bone is driven into another bone
- Pathologic: Fracture caused by disease, not stress
- Simple: No puncture through the skin

Metabolic Disease

- Osteomalacia: Softening of the bone from calcium deficiency, vitamin D deficiency, or parathyroid hormone hypersecretion; childhood rickets is one form; can cause bowlegs
- Osteoporosis: Loss of bone mass and decrease in bone density, possibly resulting from a deficiency of estrogens, protein, calcium, or vitamin D; common in postmenopausal women; can lead to brittle and broken bones

Neoplastic Disease

- Osteoma: Usually benign
- Sarcoma: Malignant

Infectious Disease

- Osteomyelitis: Bone inflammation caused by a bacterial infection, possibly from improper phlebotomy technique; very difficult to treat

Developmental Disease

- Acromegaly: Excess growth of extremities caused by overproduction of growth hormone

- Scoliosis: Curvature of the spine from side to side; can be congenital or develop in teens
- Spina bifida: Congenital disease; abnormal closing of the vertebrae, causing malformation of the spine

Joints

Trauma

- Overextension, compression, or shear of ligaments: Common sports injury; slow to heal

Infectious Disease

- Lyme disease: Inflammation of the synovial membrane caused by a bacterial infection; transmitted through tick bites

Autoimmune Disease

- Rheumatoid arthritis: Swelling and irritation of the synovial membrane
- Systemic lupus erythematosus: Chronic inflammation that affects cartilage, bones, ligaments, and tendons; more common in females than in males

Degenerative Disease

- Osteoarthritis (also called degenerative joint disease): Results from cumulative wear and tear on joint surfaces; affects about 20% of the population older than age 60 years

Metabolic Disease

- Gout: Formation of uric acid crystals in the joints, causing pain and inflammation

TABLE 6-1	Common Laboratory Tests for Bone and Joint Disorders
Test	**Disorder or Purpose**
Alkaline phosphatase (ALP)	Bone metabolism marker
Calcium	Mineral calcium imbalance
Erythrocyte sedimentation rate (ESR)	General inflammation test
Fluorescent antinuclear antibody (ANA)	Systemic lupus erythematosus (SLE)
Magnesium	Mineral magnesium imbalance
Rheumatoid factor (RF)	Rheumatoid arthritis (RA)
Synovial fluid analysis	Arthritis
Uric acid	Gout

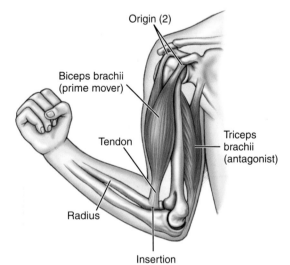

FIGURE 6-11 Muscles usually occur in antagonistic pairs, such as the triceps and biceps of the upper arm. (From Herlihy B: *The human body in health and illness,* ed. 5, St. Louis, 2015, Saunders.)

the joint. In general, the bone on one side of a joint remains stationary while the other moves. Skeletal muscles often occur in pairs, called antagonistic pairs, whose actions are opposed. The biceps, for example, flexes the elbow, and the triceps extends it (Figure 6-11). During flexion, the biceps is called the agonist, because it carries out the intended movement, and the triceps is called the antagonist, because it opposes that movement. During extension, the triceps is the agonist and the biceps is the antagonist.

Disorders of Skeletal Muscle

Disorders affecting skeletal muscle include trauma, genetic diseases of muscle proteins, metabolic diseases, autoimmune diseases, and motor neuron infection or degeneration (Box 6-2). Muscle disorders may be treated by an orthopedist, rheumatologist, or neurologist. Common laboratory tests ordered for these disorders are listed in Table 6-2.

BOX 6-2	**Disorders of the Muscular System**

Trauma
- Contusions
- Tendon injuries
- Tendonitis: From overuse, overexertion, or repetitive strain injuries

Genetic Disease
- Muscular dystrophies: Inherited defects in the proteins of the muscle cell; Duchenne's muscular dystrophy is the most common type

Metabolic Disease
- Inherited defects in metabolic function: Especially defects of the mitochondria; most are rare

Autoimmune Disease
- Myasthenia gravis: Antibodies form against the receptor for acetylcholine, preventing nerve–muscle communication
- Polymyositis and dermatomyositis

Motor Neuron Disease
- Amyotrophic lateral sclerosis (ALS; also called Lou Gehrig's disease): Degeneration of motor neurons; cause is unknown
- Poliomyelitis: Viral infection that has been virtually eradicated; new cases are caused by vaccine virus; can cause paralysis

TABLE 6-2	**Common Laboratory Tests for Muscle Disorders**

Test	Disorder or Purpose
Aldolase	Muscle disease
Aspartate aminotransferase (AST)	Muscle disease
Creatine kinase-MM (CK-MM)	Muscle damage
Creatine kinase-MB (CK-MB)	Cardiac muscle damage
Myoglobin	Muscle damage
Troponin	Cardiac muscle damage

INTEGUMENTARY SYSTEM

The integumentary system forms the outer covering of the body and includes the skin, hair, nails, and sweat glands. It is the largest organ in the body. The principal functions of the integumentary system are protection, thermoregulation (control of body temperature), and sensation. The skin forms an effective barrier against invasion by microbes and chemicals. Evaporation of sweat from the surface of the skin is the major means by which humans cool themselves. Sensory cells embedded in the skin allow the brain to receive information about the environment.

Features of the Integumentary System

Skin is a layered structure that forms by continual division of its innermost layer, the dermis (Figure 6-12). Cells of the epidermis gradually die and slough off as they move toward the outermost layers. Callus is epidermis that has extra amounts of the structural protein keratin, which provides a tough protective layer in regions subject to frequent abrasion or impact. Keratin is also the principal component of hair and nails, which are dead tissues formed from living follicles within the skin. Below the dermis is a subcutaneous layer of connective tissue, including the fat layer that provides padding and insulation. Capillary beds that lie within the dermis supply the blood for a dermal puncture.

Two main types of glands are found in the skin:
1. Sweat glands are located in the dermis, with ducts reaching up through the epidermis to form pores on the surface of the skin. Sweat cools the body by evaporation. Salt is excreted at the same time.
2. Sebaceous glands produce an oily substance called sebum that lubricates the skin and hair.

Disorders of the Integumentary System

Disorders affecting the integumentary system include trauma, infection, neoplastic disease, and inflammation (Box 6-3). Integumentary disorders are treated by a dermatologist. Common laboratory tests ordered for these disorders are listed in Table 6-3.

NERVOUS SYSTEMS

The nervous systems include the central nervous system (CNS) (the brain and spinal cord) and the peripheral nervous system (PNS) (all the neurons

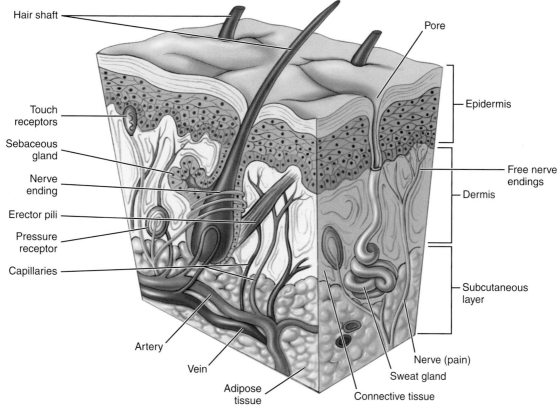

FIGURE 6-12 The integumentary system covers and protects the body. It permits sensation of the environment and regulates the internal temperature. (Modified from Herlihy B: *The human body in health and illness,* ed. 5, St. Louis, 2015, Saunders.)

BOX 6-3	Disorders of the Integumentary System

Infection
- Fungal infection
  - Athlete's foot
  - Ringworm
- Bacterial infection
  - *Staphylococcus* infection: Impetigo
  - *Streptococcus* infection: Necrotizing fasciitis ("flesh-eating" bacteria)

Neoplastic Disease
- Carcinoma
- Melanoma

Inflammation
- Acne
- Psoriasis

TABLE 6-3	Common Laboratory Tests for Integumentary Disorders	
Test	Disorder or Purpose	
Culture and sensitivity (C&S)	Bacterial or fungal infection	
Potassium hydroxide (KOH) prep	Fungal infection	
Skin biopsy	Malignancy	

the motor portion of the PNS. The CNS also directs some actions of other organs, including secretion by some glands.

Peripheral Nervous System

The PNS is composed of two major divisions: the sensory and somatic systems. Sensory neurons, called **afferents**, receive stimulation from specialized cells within their sensory organ—the eyes, nose, mouth, ears, skin, and subcutaneous tissue such as joints, muscle, and internal organs. Afferents transmit information to spinal cord neurons, allowing sensory information to ascend to the brain. Motor neurons, called **efferents**, receive information from spinal

outside the CNS) (Figure 6-13). Sensory information from the periphery is received by the CNS, where it is integrated and processed to form an understanding of experience. The CNS directs movement by sending commands to the muscles through

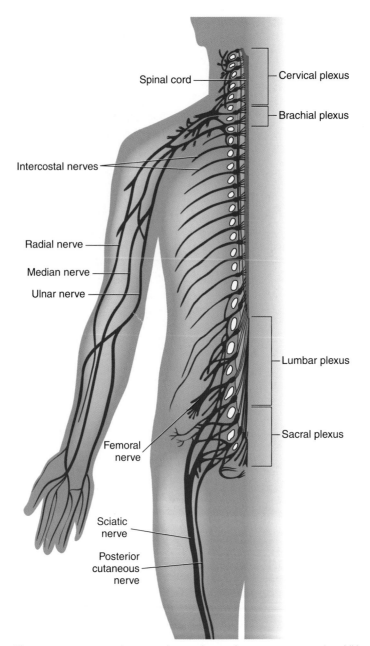

Spinal cord

Intercostal nerves

Radial nerve

Median nerve

Ulnar nerve

Femoral nerve

Sciatic nerve

Posterior cutaneous nerve

Cervical plexus

Brachial plexus

Lumbar plexus

Sacral plexus

FIGURE 6-13 The nervous system receives sensations and controls motor responses, in addition to helping maintain homeostasis.

cord neurons and carry it to the target organ, either a muscle or a gland. (A third type of neuron, the **interneuron**, conveys information between afferents and efferents and is located in the CNS.)

Neurons are bundled together in the periphery for protection. These bundles are called **nerves**. A nerve may contain only motor or only sensory neurons, or it may be a mixed nerve, containing both. Nerves also contain blood vessels, which nourish the neurons within.

Motor System

The motor system is divided into two branches: the **somatic motor system** and the **autonomic motor system**. Somatic **motor neurons** innervate skeletal muscles and can be consciously controlled. Autonomic motor neurons innervate cardiac and smooth muscle and normally cannot be consciously controlled (although indirect control is possible through focused relaxation techniques such as meditation and biofeedback). Digestive secretions are also partly controlled by the autonomic system, as are secretions from the adrenal medulla.

Motor commands of both types originate in the brain and descend through the spinal column. Spinal neurons make synapses with lower motor neurons, which branch out through the gaps between vertebrae to reach their target.

Central Nervous System

Within the CNS, bundles of neurons are called **tracts**. The spinal cord has both ascending and descending tracts. The top of the spinal cord merges into the **brainstem**, a region at the base of the skull that is vital for basic life processes, including respiration (Figure 6-14). The brainstem also connects with the **thalamus**, a major relay station for incoming sensory information. Posterior to the brainstem is the **cerebellum**, a principal site for fine-tuning of motor commands. Superior to the brainstem and partially covering the cerebellum is the **cerebrum**, which contains the **cerebral cortex**, divided into

left and right hemispheres (not shown Figure 6-14). The cerebral cortex is the site of thought, emotion, and memory. Motor control of the left side of the body begins in the right cerebral hemisphere, and the right side of the body is controlled by the left cerebral hemisphere.

In addition to the nutrients received from blood, the brain is nourished and cushioned by **cerebrospinal fluid (CSF)**, which is secreted by the brain and circulates within the **ventricles** (see Figure 6-14). The brain is surrounded by three membranes—the **pia mater**, the **arachnoid**, and the **dura mater**—that lubricate and protect the brain. Together, these constitute the **meninges**. The spinal cord is also surrounded by meninges.

Disorders of the Nervous Systems

Disorders affecting the nervous systems include trauma, stroke, infection, neoplastic diseases, degeneration, autoimmune diseases, developmental disorders, and psychiatric illnesses (Box 6-4).

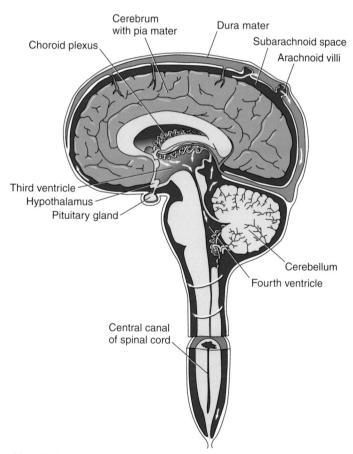

FIGURE 6-14 This sagittal section of the brain and cranium shows the brain's internal organization, plus the ventricles and three protective membranes.

| **BOX 6-4** | **Disorder of the Central Nervous System** |

Trauma
- Concussion
- Penetrating wound
- Subdural hemorrhage
- Subarachnoid hemorrhage

Stroke
- Embolic stroke: Blood clot that lodges within a cerebral vessel
- Hemorrhagic stroke: Blood vessel that bursts; usually preceded by aneurysm

Infection
- Herpes: Peripheral infection, caused by varicella-zoster virus
- Meningitis
- Polio
- Shingles: Peripheral infection, caused by varicella-zoster virus

Neoplastic Disease
- Neuroma: Benign tumor of neural tissue
- Neurosarcoma: Malignant tumor of neural tissue

Degenerative Disease
- Alzheimer's disease: Most common neurodegenerative disease, causing widespread degeneration of cortex
- Amyotrophic lateral sclerosis (ALS; also called Lou Gehrig's disease)
- Parkinson's disease: Degeneration of the basal ganglia, important for movement control

Autoimmune Disease
- Guillain-Barré syndrome: Short-term but life-threatening postinfectious attack on motor neurons
- Multiple sclerosis: Progressive attack on myelin sheath surrounding central nervous system neurons
- Myasthenia gravis

Developmental Disorders
- Cerebral palsy: Perinatal damage to motor centers of the brain; often accompanied by other impairments
- Epilepsy

Psychiatric Illness
- Bipolar disorder
- Depression
- Schizophrenia

| **TABLE 6-4** | **Common Laboratory Tests for Neurologic Disorders** |

Test (Performed on Cerebrospinal Fluid)	Disorder or Purpose
Cerebrospinal fluid (CSF) analysis	Meningitis and other neurologic disorders
Culture and Gram stain	Detection of infectious agent
Protein and glucose	Determination of variation from normal range
Cell count and differential	Detection of inflammation and immune activity

Neurologic disorders are treated by a neurologist, and psychiatric disorders are treated by a psychiatrist or other mental health professional. Common laboratory tests ordered for these disorders are listed in Table 6-4. Disorders of the CNS are most often diagnosed using imaging techniques such as magnetic resonance imaging (MRI) and computed tomography (CT) scanning.

DIGESTIVE SYSTEM

The digestive system is responsible for the absorption of nutrients into and the elimination of waste from the digestive tract. The digestive system includes the mouth, esophagus, stomach, small and large intestines, rectum, and anus, plus the accessory digestive organs, including the liver, gallbladder, and pancreas (Figure 6-15). The purpose of digestion is to break down food into molecules small enough to be absorbed by the intestines. This process includes both mechanical and chemical digestion.

The Digestion Process
Mouth to Stomach
Mechanical digestion begins in the mouth. Chewing increases the surface area of food, allowing faster chemical attack by the enzymes of the stomach and intestines. Saliva lubricates the food, allowing it to pass smoothly down the **esophagus**. Smooth muscles of the esophagus constrict in a wavelike motion called **peristalsis**, forcing the bolus of food down into the stomach. A ring of smooth muscle at the stomach's opening, called a **sphincter**, relaxes to admit the bolus of food and then contracts to prevent reflux of the stomach's contents.

The strong muscular walls of the stomach churn the food, and glands within the walls secrete hydrochloric acid and the enzyme pepsin, beginning the process of chemical digestion. This thick, soupy mixture is called **chyme**. Secretion is controlled

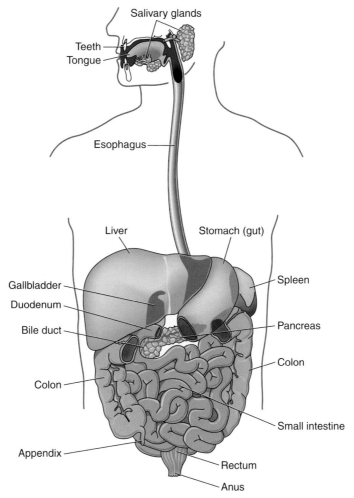

FIGURE 6-15 The digestive system extends from the mouth to the anus and includes the accessory organs of digestion.

hormonally to prevent the release of enzymes when food is not available. The stomach itself is protected from digestion by a layer of mucus.

Small Intestine

The partially digested chyme is passed by peristalsis through another sphincter into the small intestine, where further chemical digestion occurs. The pancreas secretes a large array of digestive enzymes into the small intestine, including **proteases** for breaking proteins into amino acids, **lipases** for breaking fats into fatty acids, and **carbohydrases** for breaking complex carbohydrates into simple sugars. The gallbladder releases **bile**, which also aids in the breakdown of fat. Glands in the intestinal wall release enzymes as well. The high internal surface area of the small intestine is made up of numerous finger-like projections called **villi**. These allow for rapid and efficient absorption of the digested molecules, and the rich blood supply allows nutrients to be

carried away quickly to the liver for further processing and storage. Fat is absorbed by the lymphatic system instead of the blood system.

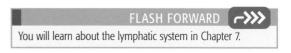

FLASH FORWARD

You will learn about the lymphatic system in Chapter 7.

Large Intestine and Elimination

The remaining material is passed through another sphincter, past the appendix, and into the large intestine, or colon. Here, much of the water is reabsorbed, and the indigestible solid material is compacted to form feces. Feces are eliminated through the anus, by strong peristaltic contraction of the smooth muscle of the rectum.

Liver

The liver is a central organ in both digestion and, more important, nutrient processing and storage.

The liver produces the bile that is stored in the gallbladder. After nutrients are absorbed by the small intestine, they pass in the bloodstream directly to the liver for further chemical action and storage. Carbohydrates are stored in the liver for immediate use, and numerous harmful substances are detoxified there. The liver has a central role in the elimination of bilirubin, a hemoglobin breakdown product. A damaged liver leads to jaundice, a condition in which unprocessed bilirubin gives a yellowish color to the skin.

Disorders of the Digestive System

Disorders affecting the digestive system include infection, inflammation, chemical damage, and autoimmune disease (Box 6-5). Digestive disorders are treated by an internal medicine specialist or gastroenterologist. Common laboratory tests ordered for these disorders are listed in Table 6-5.

URINARY SYSTEM

The urinary system includes the kidneys, the bladder, and the urethra (Figure 6-16). Through the

TABLE 6-5	Common Laboratory Tests for Digestive Disorders
Test	**Disorder or Purpose**
Amylase or lipase	Pancreatitis
Carotene	Steatorrhea (malabsorption syndrome causing fatty stools)
Complete blood count (CBC)	Appendicitis
Liver tests	Liver disease
• Alkaline phosphatase (ALP)	
• Alanine aminotransferase (ALT)	
• Aspartate aminotransferase (AST)	
• γ-Glutamyltransferase (GGT)	
• Bilirubin	
• Hepatitis B surface antigen (HBsAG)	
• Hepatitis C antibody	
• Hepatitis C virus (HCV) by polymerase chain reaction (PCR)	
• Ammonia	
Gastrin	Gastric malignancy
Occult blood	Gastrointestinal bleeding
Ova and parasites (O&P)	Parasitic infection
Stool culture	Stool pathogens

BOX 6-5	Disorders of the Digestive System

Infection
- Appendicitis: Infection and inflammation by resident bacteria; can be life threatening if appendix bursts
- Gastroenteritis: Viral or bacterial
- Giardiasis
- Hepatitis: Inflamed liver as a result of infection or injury; commonly viral (type A, B, or C)
- Tapeworm
- Ulcer: Infection by *Helicobacter pylori,* treated with antibiotics; relation to stress largely discredited

Inflammation
- Cholecystitis: Inflamed gallbladder
- Colitis: Inflamed colon; causes diarrhea
- Pancreatitis: Inflamed pancreas as a result of injury, alcohol, drugs, or gallstones
- Peritonitis: Inflamed abdominal cavity caused by a ruptured appendix, perforated ulcer, or other infectious process

Chemical Damage
- Cirrhosis of the liver: Often resulting from prolonged alcohol consumption
- Gallstones

Autoimmune Disease
- Crohn's disease: Causes intestinal cramping

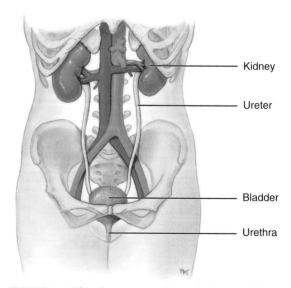

FIGURE 6-16 The urinary system collects urine from the kidneys for storage and elimination. (From Applegate E: *The anatomy and physiology learning system,* ed. 4, St. Louis, 2011, Saunders.)

Kidney

Ureter

Bladder

Urethra

production of urine, it functions to remove metabolic wastes from the circulation, maintain acid–base balance, and regulate body hydration. The kidneys also produce hormones that control blood pressure (renin) and regulate the production of red blood cells (erythropoietin).

Kidneys

Blood flows into the kidneys through the renal artery. Within the kidney, capillaries form into tight balls called glomeruli (Figure 6-17). Each **glomerulus** is enclosed within a glove-like structure known as **Bowman's capsule**. Blood pressure forces fluid out of the glomerulus, into Bowman's capsule, and then into the renal tubule. This fluid is similar in composition to the plasma it is derived from, but without most of the proteins. As it flows—through the **proximal convoluted tubule**, around the **loop of Henle**, and through the **distal convoluted tubule**—its composition changes according to the needs of the body at the time. Salts, sugar, and other small molecules are reclaimed, along with water, and returned to the capillary bed surrounding the tubule. Transport of these substances is accomplished by a combination of active transport, osmosis, and diffusion. Other substances are actively secreted back into the tubule from the capillaries. The fluid remaining in the tubule at the far end—urine—enters the **collecting duct** and drains into the bladder through the **ureter**. The entire structure, from glomerulus to collecting duct, is known as a **nephron**. The function of the nephron is regulated by hormones, especially by **antidiuretic hormone (ADH)**, produced by the posterior

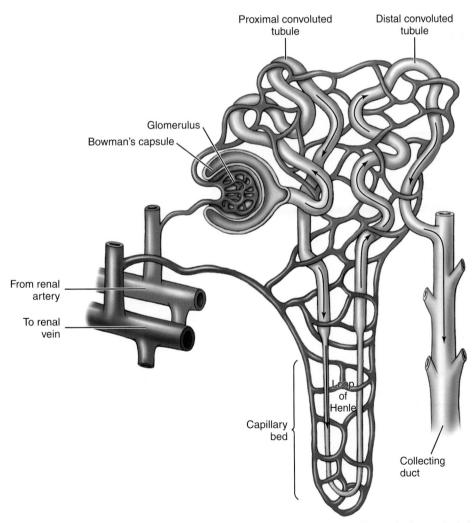

FIGURE 6-17 The nephron is the functional unit of the kidney. (Modified from Herlihy B: *The human body in health and illness,* ed. 5, St. Louis, 2015, Saunders.)

pituitary gland (described later with other endocrine glands). When more ADH is secreted, the nephron reabsorbs more water, making a more concentrated urine.

Disorders of the Urinary System

Disorders affecting the urinary system include infection and inflammation, as well as chemical disorders (Box 6-6). Renal failure—the inability of the kidneys to maintain blood homeostasis—is life threatening and must be treated with dialysis or transplantation. Urinary disorders are treated by a urologist. Common laboratory tests ordered for these disorders are listed in Table 6-6.

RESPIRATORY SYSTEM

The respiratory system includes the upper airways (nasal passages and throat) and the lower airways (trachea, larynx, bronchi, and lungs). It also in-

| BOX 6-6 | Disorders of the Urinary System |

Infection or Inflammation
- Cystitis: Inflammation of the bladder
- Glomerulonephritis: Inflammation of the glomerulus as a result of infection or immune disorder
- Pyelonephritis: Inflammation of kidney tissue as a result of a bacterial infection
- Urinary tract infection (UTI): Bacterial infection of the urinary tract

Chemical Disorder
- Renal calculi (kidney stones): Crystals of calcium oxalate, uric acid, or other chemicals form within the tubules

| TABLE 6-6 | Common Laboratory Tests for Urologic Disorders |

Test	Disorder or Purpose
Blood urea nitrogen (BUN)	Kidney disease
Creatinine	Kidney disease
Creatinine clearance	Glomerular filtration
Culture and sensitivity (C&S)	Urinary tract infection (UTI)
Electrolytes	Fluid balance
Osmolality	Fluid balance
Protein/microalbumin	Kidney disorders
Renin/angiotensin-converting enzyme (ACE)	Hypertension
Routine urinalysis	Screening for renal or metabolic disorders

volves the muscles of respiration in the abdomen, chest, and neck. The function of the respiratory system is to obtain oxygen for use by the body's cells and to expel the carbon dioxide waste from metabolic processes. The respiratory system relies on the circulatory system to transport gases to and from the lungs. **External respiration** refers to the exchange of gases in the lungs, and **internal respiration** refers to the exchange of oxygen and carbon dioxide at the cellular level.

Features of the Respiratory System
External Respiration

External respiration begins with the expansion of the chest cavity through the combined actions of the diaphragm, intercostal muscles, and accessory muscles of respiration (Figure 6-18). This expansion lowers the internal air pressure so that the higher external pressure forces air into the airways. Air entering the nostrils is warmed, moistened, and filtered by passing over mucus-covered ciliated membranes. It then passes through the throat, or **pharynx**, and enters the **trachea**, passing through the **larynx** and moving past the vocal cords. The trachea branches into left and right **bronchi**, which branch further as they enter the lungs (see Figure 6-18). These smaller branches, called **bronchioles**, continue to branch until they form sacs called **alveoli**. Oxygen from the air passes by diffusion through the thin walls of each alveolus into the capillaries that surround it. Carbon dioxide from the blood passes out by diffusion at the same time. Exhalation is accomplished principally by relaxation of the respiratory muscles, with some additional force supplied by contraction of the abdominal muscles.

The trachea contains C-shaped rings of cartilage to prevent collapse of the airway during inspiration. Trachea, bronchi, and bronchioles are lined with epithelial tissue, which secretes thin mucus for moistening and cleaning the air. This mucus traps dust, bacteria, and other particles entering the airways. Tiny hair filaments on the cell surfaces, called **cilia**, continually sweep this mucus up the airway to the throat, where it is swallowed. During infection, mucus production increases, and the mucus becomes thicker. A cough is then required to clear it.

Internal Respiration

Oxygen binds to hemoglobin in the red blood cells, forming **oxyhemoglobin**. In this form, it is carried through the circulatory system to all the body's

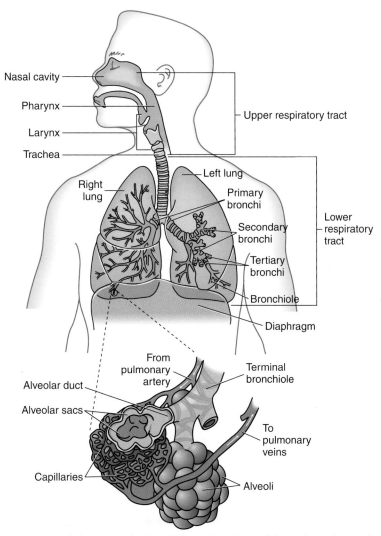

FIGURE 6-18 Structure of the lungs. The bronchial tree branches until it terminates in alveoli, where gas exchange occurs.

tissues. Because oxygen is being used in the tissues, its concentration there is decreased in relation to its concentration in the blood, and oxygen flows by diffusion out of the blood into the tissues. It passes into cells and finally to the mitochondria, which use it to react with carbon and hydrogen from food molecules, supplying energy to the cell. The waste products—carbon dioxide and water—then diffuse out of the cell. Carbon dioxide dissolves in the blood and is carried back to the lungs.

Disorders of the Respiratory System

Disorders affecting the respiratory system include infection, inflammation, obstruction, insufficient ventilation, developmental disorders, and neoplastic diseases (Box 6-7). Respiratory failure occurs when the respiratory system cannot supply adequate gas

exchange to maintain body function. It is a life-threatening condition and is treated by temporary or permanent mechanical devices to aid ventilation. Diseases of the upper respiratory tract are commonly treated by a primary care physician or an ear, nose, and throat (ENT) specialist. Disorders of the lower respiratory tract are most often treated by a pulmonologist. Common laboratory tests ordered for these disorders are listed in Table 6-7.

ENDOCRINE SYSTEM

The endocrine system comprises the glands and other tissues that produce hormones, which are released from glandular tissue directly into the circulatory system (Figure 6-19). The endocrine system functions with the nervous systems to

BOX 6-7 Disorders of the Respiratory System

Infection
- Pneumonia: Infection of the lower airway; can be viral, fungal, bacterial, or mycobacterial
- Strep throat: Infection of the throat by *Streptococcus* bacteria
- Tuberculosis: Infection by *Mycobacterium tuberculosis*
- Upper respiratory infection (URI): Infection of the nose, throat, or larynx; can be viral, fungal, or bacterial

Inflammation
- Bronchitis: Inflammation of the bronchi as a result of irritation or infection
- Emphysema: Chronic inflammation of alveoli and bronchioles; can be caused by smoking
- Pleurisy: Inflammation of the pleural membrane

Obstruction
- Asthma: Obstructed bronchi resulting from airway constriction
- Chronic obstructive pulmonary disease (COPD): Caused by emphysema
- Pulmonary edema: Fluid in the lungs

Insufficient Ventilation
- Amyotrophic lateral sclerosis (ALS; also called Lou Gehrig's disease)
- Muscular dystrophy
- Polio
- Spinal cord injury

Developmental Disorder
- Infant respiratory distress syndrome (IRDS): Collapsed alveoli; common in premature infants

Neoplastic Disease
- Lung cancer

TABLE 6-7 Common Laboratory Tests for Respiratory Disorders

Test	Disorder or Purpose
Arterial blood gases (ABGs): pH (acidity), P_{O_2} (oxygen), P_{CO_2} (carbon dioxide)	Most respiratory disorders; assess lung function
Cold agglutinins (test for antibodies that react with red blood cells at cold temperatures)	Atypical pneumonia
Electrolytes	Impaired gas exchange
Microbiologic tests • Cultures • Throat swabs • Bronchial washings	Microbial infection—pneumonia or pharyngitis
Purified protein derivative (PPD)	Skin test for tuberculosis
Respiratory syncytial virus (RSV)	Viral pneumonia

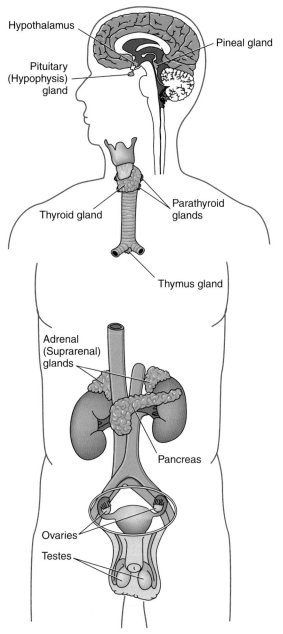

FIGURE 6-19 The glands of the endocrine system.

tightly regulate body function, maintaining homeostasis. Because of the fine degree of control required, endocrine glands are themselves regulated by other endocrine glands, in multiple control systems known as **feedback loops.** Many of these feedback loops involve the brain as well, especially the small portion of the brain known as the **hypothalamus.**

Hormones

Hormones are chemical substances released into the circulation by one group of cells that affect the function of other cells. Hormones exert their effects by binding to receptors at the target cell. Receptors may be on the surface of the target cell, in its cytoplasm, or in its nucleus. There are three principal types of hormones: **steroid hormones** (including testosterone and progesterone), **amino acid derivatives** (including thyroxine and epinephrine, which is also called adrenaline), and **peptides** (including insulin). Each type has its own mechanisms of action and duration of response. For instance, epinephrine works quickly to produce a short-lived response, whereas steroid hormones, such as testosterone, work slowly to produce long-lasting effects.

Endocrine Glands

Pituitary Gland

The pituitary gland is located at the base of the brain, just outside the cranium. It is involved in virtually every feedback loop in the endocrine system, sending hormones out and receiving hormonal messages from every other endocrine gland, including the thyroid, the adrenals, and the ovaries. For this reason, it is often called the master gland of the endocrine system. The hypothalamus secretes a variety of hormones that directly influence pituitary function.

The pituitary has two lobes: the anterior and the posterior. The anterior pituitary secretes **thyroid-stimulating hormone (TSH)**, **adrenocorticotropic hormone (ACTH)**, **follicle-stimulating hormone (FSH)**, and **luteinizing hormone (LH)**, which act on the ovaries and testes. In addition, the anterior pituitary secretes **growth hormone (GH)**, which regulates the rate of growth throughout the body; **melanocyte-stimulating hormone (MSH)**, which increases melanin pigment production in skin cells; and **prolactin**, which increases milk production in the mammary glands.

As noted earlier, the posterior pituitary produces ADH, which regulates water reabsorption by the kidney. It also produces **oxytocin**, which stimulates smooth muscle contraction in the uterus during labor and in the mammary glands during nursing.

Thyroid Gland

The thyroid gland wraps around the trachea, just below the larynx. The thyroid secretes **thyroxine**—also called T_4, because it contains four atoms of iodine—and small amounts of **triiodothyronine**, or

T_3. These two hormones regulate the basal metabolic rate, or energy consumption rate, of virtually every cell in the body. The thyroid also secretes **calcitonin**, which lowers calcium levels in body fluids.

Parathyroid Gland

The parathyroid gland is located behind the thyroid. It secretes **parathyroid hormone (PTH)**, also called **parathormone**, which regulates the amount of calcium and phosphorus in the circulation.

Thymus Gland

The thymus sits behind the sternum and plays a key role in the early development of the immune system. Among other functions, it secretes **thymosin**, which develops and maintains immunity. The thymus shrinks throughout life, and its function in adults, if any, is not clear.

Pancreas

The pancreas is located behind the stomach. It has two distinct functions. As discussed earlier, it produces digestive enzymes that are secreted into the small intestine. As an endocrine gland, it produces two hormones that regulate the level of the sugar glucose in the blood: insulin and glucagon.

Insulin promotes the uptake of glucose by the body's cells, thereby lowering blood sugar levels. It also promotes the conversion of glucose into glycogen, a storage carbohydrate, in the liver and in skeletal muscles. **Glucagon** promotes the breakdown of glycogen back into glucose and increases its release into the blood, thereby elevating blood sugar levels. The antagonistic effects of these two hormones allow tight regulation of blood glucose levels.

Adrenal Glands

There are two adrenal glands, one located above each kidney (the word *adrenal* means "above the kidney"). Each adrenal gland is composed of two parts:

- The inner **adrenal medulla** secretes the catecholamines **epinephrine** and **norepinephrine** under the direct control of the autonomic nervous system. These hormones have the familiar effects of increasing the heart rate, increasing blood flow to the skeletal muscles, and producing a subjective feeling of heightened awareness and anticipation. They are a crucial part of the fight-or-flight response.

- The outer **adrenal cortex** secretes steroid hormones. These include the **glucocorticoids**, which influence glucose metabolism; the **mineralocorticoids**, which control electrolyte balance; and androgens, or male sex hormones.

The principal glucocorticoids are **cortisol**, **cortisone**, and **corticosterone**, which decrease glucose consumption and promote fat usage. They also reduce inflammation, accounting for their use on skin rashes and other irritations. **Aldosterone** is the principal mineralocorticoid, helping regulate sodium and water balance in the kidneys.

Gonads

The gonads are the ovaries and testes. The testes produce **testosterone**, the principal male sex hormone. Testosterone promotes sperm maturation, increases protein synthesis in skeletal muscle, and causes the development of male secondary sex characteristics, including facial hair and a deep voice. The ovaries produce **estrogens** and **progesterone**, whose functions include regulation of the menstrual cycle, development of the uterus, and development of the mammary glands and other female secondary sex characteristics.

Disorders of the Endocrine System

Disorders affecting the endocrine system most often involve either hypersecretion or hyposecretion (Box 6-8). Hypersecretion is most often caused by a tumor of the glandular tissue or excess administration (as with insulin); hyposecretion may result from genetic disease, autoimmunity, or nutritional

TABLE 6-8	Common Laboratory Tests for Endocrine Disorders
Test	Disorder or Purpose
Calcium	Parathyroid function
Catecholamines (epinephrine, norepinephrine)	Adrenal function
Cortisol	Adrenal cortex function and Addison disease
Fasting glucose or fasting blood sugar (FBS)	Diabetes mellitus
Follicle-stimulating hormone (FSH)	Infertility
Growth hormone (GH)	Pituitary function
Luteinizing hormone (LH)	Infertility
Parathyroid hormone (PTH)	Parathyroid function
Phosphorus	Parathyroid function
Triiodothyronine (T_3), thyroxine (T_4), and thyroid-stimulating hormone (TSH)	Graves disease and Hashimoto thyroiditis
Testosterone	Infertility
Thyroid function studies	Thyroid disorder
Vitamin D	Parathyroid function

deficiency. Diseases of the endocrine system are treated by an endocrinologist. Common laboratory tests ordered for these disorders are listed in Table 6-8.

REPRODUCTIVE SYSTEMS

The reproductive systems include the **gonads**— ovaries or testes—plus the accessory structures required for successful reproduction. The reproductive system in men produces and ejaculates sperm. In women, the reproductive system produces mature eggs, allows for their fertilization, and hosts and nourishes the embryo as it develops.

Male Reproductive System

The testes are the site of sperm, as well as testosterone, production (Figure 6-20). The testes are enclosed by the **scrotum**. Sperm pass from the testis into the **epididymis**, a coiled tube atop the testis, where they mature. Mature sperm pass into the **vas deferens**, where they are stored before ejaculation. Sexual arousal causes contraction of the smooth muscle lining, the vas deferens, propelling sperm into the **urethra**. Fluid from several glands is secreted into the urethra as well, to nourish and protect the sperm and provide a fluid medium for them to swim in. Glands supplying fluid are the **prostate**, the **seminal vesicles**, and the **bulbourethral glands**. The sperm and fluid together constitute **semen**. The urethra passes through the **penis**,

BOX 6-8	Disorders of the Endocrine System

Hypersecretion
- Acromegaly or gigantism: Excess growth hormone (GH), commonly due to pituitary tumor
- Cushing's disease: Excess cortisol and adrenocorticotropic hormone
- Graves' disease: Excess thyroid hormone
- Hyperinsulinism: Most often resulting from insulin overdose or tumor

Hyposecretion
- Addison's disease: Loss of adrenal cortex function
- Diabetes insipidus: Lack of antidiuretic hormone
- Diabetes mellitus: Lack of insulin production; autoimmune destruction of pancreatic islet cells
- Hypothyroidism: Lack of thyroxine (T_4); can be caused by iodine deficiency (goiter); can lead to myxedema or death
- Pituitary dwarfism: Lack of GH

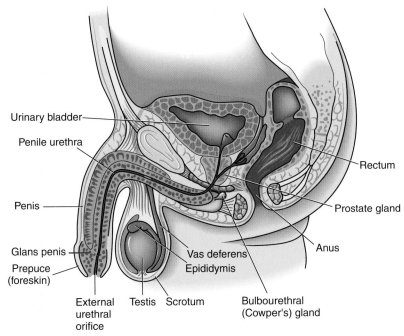

FIGURE 6-20 The male reproductive system.

whose spongy muscular tissue swells with blood during erection. Ejaculation occurs when strong peristaltic contractions of urethral smooth muscle propel the semen out of the urethra.

Female Reproductive System

The **ovaries** produce eggs during early development. Beginning at puberty, one or more eggs mature each month, under the influence of the pituitary hormones FSH and LH. At the same time, estrogens and progesterone produced by the ovaries induce changes in the uterine lining in preparation for implantation of a fertilized egg, including tissue buildup and increased blood flow. **Ovulation**, or release of the egg, is triggered by a sharp spike in LH levels. The egg enters the **fallopian tube** (Figure 6-21), where it is conveyed toward the **uterus** by cilia on the surface of the cells lining the tube. Fertilization occurs within the fallopian tube. Fertilization can occur only when a sperm swims up

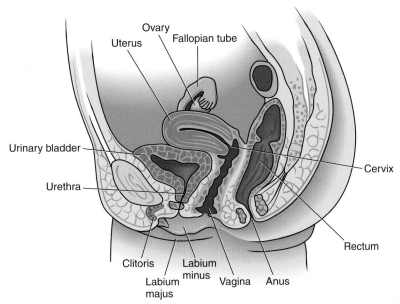

FIGURE 6-21 The female reproductive system.

the **vagina**, through the **cervix**, through the uterus, and into the fallopian tube containing the egg and then unites with the egg, all within the 2 to 4 days after ovulation in which the egg remains viable.

Implantation of the fertilized egg in the wall of the uterus induces changes that lead to the development of the placenta. Among other hormones, the placenta releases **human chorionic gonadotropin (hCG)**, which can be detected by early pregnancy tests. Without hCG, the uterine lining begins to deteriorate shortly after ovulation, culminating in menstruation. An unfertilized egg passes out of the uterus at that time.

Disorders of the Reproductive Systems

Disorders of the male reproductive system are treated by a urologist or an endocrinologist. Disorders of the female reproductive system are treated by an obstetrician/gynecologist or an endocrinologist (Box 6-9). Infertility may be treated by a specialist. Common laboratory tests ordered for these disorders are listed in Table 6-9.

TABLE 6-9	Common Laboratory Tests for Reproductive Disorders
Test	Disorder or Purpose
Culture and sensitivity (C&S)	Microbial infection
Estradiol	Assess ovarian or placental function
Estrogen	Assess ovarian function
Fluorescent treponemal antibody absorption test (FTA-ABS)	Syphilis
Human chorionic gonadotropin (hCG)	Assess for pregnancy or ectopic pregnancy
Pap smear	Cervical or vaginal carcinoma
Prostate-specific antigen (PSA)	Prostate cancer
Rapid plasma reagin (RPR)	Syphilis
Semen analysis	Infertility; assess effectiveness of vasectomy
Testosterone	Evaluation of testicular function

REVIEW FOR CERTIFICATION

Cells are the smallest unit of structure and function in the body and are made up of numerous subcellular structures, including the nucleus, the mitochondria, and the plasma membrane. Cells of similar function combine to make tissue. The four tissue types—epithelial, connective, muscle, and nerve—combine to create organs, which in turn combine to create organ systems and, ultimately, the functioning body. Anatomic terminology is used to describe the relationships of body parts. Each of the body systems—skeletal, muscular, integumentary, nervous, digestive, urinary, respiratory, endocrine, and reproductive—has its own set of organs and interactions that contribute to its function, as well as its own set of disorders. A summary table of common laboratory tests, arranged by body system, is presented in Table 6-10.

BOX 6-9	Disorders of the Reproductive System

Male Reproductive System
- Benign prostatic hyperplasia
- Prostate cancer
- Sexually transmitted infections (STIs)
  - Gonorrhea
  - Genital herpes
  - Syphilis
  - Human immunodeficiency virus (HIV)
- Sperm malformation

Female Reproductive System
- Cancer
  - Vaginal
  - Cervical
  - Uterine
- Fibroids: Benign uterine tumors

- Ovarian endometriosis: Endometrial tissue migrates to areas outside the uterus
- Pelvic inflammatory disease (PID): Infections in the pelvic region that cause infertility; can be caused by *Chlamydia* or other microorganisms
- Premenstrual syndrome (PMS)
- STIs
  - Gonorrhea
  - Genital herpes
  - Syphilis
  - HIV
  - *Chlamydia* infection
  - Trichomoniasis
- Toxic shock syndrome (TSS): *Staphylococcus* infection associated with use of superabsorbent tampons

TABLE 6-10   Summary of Common Laboratory Tests by Body System

Test	Disorder or Purpose
Bone and Joints	
Alkaline phosphatase (ALP)	Bone metabolism marker
Anticitrullinated protein (rheumatoid factor [RF])	Rheumatoid arthritis (RA)
Calcium	Mineral calcium imbalance
Erythrocyte sedimentation rate (ESR)	General inflammation test
Fluorescent antinuclear antibody (ANA)	Systemic lupus erythematosus (SLE)
Magnesium	Mineral magnesium imbalance
Synovial fluid analysis	Arthritis
Uric acid	Gout
Digestive System	
Amylase, lipase	Pancreatitis
Carotene	Steatorrhea (malabsorption syndrome causing fatty stools)
Complete blood count (CBC)	Appendicitis
Gastrin	Gastric malignancy
Liver tests	Liver disease
• ALP	
• Alanine aminotransferase (ALT)	
• Aspartate aminotransferase (AST)	
• γ-Glutamyltransferase (GCT)	
• Bilirubin	
• Hepatitis B surface antigen (HBsAG)	
• Hepatitis C antibody	
• Hepatitis C virus by polymerase chain reaction	
• Ammonia	
Occult blood	Gastrointestinal bleeding
Ova and parasites (O&P)	Parasitic infection
Stool culture	Stool pathogens
Endocrine System	
Calcium	Parathyroid function
Catecholamines (epinephrine, norepinephrine)	Adrenal function
Cortisol	Adrenal cortex function and Addison disease
Fasting glucose or fasting blood sugar (FBS)	Diabetes mellitus
Follicle-stimulating hormone (FSH)	Infertility
Growth hormone (GH)	Pituitary function
Luteinizing hormone (LH)	Infertility
Parathyroid hormone (PTH)	Parathyroid function
Phosphorus	Parathyroid function
Testosterone	Infertility
Triiodothyronine (T_3), thyroxine (T_4), and thyroid-stimulating hormone (TSH)	Graves disease and Hashimoto thyroiditis
Thyroid function studies	Thyroid disorder
Vitamin D	Parathyroid function
Integumentary System	
Culture and sensitivity (C&S)	Bacterial or fungal infection
Potassium hydroxide (KOH) prep	Fungal infection
Skin biopsy	Malignancy
Muscle	
Aldolase	Muscle disease
Aspartate aminotransferase (AST)	Muscle disease
Creatine kinase (CK-MM)	Muscle damage
CK isoenzymes (CK-MM, CK-MB)	Cardiac muscle damage

Continued

TABLE 6-10	Summary of Common Laboratory Tests by Body System—cont'd
Test	Disorder or Purpose
Lactate dehydrogenase	Cardiac muscle damage
Myoglobin	Muscle damage
Troponin	Cardiac muscle damage
Nervous System	
Cell count and differential	Infection
Cerebrospinal fluid (CSF) analysis	Meningitis, other neurologic disorders
CK isoenzymes (CK-BB)	Brain damage (causes elevations)
Culture and Gram stain	Infection
Protein and glucose	Disorders of the nervous system
Reproductive System	
Culture and sensitivity (C&S)	Microbial infection
Estradiol	Assess ovarian or placental function
Estrogen	Assess ovarian function
Fluorescent treponemal antibody absorption test (FTA-ABS)	Syphilis
Human chorionic gonadotropin (hCG)	Assess for pregnancy or ectopic pregnancy
Pap smear	Cervical or vaginal carcinoma
Prostate-specific antigen (PSA)	Prostate cancer
Rapid plasma reagin (RPR)	Syphilis
Semen analysis	Infertility; assess effectiveness of vasectomy
Testosterone	Evaluation of testicular function
Respiratory System	
Arterial blood gases (ABGs): pH (acidity), P_{O_2} (oxygen), P_{CO_2} (carbon dioxide)	Most respiratory disorders; assess lung function
Cold agglutinins (test for antibodies that react with red blood cells at cold temperatures)	Atypical pneumonia
Electrolytes	Impaired gas exchange
Microbiologic tests	Microbial infection—pneumonia or pharyngitis
• Cultures	
• Throat swabs	
• Bronchial washings	
Purified protein derivative (PPD)	Skin test for tuberculosis
Respiratory syncytial virus (RSV)	Viral pneumonia
Urologic System	
Blood urea nitrogen (BUN)	Kidney disease
Creatinine	Kidney disease
Creatinine clearance	Glomerular filtration
Culture and sensitivity (C&S)	Urinary tract infection (UTI)
Electrolytes	Fluid balance
Osmolality	Fluid balance
Protein/microalbumin	Kidney disorders
Renin/angiotensin-converting enzyme (ACE)	Hypertension
Routine urinalysis	Screening for renal or metabolic disorders

BIBLIOGRAPHY

Hall JE: *Guyton and Hall textbook of medical physiology,* ed. 12, Philadelphia, 2011, Saunders.

Patton KT, Thibodeau GA: *Anatomy & physiology,* ed. 8, St. Louis, 2013, Mosby.

STUDY QUESTIONS

See answers in Appendix F.

1. What is homeostasis?

2. Name the four basic types of tissues that compose the human body, and give an example of each.

Match each term to its description:

3. Nucleus
4. Plasma membrane
5. Mitochondria
6. Cytoplasm

a. regulates the flow of materials in and out of the cell
b. "power plants" of the cell
c. contains DNA
d. cellular material

7. Describe the anatomic position.

8. What are body cavities?

Match each position to its description:

9. Ventral
10. Posterior
11. Lateral
12. Medial
13. Prone
14. Supine
15. Extension
16. Inferior

a. lying on the abdomen facing down
b. toward the side
c. toward the middle
d. straightening the joint
e. front surface of the body
f. below
g. back surface of the body
h. lying on the back

17. Name and describe the three body planes.

18. What is hematopoiesis?

19. Name three laboratory tests, and the disorders they test for, that are used to assess for bone and joint disorders.

20. _____ is a bone infection that can be caused by improper phlebotomy technique.

21. Name four laboratory tests that are used to assess for muscle disorders.

22. What are the divisions of the CNS?

23. Name five laboratory tests that are used to assess for digestive disorders.

24. Describe the difference between external and internal respiration.

25. What does the endocrine system do?

26. Name the three types of joints, and give an example of each.

CERTIFICATION EXAMINATION PREPARATION

See answers in Appendix F.

1. The term to define the overall well-being of the body is
   a. hemolysis.
   b. hemostasis.
   c. homeostasis.
   d. hematopoiesis.

2. The functional unit of the nervous systems is
   a. nephron.
   b. neuron.
   c. neoplasm.
   d. nucleus.

3. ATP is found in which part of the cell?
   - a. Mitochondria
   - b. Cytoplasm
   - c. Nucleus
   - d. Plasma membrane

4. Which type of muscle tissue is involved in hemostasis?
   - a. Skeletal
   - b. Smooth
   - c. Epithelial
   - d. Striated

5. Blood is considered which type of tissue?
   - a. Nerve
   - b. Connective
   - c. Muscle
   - d. Epithelial

6. In which system does hematopoiesis occur?
   - a. Skeletal
   - b. Nervous
   - c. Muscular
   - d. Digestive

7. Which is *not* a laboratory test that assesses for muscle disorders?
   - a. AST
   - b. Troponin
   - c. C&S
   - d. Myoglobin

8. Which is *not* a laboratory test that assesses for disorders of the integumentary system?
   - a. C&S
   - b. KOH prep
   - c. BUN
   - d. Skin biopsy

9. Hepatitis involves the
   - a. heart.
   - b. liver.
   - c. brain.
   - d. ovaries.

10. Which laboratory test is *not* useful in the assessment of liver problems?
   - a. AST
   - b. GGT
   - c. ALP
   - d. All are important

11. _____ promotes the breakdown of glycogen back to glucose.
   - a. Insulin
   - b. Glucagon
   - c. Thymosin
   - d. Calcitonin

12. Pancreatitis can be screened for by performing which laboratory test?
   - a. Amylase
   - b. CSF
   - c. Myoglobin
   - d. Occult blood

13. The functional unit of the kidney is known as the
   - a. neuron.
   - b. medulla.
   - c. thalamus.
   - d. nephron.

14. Microbiology may perform the following laboratory test for urologic disorders:
   - a. BUN.
   - b. PPD.
   - c. C&S.
   - d. FBS.

15. ABGs typically test for
   - a. digestive disorders.
   - b. urinary disorders.
   - c. respiratory disorders.
   - d. muscular disorders.

16. The hormone that regulates the amount of calcium and phosphorus in the circulation is
   - a. insulin.
   - b. thymosin.
   - c. oxytocin.
   - d. parathyroid hormone.

17. Which hormone regulates water reabsorption by the kidney?
   - a. ACTH
   - b. TSH
   - c. ADH
   - d. MSH

18. The hormone that can be detected by early pregnancy tests is
   - a. hCG.
   - b. ADH.
   - c. GH.
   - d. MSH.

19. Thyroxine is otherwise known as
   - a. T_3.
   - b. T_4.
   - c. TSH.
   - d. T_1.

20. Hormones are produced by which body system?
   - a. Integumentary
   - b. Endocrine
   - c. Digestive
   - d. Respiratory

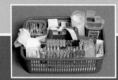

CHAPTER 7 Circulatory, Lymphatic, and Immune Systems

The circulatory system transports blood containing oxygen and nutrients throughout the body and picks up metabolic waste products for disposal. Beginning at the heart, blood passes from arteries, to capillaries, to veins, and then back to the heart. The structure of each type of blood vessel is adapted to its function within the system. In addition to its role in nutrient and waste transport, blood transports hormones and enzymes, as well as clotting factors that minimize blood leakage in the event of injury. Hemostasis ensures that a rupture in a blood vessel is repaired quickly. A separate but linked circulatory system, the lymphatic system, redistributes intercellular fluid and provides an important route of transport for cells of the immune system. The immune system fights foreign invaders through a combination of cellular and chemical defenses.

OUTLINE

Circulatory System
  Heart
  Circulation Through the Heart
  Contraction of the Heart and
    Blood Pressure
  Blood Vessels

Blood
Hemostasis
Blood Disorders
Lymphatic System
Lymphatic Vessels
Lymph Organs

Lymphatic System Disorders
Immune System
Nonspecific Immunity
Specific Immunity
Immune System Disorders
Review for Certification

OBJECTIVES

After completing this chapter, you should be able to:

1. Describe the circulation of blood from the heart to the lungs and other body tissues.
2. Differentiate arteries, veins, and capillaries.
3. Locate the major arteries and veins of the human body.
4. Define systole, diastole, and sphygmomanometer.
5. List and define at least 10 diseases of the heart and blood vessels.
6. Describe the components of whole blood.
7. Describe the three cellular elements of the blood, including their major functions.
8. Explain the process of hemostasis.

9. For red blood cells (RBCs), white blood cells (WBCs), and hemostasis, list at least three diseases that affect each.
10. Describe laboratory tests that may be used to detect diseases of RBCs, WBCs, and hemostasis.
11. Differentiate lymphatic circulation from that of blood.
12. Explain the functions of the lymphatic system.
13. Differentiate among nonspecific, humoral, and cellular immunity.
14. Describe the functions of T and B cells.

KEY TERMS

acquired immunodeficiency
  syndrome (AIDS)
adhesion
aggregation
albumin
allergy
antibodies
anticoagulant
antigens
aorta

aortic semilunar valve
arteries
arterioles
atria
autoimmunity
B cells
basilic vein
basophils
bicuspid valve
CD_4^+ cells

cellular immunity
cephalic vein
common pathway
complement
coronary arteries
cytokines
cytotoxic T cells
diastole
disseminated intravascular
  coagulation (DIC)

electrolytes
endocardium
eosinophils
epicardium
erythrocyte
extrinsic pathway
fibrin
fibrin degradation products
  (FDPs)
fibrinogen

KEY TERMS—cont'd

fibrinolysis	lymphocytes	platelets	sphygmomanometer
formed elements	lymphoma	polymorphonuclear (PMN)	stroke
granulocytes	major histocompatibility	leukocytes	systemic circulation
helper T cells	complex (MHC)	primary hemostasis	systole
human leukocyte antigens	median cubital vein	prothrombin	T cells
(HLAs)	megakaryocytes	pulmonary arteries	terminal lymphatics
humoral immunity	memory cells	pulmonary circulation	thoracic duct
immunization	memory T cells	pulmonary semilunar	thrombin
immunoglobulins	mitral valve	(pulmonic) valve	thrombocytes
inflammation	monocytes	pulmonary trunk	tissue plasminogen
interferons	mononuclear leukocytes	pulmonary veins	activator (t-PA)
interleukins	myocardial infarction (MI)	reticulocyte	tricuspid valve
interstitial fluid	myocardium	right atrioventricular (AV)	tunica adventitia
intrinsic pathway	natural killer (NK) cells	valve	tunica intima
ischemia	neutrophils	right lymphatic duct	tunica media
left atrioventricular (AV)	pericardium	secondary hemostasis	vascular spasm
valve	phagocytes	segmented neutrophils	veins
leukemia	plasma	(segs)	venae cavae
leukocytes	plasma cells	serum	venules
lymphedema	plasmin	severe combined immune	
lymph nodes	plasminogen	deficiency (SCID)	

ABBREVIATIONS

AIDS acquired immunodeficiency syndrome
ANA antinuclear antibody
APL antiphospholipid antibody
aPTT activated partial thromboplastin time
AV atrioventricular
CBC complete blood count
DIC disseminated intravascular coagulation
DVT deep vein thrombosis
FDPs fibrin degradation products
HIV human immunodeficiency virus
HLAs human leukocyte antigens
MHC major histocompatibility complex

MI myocardial infarction
NK natural killer
PMN polymorphonuclear
PT prothrombin time
RBCs red blood cells
SCID severe combined immune deficiency
segs segmented neutrophils
stat short turnaround time
TIBC total iron-binding capacity
t-PA tissue plasminogen activator
WBCs white blood cells

CIRCULATORY SYSTEM

The circulatory system is a system of closed tubes. Circulation occurs in two large loops: the pulmonary circulation and the systemic circulation. The **pulmonary circulation** carries blood between the heart and the lungs for gas exchange, and the **systemic circulation** carries blood between the heart and the rest of the body's tissues. In both cases, **arteries** carry blood from the heart to capillary beds, where exchange occurs. **Veins** return blood to the heart.

Heart

The heart is a muscular double pump whose contractions push blood through the circulatory system. It is located in the thoracic cavity behind and slightly to the left of the sternum, between the lungs. The heart is surrounded by a thin membranous sac, the **pericardium**, which supports and lubricates the heart during contraction. The outer layer of the heart, the **epicardium**, consists of epithelial cells and underlying fibrous connective tissue. The **coronary arteries**, which supply oxygen to the heart, are embedded in this layer. The middle layer, the **myocardium**, is composed of cardiac muscle, whose cells make extensive contacts with adjacent cells to allow electrical activity to spread easily from one cell to the next. The innermost layer, the **endocardium**, is made up of endothelial cells, modified epithelium that is continuous with the endothelium lining the blood vessels that enter and exit the heart's chambers.

The four chambers of the heart are the left and right **atria** (singular: atrium) and the left and right ventricles (Figure 7-1). The atrial septum divides the two atria, and the interventricular septum divides the two ventricles.

The heart has four valves that prevent the backflow of blood. The **right atrioventricular (AV) valve**, also called the **tricuspid valve**, separates the right atrium and the right ventricle, and the **pulmonary semilunar (pulmonic) valve** separates the right ventricle from the **pulmonary arteries**. The **left atrioventricular (AV) valve**, also called the **bicuspid valve** or **mitral valve**, separates the left atrium from the left ventricle, and the **aortic semilunar valve** separates the left ventricle from the **aorta**.

Circulation Through the Heart

Deoxygenated blood from the systemic circulation collects in the superior and inferior **venae cavae** (singular: vena cava), which empty into the right atrium (Figure 7-2). Contraction of the right atrium forces blood through the tricuspid valve into the right ventricle. Contraction of the right ventricle forces blood out through the pulmonary semilunar valve, through the **pulmonary trunk**, and into the left and right pulmonary arteries. Blood then travels to the lungs, picking up oxygen and releasing carbon dioxide in the capillaries surrounding the alveoli. Returning to the heart via the left and right **pulmonary veins**, oxygenated blood enters the left atrium. Contraction of the left atrium forces blood through the mitral valve into the left ventricle. Contraction of the left ventricle forces blood through the aortic semilunar valve into the aorta. The aorta rises up from the top of the heart before turning and descending through the thoracic and abdominal cavities. Many of the major arteries in the body branch directly from the aorta. Arteries branch further into arterioles, which lead to capillary beds within the tissues, where the blood releases its oxygen. Blood becomes deoxygenated as it passes

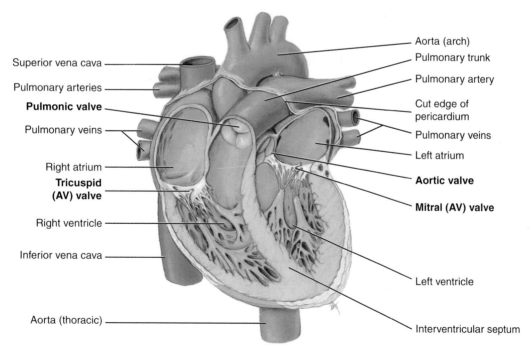

FIGURE 7-1 The heart is a muscle composed of four chambers, separated by valves. (From Applegate E: *The anatomy and physiology learning system,* ed. 4, St. Louis, 2011, Saunders.)

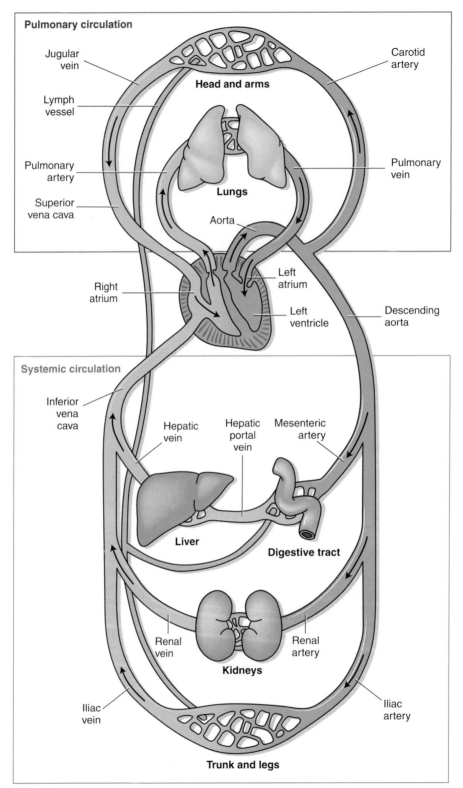

FIGURE 7-2 Blood flow through the heart. Blood from the body enters the right atrium and passes into the right ventricle, where it is pumped to the lungs. It reenters the left atrium and passes into the left ventricle, where it is pumped to the rest of the body.

through the capillaries and then enters venules, which link to form veins. Major veins empty into the venae cavae, which return blood to the right atrium, completing the cycle.

Contraction of the Heart and Blood Pressure

Each heartbeat cycle includes a contraction and a relaxation of each chamber. The contraction, called systole, develops pressure and forces blood through the system. The relaxation, called diastole, allows the chamber to fill again. The two atria contract together, as do the two ventricles. Atrial systole occurs slightly before ventricular systole and is not as forceful. The familiar "lubb-dupp" sound of the heartbeat is actually the sound of the valves closing—the "lubb" is the closing of the two AV valves at the start of ventricular systole, and the "dupp" is the closing of the two semilunar valves as arterial backpressure forces them shut at the start of ventricular diastole.

Blood in the circulatory system is under pressure, even during ventricular diastole. Blood pressure, measured by a sphygmomanometer, (SFIG-mo-man-OM-uh-ter)is the measure of the force of blood on the arterial walls. Blood pressure is given as the ratio of ventricular systole to diastole.

Blood pressure differs markedly at different points in the circulatory system, and for this reason, it is always measured from the brachial artery at the upper arm.

Blood Vessels

In general, blood vessels (except for capillaries) have three discrete layers surrounding the lumen, or the space in which blood flows (Figure 7-3). The tunica adventitia, or outer layer, is composed of connective tissue; the tunica media, or middle layer, is made of smooth muscle; and the tunica intima, or inner layer, is composed of a single layer of endothelial cells.

Arteries

Arteries carry blood from the heart. Arteries are built to withstand the high blood pressure generated by ventricular contraction. They have a thick muscular wall, which can expand when blood is pumped into them and then contract to maintain flow and pressure during diastole. Arteries are located deeper than veins, but they can be found by feeling for the pulse. Arteries branch into smaller vessels called arterioles, which ultimately branch

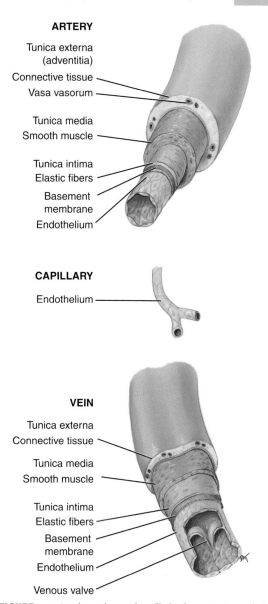

FIGURE 7-3 Arteries, veins, and capillaries have structures that correlate with their functions. (From Applegate E: *The anatomy and physiology learning system,* ed. 4, St. Louis, 2011, Saunders.)

to form capillaries. Figure 7-4 indicates the names and locations of the major arteries.

A myocardial infarction (MI, or heart attack) occurs when the heart receives inadequate blood supply through the coronary arteries. This often occurs when the arteries become clogged with built-up atherosclerotic plaques. The resulting lack of oxygen, termed ischemia, causes damage to the muscle. The damaged cardiac muscle releases a number of proteins into the circulation, which can be used for diagnosis and to determine the timing of

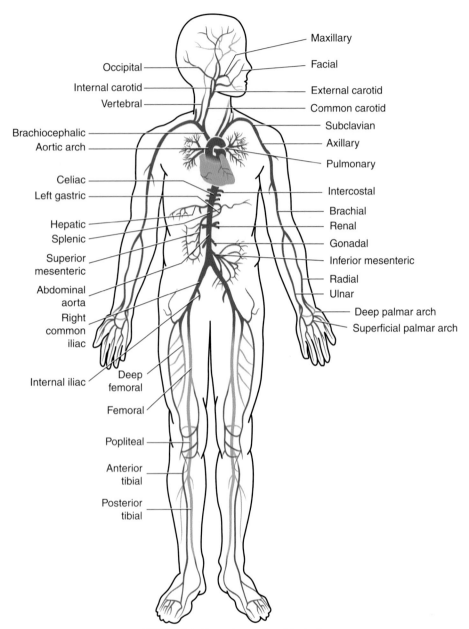

FIGURE 7-4 The major arteries of the body.

the MI. Tests used are indicated in Box 7-1. Other disorders of the heart and blood vessels are listed in Table 7-1.

Capillaries

Capillaries are composed only of the tunica intima, a single layer of endothelial cells. This allows rapid diffusion of gases and nutrients between tissues and blood across the capillary membrane. Capillaries form meshworks, called capillary beds, which

BOX 7-1	Tests Used to Diagnose a Myocardial Infarction

- CK total: Creatine kinase total
- CK-MB fraction: Creatine kinase MB fraction
- Myoglobin
- Troponin T (TnT)
- Troponin I

TABLE 7-1	Disorders of the Heart and Blood Vessels
Disorder	Description
Arteries	
Aneurysm	A bulge in a vessel, usually an artery, caused by weakening of the wall or hypertension; without surgical correction, aneurysms may burst
Arteriosclerosis	Accumulation of fatty deposits on the tunica intima of arteries, causing thickening and toughening of the arterial wall; loss of elasticity increases strain on the artery and may lead to myocardial infarction (MI) or stroke
Stroke	A loss of blood to the brain as a result of either hemorrhage or, more commonly, blocked circulation
Heart	
Bacterial infection	Pericarditis (infection of the pericardium) and endocarditis (infection of the endocardium)
Congestive heart failure	Inadequate heart output, leading to edema of the peripheral tissues
Coronary artery disease	Any type of degenerative change in the coronary arteries including coronary atherosclerosis
MI	Death of heart muscle cells as a result of an interruption in blood supply; also known as a heart attack
Rheumatic heart disease	Autoimmune disease affecting cardiac tissue; caused by a previous streptococcal infection elsewhere in the body
Valvular heart disease	Thickening and calcification of a valve that causes stenosis, or narrowing of the passage through the valve, and incomplete closure; causes heart murmur and may lead to congestive heart failure
Veins	
Hemorrhoids	Swollen veins in the walls of the anus, often resulting from prolonged exertion or pressure during defecation
Varicose veins	Veins that are tortuous and dilated because of swelling and loss of function of valves; often caused by prolonged sitting or standing

permeate the tissues. On average, no cell is farther than a few cells from a capillary. In its chemical composition, capillary blood is more similar to arterial blood than to venous blood, especially in warmed tissue, where blood flow is rapid.

Veins

Veins carry blood back toward the heart. Capillary blood enters **venules**, the smallest veins. Venules join to form larger veins. Veins have thinner walls and less muscle than arteries do, because they do not experience large fluctuations in blood pressure. To help prevent backflow of blood, veins have valves within them at various points along their length that are pushed closed when blood flows back against them (Figure 7-5). Veins are closer to the surface than are arteries. Most blood tests are performed on venous blood because of the easier access and because venipuncture is safer than arterial puncture. The major veins are illustrated in Figure 7-6.

Circulatory Anatomy of the Antecubital Fossa

The antecubital fossa is the area just distal to the elbow joint where blood is usually drawn. This area is easily accessible and contains several prominent

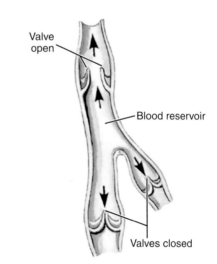

FIGURE 7-5 Valves in veins prevent backflow of blood. (From Thibodeau GA, Patton KT: *Anatomy and physiology,* ed. 5, St. Louis, 2003, Mosby.)

veins that are usually located a safe distance from nerves and arteries, making it an ideal location for venipuncture. Becoming familiar with the anatomy of this area will help you draw blood safely and confidently.

The capillary beds of the hand drain into a network of veins that pass into the forearm. These

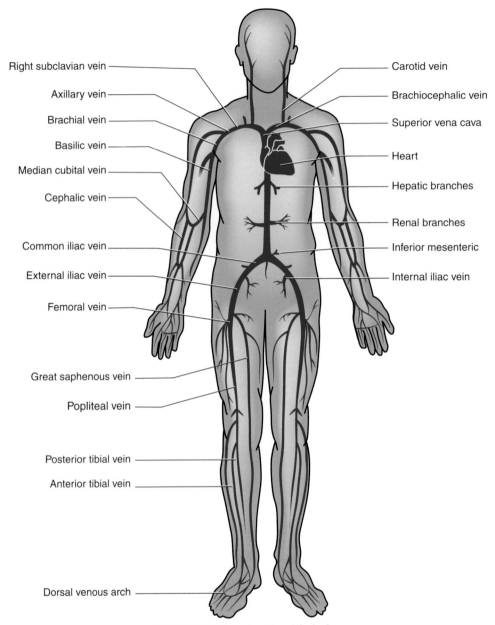

FIGURE 7-6 The major veins of the body.

collect to form several major veins (Figure 7-7). On the anterior surface (where blood is drawn), the most prominent of these are the **cephalic vein**, the **median cubital vein**, and the **basilic vein**. The median cubital vein splits just below the elbow, sending one branch to the basilic vein and one branch to the cephalic vein. Thus these veins form a rough letter M in this region. Blood is typically drawn from one of the veins forming part of this M. In other patients, the veins will resemble the letter H.

It is important to note that the exact anatomy of this region may vary considerably from person to person. Veins may branch multiple times, some smaller veins may be absent, or they may be located in unusual places. For the phlebotomist, this rarely causes problems, as long as a prominent vein can be found for drawing blood.

Problems can arise, however, from the location of other structures in the antecubital fossa. The brachial artery passes through the elbow, splitting into the radial and ulnar arteries. These are located deeper than the veins, though, and the skilled phlebotomist rarely has any trouble avoiding them. A more common (although still rare) complication

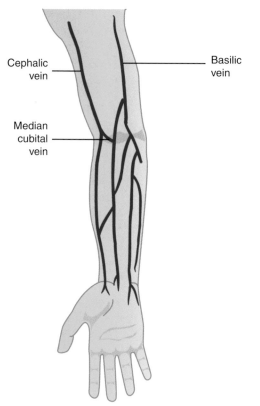

FIGURE 7-7 Veins of the antecubital fossa in the right arm. (From Bonewit-West K: *Clinical procedures for medical assistants,* ed. 9, St. Louis, 2015, Saunders.)

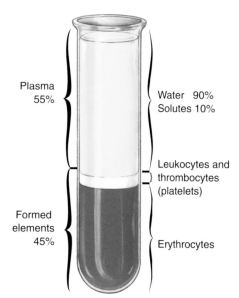

FIGURE 7-8 Composition of blood. (From Applegate E: *The anatomy and physiology learning system,* ed. 4, St. Louis, 2011, Saunders.)

arises from the position of two nerves that also pass through this busy intersection. The external cutaneous nerve passes close to the cephalic vein, and the internal cutaneous nerve passes close to the basilic vein. In many patients the nerves are no deeper than the veins, and in some patients the nerves may pass over, rather than under, the veins. Contacting the nerve with the needle causes an intense, sharp pain and may lead to long-term nerve damage.

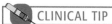

CLINICAL TIP

When possible, draw from the medial cubital vein to reduce the likelihood of complications.

FLASH FORWARD ↱ >>>

You will learn more about nerve and artery complications in Chapter 11.

Blood

An average adult has 5 to 6 L of blood. Blood is composed of **plasma**—the fluid portion—and cellular components, called the **formed elements** (Figure 7-8).

Plasma

Plasma constitutes 55% of the volume of blood. It is 90% water, with the rest made up of dissolved proteins, amino acids, gases, electrolytes, sugars, hormones, lipids, and vitamins, plus waste products such as urea, destined for excretion.

The most significant elements of plasma are **albumin**, a plasma protein responsible for osmotic pressure and transport of many types of molecules; the **immunoglobulins**, or **antibodies**, which are important parts of the immune system; and **fibrinogen**, responsible for blood clotting. Other proteins include hormones, such as insulin, and transport proteins, such as transferrin, which carries iron. Plasma also contains **complement**, a group of immune system proteins that, when activated, destroy target cells by puncturing their membranes. **Electrolytes** include the major ions of plasma—sodium (Na^+) and chloride (Cl^-), plus potassium (K^+), calcium (Ca^{2+}), magnesium (Mg^{2+}), bicarbonate (HCO_3^-), phosphate (PO_4^{3-}), and sulfate (SO_4^{2-}) ions.

A plasma sample is collected in a tube containing an **anticoagulant**, a chemical that keeps blood from clotting. The sample is spun at high speed in a centrifuge, which separates the plasma from the cells. The plasma is the straw-to-yellow color fluid that floats on top of the cells in the sample.

Plasma samples are collected in tubes with a top that is one of these colors: light blue, royal blue, pink, pearl, gray, green, light green, or tan. Plasma samples are used for short turnaround time (stat) chemistry tests, because when results are needed immediately, there is not time to allow coagulation. These samples are collected in a green-top tube. They are also used for coagulation tests, which are collected in a blue-top tube.

FLASH FORWARD

You will learn more about blood specimen collection in Chapter 8.

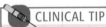

CLINICAL TIP

If 3 mL of plasma is needed for a test, 6 mL of whole blood should be drawn, because blood is about half plasma.

Serum

Plasma without its clotting factors is called **serum**. Serum is formed when a blood sample is collected in a glass or plastic container that has no additives and is induced to clot (a *serum separator tube* is used for this purpose). The conversion of fibrinogen to fibrin forms strands that trap all of the cellular elements. After clotting, the serum is separated from the clotted material by centrifugation. A serum sample is used for many types of tests, because clotting would interfere with the results. Serum samples are collected in tubes with a top that is one of these colors: orange, royal blue, red, gold, or tiger-speckled (red and gold).

Formed Elements

The formed elements constitute 45% of blood volume. Of these, 99% are red blood cells (RBCs), with white blood cells (WBCs) and platelets making up the rest. All blood cells are formed in the bone marrow from the division of long-lived progenitors called stem cells.

Red Blood Cells

RBCs carry hemoglobin, the iron-containing oxygen transport protein that gives blood its red color (Figure 7-9). There are 5 million RBCs in a microliter (μL) of whole blood (1 μL = 10^{-6} L). An RBC initially contains a cell nucleus, but this is expelled shortly after formation, at which stage the RBC is known as a **reticulocyte**. (The reticulocyte count, a common laboratory test, provides the physician with an indirect measure of how well the bone marrow is producing RBCs.) Once released into

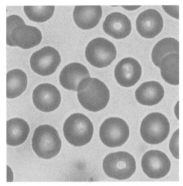

FIGURE 7-9 Wright-stained red blood cells as seen through a light microscope. (From Rodak BF, Carr JH: *Clinical hematology atlas,* ed. 4, St. Louis, 2013, Saunders.)

the peripheral circulation, within a day or two, it matures into an **erythrocyte**.

A single RBC remains in the peripheral circulation about 120 days before being removed by the liver, bone marrow, or spleen. RBC destruction results in three major breakdown products: iron, amino acids, and bilirubin. The iron and amino acids are recycled. The only waste product, bilirubin, is transported to the liver for elimination from the body. The iron-containing heme groups are recycled to make new hemoglobin for packing into new RBCs.

White Blood Cells

White blood cells (WBCs) or **leukocytes** protect the body against infection. WBCs are produced in the bone marrow and lymph nodes and undergo a complex maturation process, which may involve the thymus and other organs. There are 5000 to 10,000 WBCs in 1 μL of whole blood. At any time, most WBCs are not in the blood but in peripheral tissues and lymphatic system.

An important feature of all WBCs is their ability to recognize specific molecules on the surface of infectious agents and to distinguish them from markers on the body's own cells. This molecular recognition is responsible for the extraordinary ability of the immune system to protect the body against the daily threat of attack from bacteria, viruses, and other infectious organisms.

Two major categories of leukocytes exist: granulocytes and mononuclear leukocytes. **Granulocytes** get their name because of the presence of visible granules in their cytoplasm. The granulocytes include neutrophils, eosinophils, and basophils. **Mononuclear leukocytes** have larger, unsegmented nuclei. They include lymphocytes and monocytes. They all contain powerful chemicals that destroy foreign cells and signal other parts of the immune system.

Neutrophils, so called because their granules do not take up either acidic or basic dyes, make up 40% to 60% of all leukocytes in the blood (Figure 7-10, *A*). They are **phagocytes**, whose role is to attack and digest bacteria, and their numbers increase during a bacterial infection. They are often the first WBCs on the scene of an infection, and their rather short life span (approximately 3 to 4 days) is further shortened when they engulf and digest bacterial and cellular debris. Neutrophils are also called **polymorphonuclear (PMN) leukocytes**, or **segmented neutrophils (segs)**, because of their highly divided and irregularly shaped nuclei.

Eosinophils take up the dye eosin, which stains their granules an orange-red (Figure 7-10, *B*). They represent 1% to 3% of all circulating leukocytes. Eosinophils are also phagocytic, and their principal targets are parasites and antibody-labeled foreign molecules rather than cells. Their numbers increase in the presence of allergies, skin infections, and parasitic infections.

Basophils stain darkly with basic dyes and are deep purple in a standard blood smear (Figure 7-10, *C*). They account for less than 1% of leukocytes in the blood. Basophils are phagocytic. They also release histamine, a chemical that swells tissue and causes allergic reactions. Basophils produce heparin as well, which is an anticoagulant. Increased

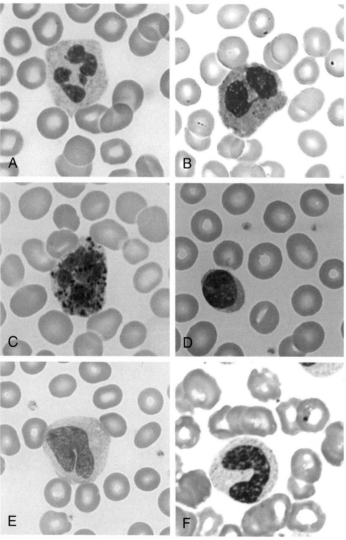

FIGURE 7-10 Wright-stained smears. **A,** Neutrophil. **B,** Eosinophil. **C,** Basophil. **D,** Lymphocyte. **E,** Monocyte. **F,** Band neutrophil. (From Rodak BF, Carr JH: *Clinical hematology atlas,* ed. 4, St. Louis, Saunders, 2013.)

numbers of basophils are usually associated with some kind of **leukemia**.

Lymphocytes make up 20% to 40% of all circulating leukocytes, but this is a small fraction of their total number, most of which reside in lymph nodes (Figure 7-10, *D*). Lymphocytes circulate between the lymphatic system and the circulatory system, and their numbers may increase during viral infection. Lymphocytes include **B cells**, which produce antibodies; **natural killer (NK) cells**, which destroy both foreign and infected cells; and **T cells**, which control cellular immunity.

Monocytes are large phagocytic cells that make up 3% to 8% of all circulating leukocytes (Figure 7-10, *E*). Monocytes pass from the circulatory system into the peripheral tissues, where they transform into macrophages and act as roving sentries. Their signals help activate B cells to make antibodies.

Platelets

Platelets are created in the bone marrow from **megakaryocytes**, which package and release them into the circulation. Although they are also called **thrombocytes**, platelets are not actually cells; they are simply membrane-bound packets of cytoplasm (Figure 7-11). Platelets play a critical role in blood coagulation, as discussed later. Every 1 μL of blood contains approximately 200,000 platelets, each of which remains in circulation for 9 to 12 days.

Hemostasis

Hemostasis refers to the processes by which blood vessels are repaired after injury. It occurs in a series of steps, from muscular contraction of the vessel walls, through clot formation, to removal of the clot when the vessel repairs itself.

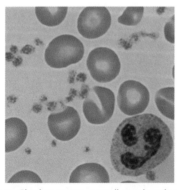

FIGURE 7-11 Platelets appear as small, purple-stained dots. The larger cell in the bottom right-hand corner is a neutrophil. (From Rodak BF, Carr JH: *Clinical hematology atlas,* ed. 4, St. Louis, 2013, Saunders.)

Vascular Phase

Rupture of a vein or artery causes an immediate **vascular spasm**, or contraction of the smooth muscle lining the vessel. This reduces the vessel diameter, substantially reducing the blood loss that would otherwise occur. This contraction lasts about 30 minutes. For capillaries, this may be enough to allow the wound to seal.

Platelet Phase

Exposure of materials beneath the endothelial lining causes platelets to stick to the endothelial cells almost immediately, a process known as **adhesion**. Additional platelets then stick to these, a process known as **aggregation**. Aggregating platelets become activated, releasing factors that promote fibrin accumulation in the next phase. The combination of the vascular phase and the platelet phase is called **primary hemostasis**. The next phase, coagulation, is known as **secondary hemostasis**.

Coagulation Phase

Coagulation involves a complex and highly regulated cascade of enzymes and other factors whose activation ultimately results in formation of a blood clot—a meshwork of fibrin, platelets, and other blood cells that closes off the wound. The coagulation cascade begins from 30 seconds to several minutes after the injury.

Coagulation is initiated through two different pathways that feed into a single common pathway (Figure 7-12). The **extrinsic pathway** begins with the release of tissue factor by endothelial cells, which combines with calcium ions and coagulation factor VII from the plasma to form an active enzyme. The **intrinsic pathway** is initiated when other plasma coagulation factors contact the materials exposed when the blood vessel is damaged (similar to platelet adhesion). A series of reactions takes place to form an enzyme that can initiate the **common pathway**.

Enzymes from both pathways then enter the common pathway, reacting with factors X and V to convert circulating inactive **prothrombin** (also called factor II) to active **thrombin**. Once activated, thrombin converts circulating fibrinogen to fibrin. **Fibrin** is a fibrous protein whose strands adhere to the platelets and endothelial cells at the wound, forming a dense fibrous network that, in turn, traps other cells. Platelets then contract and pull the edges of the wound closer together, allowing endothelial cells grow across the wound and repairing the damaged lining.

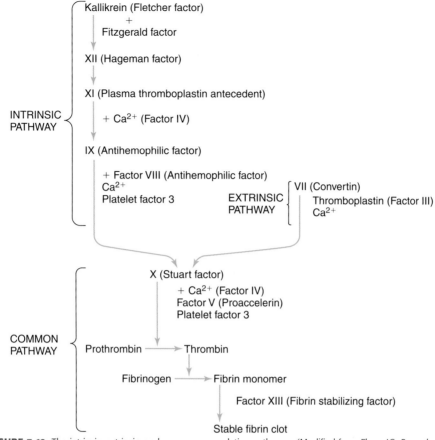

FIGURE 7-12 The intrinsic, extrinsic, and common coagulation pathways. (Modified from Flynn JC: *Procedures in phlebotomy*, ed. 4, St. Louis, Saunders, 2012.)

Fibrinolysis

As the wound is closed and tissue repair commences, fibrin itself is broken down slowly, a process called **fibrinolysis.** This creates **fibrin degradation products (FDPs).** FDPs are monitored to diagnose **disseminated intravascular coagulation (DIC),** a condition in which blood clots abnormally in the circulatory system. DIC is a potential complication of pregnancy, as well as other conditions.

Fibrinolysis is controlled by **plasmin,** an enzyme made from **plasminogen** by **tissue plasminogen activator (t-PA).** Synthetic t-PA is used to dissolve blood clots in **stroke,** MI, pulmonary embolism, and other conditions. Urokinase and streptokinase are also used to activate plasminogen in these conditions.

Blood Disorders

Blood disorders and the tests for them are outlined in Table 7-2. Knowing these disorders and tests will improve your ability to interact with your professional colleagues. However, it is important to remember that, as a phlebotomist, you may not know the actual reason any particular test is ordered for any particular patient. You should not discuss the purpose of a test with a patient—that is the role of the doctor.

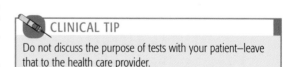

CLINICAL TIP

Do not discuss the purpose of tests with your patient—leave that to the health care provider.

LYMPHATIC SYSTEM

The lymphatic system includes the lymphatic vessels, the lymph nodes, and several associated organs, plus the lymph fluid flowing in the lymphatic vessels and the leukocytes that reside in the lymph nodes and elsewhere (Figure 7-13). The lymphatic system returns tissue fluid to the circulatory system—in the process, screening it for signs of infection—and provides a passageway for lymphocytes patrolling the tissues.

TABLE 7-2	Blood Disorders	
Disorder	Description	Tests
Hemostasis, Platelets, and Clotting		
Hemophilias	Group of inherited disorders marked by deficient clotting factor production and increased bleeding; the most common is hemophilia A, a deficiency in clotting factor VIII	Activated partial thromboplastin time (aPTT) or prothrombin time (PT) and clotting factor activity (factor VIII activity)
Disseminated intravascular coagulation (DIC)	Activation of the clotting system throughout the circulatory system in response to bacterial toxins, trauma, or other stimuli; fibrin is eventually degraded, but small clots may form, damaging tissue; fibrinogen deficiency may follow	Fibrin degradation product (FDP) D-Dimer Fibrinogen
Thrombocytopenia	Decreased number of platelets	Complete blood count (CBC)
Thrombosis or deep vein thrombosis (DVT)	Localized activation of the clotting system, called thrombophlebitis in veins; an embolus is a piece of clot that has broken off and entered the circulation	Protein C Protein S
Red Blood Cells (RBCs) and Hemoglobin		
Anemia	Decrease in number of RBCs or amount of hemoglobin in the blood	Reticulocyte count Iron studies: ferritin and total iron-binding capacity (TIBC) Vitamin B_{12} and folate levels CBC
Polycythemia	Increase in total number of blood cells, especially RBCs; treated with therapeutic phlebotomy	CBC
Sickle cell disease	Inherited hemoglobin disorder, resulting in sickle-shaped RBCs; requires inheritance from both parents (autosomal recessive inheritance)	Sickle cell solubility Hemoglobin electrophoresis CBC
Thalassemia	Group of inherited hemoglobin disorders resulting in decreased production of hemoglobin and anemia	Hemoglobin electrophoresis CBC
White Blood Cells (WBCs)		
Bacterial infection	WBCs respond to many kinds of infection and inflammations	CBC with differential Bacterial cultures
Human immunodeficiency virus (HIV) infection	Infection of helper T cells by HIV; can lead to acquired immunodeficiency syndrome (AIDS)	Anti-HIV antibody Western blot T cell count: CD3, CD4, and CD8
Leukemia	Malignant neoplasm in the bone marrow, causing increased production of WBCs	CBC with differential Cell marker studies
Mononucleosis	Increased numbers of reactive lymphocytes in response to infection with the Epstein-Barr virus	CBC Monospot or heterophile antibody
Disorders of the Immune System		
Rheumatoid arthritis	Body produces antibodies that attack the membranes lining the joints	Rheumatoid factor Anticitrullinated peptide (anti-CCP)
Systemic lupus erythematosus	Body produces antibodies that attack a variety of tissues and organs: joints, lungs blood cells, nerves, and kidneys	Antiphospholipid antibodies (APLs) Antinuclear antibodies (ANA)
Multiple sclerosis	Body produces antibodies that attack nerve cells	No blood test Spinal tap and magnetic resonance imaging
Severe combined immune deficiency (SCID)	Genetically inherited disease in which the immune system is severely impaired	Immunoglobulin quantitation

Lymphatic Vessels

In contrast to arteries and veins, which form a complete circulatory loop, lymphatic vessels are closed at their distal ends. These closed-end tubes, called **terminal lymphatics**, are slightly larger than capillaries and permeate the tissues (except for the central nervous system), although not as extensively as capillaries do. The wall of a terminal lymphatic vessel is an endothelial layer that is one cell thick.

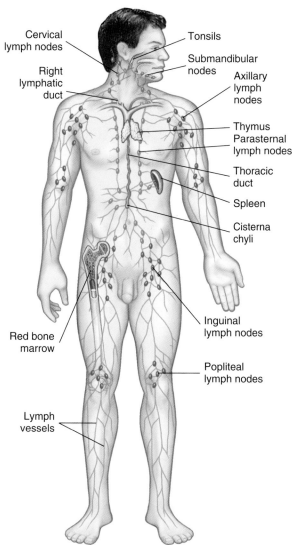

Cervical
lymph nodes

Tonsils

Submandibular
nodes

Right
lymphatic
duct

Axillary
lymph
nodes

Thymus
Parasternal
lymph nodes

Thoracic
duct

Spleen

Cisterna
chyli

Inguinal
lymph nodes

Red bone
marrow

Popliteal
lymph nodes

Lymph
vessels

FIGURE 7-13 The lymphatic system permeates the body, collecting interstitial fluid and returning it to the circulation. Lymph nodes are important components of the immune system. (From Patton KT, Thibodeau GA: *The human body in health & disease,* ed. 6, St. Louis, Mosby, 2014.)

Small lymphatic vessels feed into larger ones and finally into the thoracic duct and right lymphatic duct. These empty into the venous system just distal to the superior vena cava. Along the way, valves within the lymphatic vessels keep fluid moving in one direction.

Lymphatic fluid is derived from the fluid between cells, called interstitial fluid. Interstitial fluid is a combination of plasma that has been forced out of capillaries by blood pressure and cellular fluid exiting the cells through osmosis. Lymphatic fluid thus carries the chemical signature of the peripheral fluid as a whole. Most important,

it contains proteins and other molecules released by infectious agents, which are carried to the lymph nodes for examination by WBCs. Lymphatic fluid is also important for the transport of fat—terminal lymphatics in the intestine absorb dietary fat, keeping it out of the capillary circulation.

Lymph Organs

Lymph nodes are chambers located along the lymphatic vessels and are populated by lymphocytes. Lymph nodes are especially common in the digestive, respiratory, and urinary tracts. The tonsils are particularly large lymph nodes. Lymphocytes in the nodes screen the lymph fluid for signs of infection. In addition, macrophages journey to the lymph nodes from infection sites, carrying molecular samples for examination by B and T cells.

The other organs of the lymphatic system include the spleen and the thymus. In the spleen, worn-out RBCs are recycled by macrophages, and blood is examined by resident B and T cells. The thymus is principally involved in maturation of the immune system during development and early life.

Lymphatic System Disorders

Lymphedema is an accumulation of interstitial fluid in tissues as a result of a blocked lymphatic vessel. Elephantiasis is a severe form of lymphedema, caused by a mosquito-borne parasite that colonizes the lymphatic vessels. Lymphoma is a tumor of a lymph gland. Hodgkin's disease is a type of lymphoma.

Because they provide passageways for mobile cells, lymphatic vessels provide a route for the spread of metastatic cancer cells, which may either take up residence in a lymph node or pass out of the lymphatic system to invade surrounding tissue. For this reason, biopsy of nearby lymph nodes is often performed to determine whether a cancer has metastasized.

IMMUNE SYSTEM

The immune system involves the coordinated action of many cell types, along with the circulating proteins of antibodies and complement. In addition, it includes physical barriers to the entry of infection, such as the skin and the epithelial lining of the lungs, gut, and urinary tract.

Nonspecific Immunity

Nonspecific immunity refers to defense against infectious agents independent of the specific chemical markers on their surfaces. This includes physical barriers, the complement system, and phagocytes (monocytes and neutrophils), which engulf and destroy foreign cells without regard to their exact identity.

Inflammation is a coordinated, nonspecific defense against infection or irritation. It combines increased blood flow and capillary permeability, activation of macrophages, temperature increase, and the clotting reaction to wall off the infected area. These actions also activate the mechanism of specific immunity.

Specific Immunity

Specific immunity involves the molecular recognition of particular markers, called antigens, on the surface of a foreign agent. Recognition of these antigens in the appropriate context triggers activation of T and B cells, while also increasing the activity and accuracy of nonspecific defenses, such as complement and macrophages.

In one form of antigen recognition, antigens are taken up by a macrophage, which displays them on its surface in a receptor complex controlled by genes in the major histocompatibility complex (MHC). The proteins in these complexes are also known as human leukocyte antigens (HLAs). The antigen complex is presented to T cells, which are activated when they recognize the HLA–antigen combination. Activated T cells influence the production of both cytotoxic T cells, which recognize antigens and destroy both foreign and infected host cells, and memory T cells, which are primed to respond more rapidly if the antigen is encountered again later in life. Other T cells, called helper T cells, are important regulators of the entire immune response. They are needed to make both antibodies and cytotoxic T cells. Helper T cells are also known as T4 or CD4+ cells, named after one of their surface receptors; these are the cells infected by human immunodeficiency virus (HIV). T cell–based immunity is also called cellular immunity.

Antigens can be recognized in another way. An antigen can bind to an antibody, a product of a B cell. Each B cell makes an antibody of a slightly different shape, allowing recognition of an enormous variety of antigens. If the antibody shape is complementary to the antigen shape, it will activate the B cell under the influence of helper T cells and macrophages to undergo rapid cell division. Most of the offspring are plasma cells, which produce and release large numbers of antibodies into the lymphatic system and, ultimately, into the circulation.

These antibodies bind to antigens at the site of infection and elsewhere, directly inactivating them; they also act as flags for targeting by macrophages. The remaining B-cell offspring become memory cells, which serve a similar function to memory T cells. This is the basis of immunization. Antibody-based immunity is also called humoral immunity, after *humor*, the antiquated term for a body fluid.

In addition to the direct contact between cells, immune cells communicate through cytokines, chemical messengers that include interferons and interleukins. Functionally, these molecules are hormones, released by one cell to influence the behavior of another.

Immune System Disorders

Autoimmunity is an attack by the immune system on the body's own tissues. Autoimmune disorders include rheumatoid arthritis, systemic lupus erythematosus, myasthenia gravis, and multiple sclerosis. Allergy is an inappropriately severe immune reaction to an otherwise harmless substance. Severe combined immune deficiency (SCID) is an inherited disorder marked by an almost total lack of B and T cells. Acquired immunodeficiency syndrome (AIDS) is caused by HIV infection.

REVIEW FOR CERTIFICATION

The pulmonary circulation carries blood between the heart and lungs for gas exchange, and the systemic circulation carries blood between the heart and the rest of the body's tissues.

The heart is a muscular double pump located in the thoracic cavity. It is surrounded by the pericardium. The epicardium, myocardium, and endocardium are the three layers of the heart. Blood from the systemic circulation passes from the venae cavae into the right atrium and through the tricuspid valve into the right ventricle. From there, blood passes out through the pulmonary semilunar valve, through the pulmonary trunk, into the left and right pulmonary arteries, and on to the lungs. It returns via the pulmonary veins to the left atrium and then through the mitral valve into the left ventricle. It passes out through the aortic semilunar valve into the aorta, which branches to form the major arteries. Arteries branch further into arterioles, which lead to capillary beds within the tissues, where oxygen exchange occurs. Blood then enters venules and veins, which empty into the venae cavae. Blood pressure is higher in the arteries than in the veins. Arteries are thick and muscular; veins are thinner and contain valves to prevent backflow. Capillaries are composed of a single layer of endothelial cells.

Blood is composed of plasma and cellular components. RBCs carry hemoglobin. WBCs protect the body against infection. There are five types of WBCs: neutrophils, eosinophils, basophils, lymphocytes, and monocytes. Platelets play a critical role in blood coagulation. Serum is plasma minus its clotting factors. Hemostasis occurs in four phases: the vascular phase (muscular contraction of the vessel walls), the platelet phase, the coagulation phase (clot formation), and fibrinolysis (removal of the clot). The coagulation phase includes the intrinsic and extrinsic pathways, which unite to enter the common pathway.

The lymphatic system returns interstitial fluid to the circulatory system through lymphatic ducts, screening it for signs of infection at lymph nodes. Lymph organs include the tonsils, the spleen, and the thymus.

Nonspecific immunity includes physical barriers, the complement system, inflammation, and phagocytes. Specific immunity involves recognition of antigens, which triggers activation of T cells (cellular immunity) and B cells (humoral immunity).

BIBLIOGRAPHY

Hall JE: *Guyton and Hall textbook of medical physiology,* ed. 12, Philadelphia, 2011, Saunders.

Horowitz SH: Venipuncture-induced causalgia: Anatomic relations of upper extremity superficial veins and nerves, and clinical considerations, *Transfusion* 40(9):1036–1040, 2000.

Ogden-Grable H, Gill GW: Phlebotomy puncture juncture: Preventing phlebotomy errors—Potential for harming your patients, *Laboratory Medicine* 36(7):430–433, 2005. Retrieved from www.medscape.com/viewarticle/509098_print.

Keohane EM, Smith LJ, Walenga JM: Rodak's Hematology: *Clinical principles and applications,* ed. 5, St. Louis, 2016, Saunders.

Turgeon ML: *Clinical hematology: Theory and procedures,* ed. 5, Philadelphia, 2012, Lippincott Williams & Wilkins.

STUDY QUESTIONS

See answers in Appendix F.

1. Describe the different functions of the circulatory system.

2. Discuss the difference between pulmonary and systemic circulation.

3. Explain the functional difference between veins and arteries.

4. Name the four valves of the heart.

5. Contraction of the heart is known as _____, and relaxation is known as _____.

6. Name the three layers surrounding the lumen of veins and arteries.

7. The yellow liquid portion of whole blood, containing fibrinogen, is known as _____.

8. The formed elements constitute _____% of blood volume.

9. What is the role of a phagocyte?

10. Which type of lymphocyte produces antibodies?

11. Describe the two pathways in the coagulation cascade.

12. Define and give an example of autoimmunity.

13. Describe the lymph organs and their functions. Give one lymphatic system disorder, and explain its due process.

14. Name the types of immunity, how they differ, and how they are similar.

15. Explain the function of enzymes in the coagulation process.

CERTIFICATION EXAMINATION PREPARATION

See answers in Appendix F.

1. In the circulatory system, gas exchange occurs in the
   a. capillaries.
   b. veins.
   c. arteries.
   d. venules.

2. Which blood vessels are a single cell in thickness?
   a. Capillaries
   b. Veins
   c. Arteries
   d. Arterioles

3. Veins and arteries are composed of how many layers?
   a. 1
   b. 2
   c. 3
   d. 4

4. A characteristic of arteries is
   a. they are composed of a single layer of endothelial cells.
   b. they have a thick muscle layer lining the lumen.
   c. they have valves along the lumen.
   d. they carry blood toward the heart.

5. An average adult has _____ L of blood.
   a. 1 to 2
   b. 3 to 4
   c. 5 to 6
   d. 7 to 8

6. Plasma constitutes _____ % of total blood volume.
   a. 45
   b. 55
   c. 80
   d. 92

7. Another name for a WBC is
   a. leukocyte.
   b. reticulocyte.
   c. erythrocyte.
   d. electrolyte.

8. The main function of leukocytes is to
   a. transport hemoglobin.
   b. transport lipids.
   c. protect the body against infection.
   d. recycle RBCs.

9. Which leukocyte is known as a phagocyte?
   a. Lymphocyte
   b. Neutrophil
   c. Eosinophil
   d. Basophil

10. Platelets remain in the circulation for
    a. 2 to 5 days.
    b. 9 to 12 days.
    c. 10 to 20 days.
    d. 1 month.

11. Which cellular component is responsible for the transport of hemoglobin?
    a. WBCs
    b. RBCs
    c. Electrolytes
    d. Plasma

12. Which laboratory test does not assist in diagnosing HIV infection?
    a. Western blot
    b. T-cell count
    c. aPTT
    d. Anti-HIV antibody

13. A group of inherited disorders marked by increased bleeding times is known as
    a. anemias.
    b. leukemias.
    c. polycythemias.
    d. hemophilias.

14. Which organ is not included in the lymphatic system?
    a. Liver
    b. Spleen
    c. Thymus
    d. Tonsils

15. Helper T cells are needed to make
    a. antigens.
    b. antibodies.
    c. cytokines.
    d. interleukins.

UNIT 3
Specimen Collection

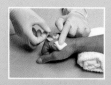

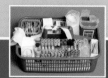

CHAPTER 8   Venipuncture Equipment

Equipment for routine venipuncture includes materials needed for the safe and efficient location of a vein and collection of a blood sample, plus equipment to ensure the safety and comfort of both the patient and the user. Most venipuncture procedures are performed with a double-ended multisample needle that delivers blood into an evacuated tube with a color-coded stopper. The stopper indicates the additives used in the tube. Learning what each color signifies, and in what order different-colored tubes should be drawn, is essential for a phlebotomist.

OUTLINE

OBJECTIVES

After completing this chapter, you should be able to:

1. List the equipment that should be available for venipuncture.
2. Describe the purpose of a tourniquet, and list types that may be used to locate a vein.
3. Differentiate between an antiseptic and a disinfectant, and list those that may be used for blood collection.
4. Locate the bevel, shaft, hub, and point of a needle, and describe safety features that may be included.
5. Define needle gauge, and explain the use of different gauges.
6. Name the parts of a syringe, and describe how the syringe system differs from the evacuated tube system.

7. Explain when a syringe system or winged infusion set (butterfly) is used in blood collection.
8. Describe the proper use of the tube holder (needle adapter).
9. Differentiate whole blood, serum, and plasma, and list at least one use for each.
10. Describe at least nine additives, including their mode of action and uses.
11. List at least 10 colors for tube tops. Identify the additive(s) in each, and state one use for each.
12. State the correct order of draw for both evacuated tube collection and syringe collection.
13. Describe the proper disposal of a used needle.

KEY TERMS

additives	gauge	needle adapter	tube advancement mark
antiseptic	glycolysis	order of draw	tube holder
bacteriostatic	inpatients	outpatients	whole blood
butterfly	Luer adapter	polymer gel	winged infusion set
clot activators	lumen	thixotropic gel	
disinfectant	multisample needle	tourniquet	

ABBREVIATIONS

ABGs arterial blood gases

CBC complete blood count

CDC Centers for Disease Control and Prevention

CLSI Clinical and Laboratory Standards Institute

EDTA ethylenediaminetetraacetic acid

FBS fasting blood sugar (glucose)

HLA human leukocyte antigen

MRSA methicillin-resistant *Staphylococcus aureus*

OSHA Occupational Safety and Health Administration

PSTs plasma separator tubes

RBCs red blood cells

SPS sodium polyanetholesulfonate

SSTs serum separator tubes

stat short turnaround time

WHAT WOULD YOU DO?

You are performing the last draw of your shift at Plainview Hospital. It's been a long day and you are look-ing forward to meeting your friends for pizza right after work. The patient is prepped, the tourniquet is on, and you reach for the red-topped tube, the last one in your tray. As you are about to insert the multisample needle into the tube, you notice the expiration date—it just expired. Should you go ahead and perform the draw anyway, since the tube contains no additives that might go bad over time and the vacuum is almost certainly still good? Or should you stop the draw and ask the patient to wait while you go get another tube?

PHLEBOTOMY EQUIPMENT

As a phlebotomist, your primary duty is to collect blood and prepare it properly for delivery to the laboratory. Your collection equipment includes the needles and tubes that allow you to collect a pa-tient's blood, plus materials to ensure that a vein can be located, the puncture site is clean, and the sample is labeled and transported correctly. In ad-dition, your equipment includes materials that protect you from potential blood hazards and that allow you to bandage the puncture site after collec-tion. A list of commonly stocked equipment is provided in Box 8-1.

ORGANIZING AND TRANSPORTING EQUIPMENT

Phlebotomists use a portable tray to carry all neces-sary equipment. Like a carpenter's toolbox, the tray is a compact, efficient way to store and transport the tools of the trade to a work site (Figure 8-1).

You are responsible for making sure that your tray is well stocked, clean, and organized at all times. You should empty the tray and disinfect it with a bleach solution once a week, or more often if necessary. A 10% bleach solution works well as a disinfectant. Commercial products are also avail-able and may be preferred by your institution.

> **◀◀↰ FLASHBACK**
>
> You learned about using a dilute bleach solution for infection control in Chapter 4.

BOX 8-1	**Equipment Used in Routine Venipuncture**

- Antiseptic cleaning solution
- Bandages
- Collection tubes
- Gauze pads
- Gloves
- Marking pens
- Needle disposal containers
- Needle holders
- Needles
- Syringes with transfer device
- Tourniquets
- Winged infusion sets (butterflies)

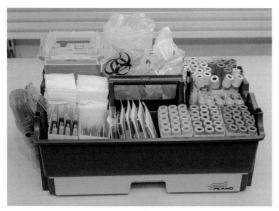

FIGURE 8-1 Phlebotomy tray.

You will encounter patients in two primary settings: inpatient and outpatient. **Inpatients** have been admitted to a hospital, and you usually draw their blood at the bedside. A wheeled cart is sometimes used to transport large quantities of supplies when you are scheduled to collect samples from many patients, but the cart should remain in the hospital corridor to reduce the risk of spreading infection from one patient to another. Bring only the tray into the room. Once in the patient's room, do not place your tray on the patient's bed, where it could easily be overturned, or on the patient's bedside table used for eating. Instead, *place the tray on a flat, solid surface such as a nightstand.* Always keep extra supplies within reach, however. You may need them during a draw; for instance, you may need to replace a tube while the needle is still in the patient's arm (which can happen if you get a defective tube).

> **CLINICAL TIP**
> Never place your tray on the patient's bed or eating table.

Outpatients usually come to you at a phlebotomy drawing station in a clinic or hospital. The

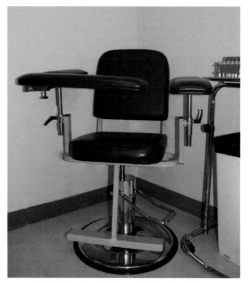

FIGURE 8-2 Phlebotomy drawing station.

drawing station includes a special phlebotomy chair with an adjustable armrest (Figure 8-2). The armrest locks to prevent the patient from falling out in the event of fainting. A bed may also be available for patients with a history of fainting. Supplies may be available at the drawing station, or you may need to bring your tray to it.

LOCATING VEINS

To draw blood, you first need to locate a vein. Applying a **tourniquet** is the most common way to do this. A tourniquet prevents venous blood flow out of the arm, causing the veins to bulge. Various types of tourniquets are shown in Figure 8-3.

The most common type of tourniquet is a simple strip of latex or nonlatex material tied around the upper arm. Nonlatex tourniquets are made from synthetic rubber or nitrile. Latex has the advantage of being inexpensive and therefore disposable, but,

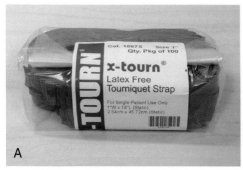
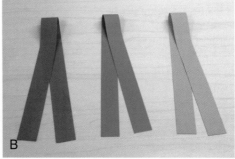

FIGURE 8-3 Various types of tourniquets.

due to increased latex sensitivity, may not be used in some facilities. Clinical and Laboratory Standards Institute (CLSI) standards indicate that once a tourniquet has been used, it should be disposed of to reduce the risk of pathogen transmission between patients, including skin pathogens such as methicillin-resistant *Staphylococcus aureus* (MRSA).

A blood pressure cuff may also be used as a tourniquet when veins are hard to find. It too allows you to temporarily relieve pressure and then reapply it. The cuff is inflated to a pressure above the diastolic but below the systolic reading. Using the cuff requires special training beyond your normal phlebotomy training and should only be done with approval of your supervisor.

Devices are available that shine a bright light through the patient's skin. When such a device is positioned properly, veins are visible as dark lines within the tissue. This works especially well for finding veins in the hand and foot.

CLEANING THE PUNCTURE SITE

Antiseptics and disinfectants are used to reduce the risk of infection. By convention, antiseptic refers to an agent used to clean living tissue. Disinfectant refers to an agent used to clean a surface other than living tissue.

> ◀◀◀↩ **FLASHBACK**
> You learned about infection control in Chapter 4.

An antiseptic prevents sepsis, or infection. Antiseptics are used to clean the patient's skin before routine venipuncture collection to prevent contamination by normal skin bacteria. The most commonly used antiseptic is 70% isopropyl alcohol (rubbing alcohol). Isopropyl alcohol is bacteriostatic, meaning that it inhibits the growth or reproduction of bacteria but does not kill them. For maximal effectiveness, the antiseptic should be left in contact with the skin for 30 to 60 seconds. You should not fan or blow on the site to speed drying—this may introduce more bacteria. Prepackaged alcohol "prep pads" are the most commonly used product.

Other antiseptics are often used for blood cultures or arterial punctures. Povidone–iodine solution (Betadine) is sometimes used. However, iodine interferes with some chemistry test results and cannot be used routinely. Chlorhexidine gluconate or benzalkonium chloride (Zephiran Chloride) is available and is used for blood cultures and for patients sensitive to iodine. Chlorhexidine gluconate should not be used on infants younger than 2 months.

PROTECTING THE PUNCTURE SITE

After drawing blood, you need to stop the bleeding by applying pressure to the puncture site. This is done with a 2- × 2-inch gauze pad, folded into quarters. Bleeding usually stops within several minutes, although patients on aspirin or anticoagulant medications may require 10 to 15 minutes. When bleeding stops, the gauze can be replaced with an adhesive hypoallergenic bandage. Alternatively, you can tape the gauze in place using an adhesive bandage. Use of cotton balls instead of gauze is not recommended. Cotton fibers may get trapped in the clot and, when pulled off the puncture site, they may tear the clot and restart bleeding. For sensitive or fragile skin, Coban is a good alternative, since it sticks only to itself, not to skin. It is wrapped all the way around the arm and back onto itself.

NEEDLES

In routine venipuncture, a needle inserted into a vein allows blood to flow out into an evacuated collection tube or syringe. A critical part of your job as a phlebotomist is knowing which needle and which tube to use in each situation.

All needles used for phlebotomy are sterile, disposable, and used only once. Inspect each needle package before opening it to be sure that the seal has not been broken. If it has, discard it. Next, inspect the needle itself to be sure that it has no manufacturing defects. The needle should be straight, sharp, beveled, and free of nicks or burrs. Discard any defective needle.

Features of Needles

All needles have several features you should be familiar with (Figure 8-4).

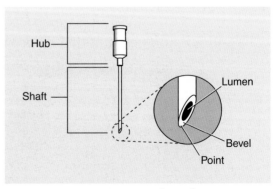

FIGURE 8-4 Parts of a needle.

Point

A sharp needle provides smooth entry into the skin with a minimum of pain.

Bevel

The bevel, or angle, eases the shaft into the skin and prevents the needle from coring out a plug of tissue.

Shaft

Shafts differ in both length and gauge. The needles used for routine venipuncture range from ¾ inches for "butterflies" (see below) to 1 to 1½ inches long for standard needles. Factors that influence the choice of length include location and depth of the vein, and the experience and preference of the phlebotomist. Some phlebotomists prefer a longer needle because it is easier to manipulate; others prefer a shorter needle because it makes patients less uneasy.

The **gauge** describes the diameter of the needle's **lumen**, the hollow tube within the shaft. The smaller the gauge number, the larger the lumen diameter; the larger the number, the smaller the lumen. Needle packs are color coded by gauge for easy identification. The choice of gauge is not a matter of personal preference; it depends on the type of collection and the condition of the patient. The largest-diameter needles routinely used in phlebotomy are 21 to 22 gauge. The blood bank uses 16- to 18-gauge needles to collect blood from donors for transfusions. The smallest needles commonly used are 23 gauge, for collection from small, fragile veins. A typical gauge for routine adult collection is 21 gauge. Large needles deliver blood more quickly but are more damaging to the tissue and may collapse the vein. Small needles are less damaging to tissue, but collection is slower, and the blood cells may be hemolyzed as they pass through the narrower opening. Learning the most appropriate gauge for each clinical situation is part of your training as a phlebotomist.

Hub

The needle attaches to the collecting tube or syringe at its hub.

Multisample Needles

For most collections, you use a double-ended needle. While one tip of the needle penetrates the patient's skin, the second tip pierces the rubber cap of an evacuated collection tube. The most common double-ended needle is the **multisample needle** (Figure 8-5), which has a retractable rubber sleeve that covers the second tip when it is not inserted into a tube. A multisample

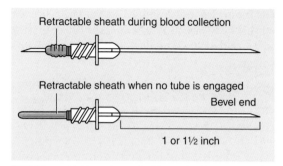

FIGURE 8-5 Multisample needle. The cap has been removed for clarity.

needle remains in place in the patient's vein while one tube is replaced with another. The sleeve keeps blood from leaking onto or into the adapter or tube holder while you are changing tubes.

Safety Syringes and Safety Syringe Needles

A syringe (Figure 8-6) is sometimes useful for patients with fragile or small veins, when the vacuum of the collection tube is likely to collapse the vein. Because suction can be applied gradually, by slowly drawing back the plunger, a syringe provides a controlled, gentle vacuum for fragile veins. A syringe needle (also called a hypodermic needle) (see Figure 8-4) fits onto the syringe barrel. The needles come in a range of sizes. The most common size is 22 gauge, 1 inch long. Syringe needles have an advantage over multisample

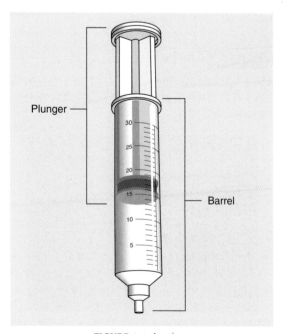

FIGURE 8-6 A syringe.

needles in that blood appears in the hub when the vein has been entered. A safety transfer device must be used with the syringe needle whenever drawing with a syringe.

FLASH FORWARD

The use of syringes for venous collection is discussed in Chapter 9.

Winged Infusion Sets or Butterflies

The **winged infusion** set (Figure 8-7), also called a winged collection set or **butterfly**, is used for venipuncture on small veins, such as those in the hand, and in elderly or pediatric patients. Without the bulk of a syringe or collection tube in the way, the butterfly needle allows you great flexibility in placing and manipulating the needle.

The most common needle size is 23 gauge, ¾ inch long. The needle is held by a plastic butterfly-shaped grip and is connected to flexible latex tubing. By using an appropriate adapter, when necessary, the tubing can be connected to either an evacuated collection tube or a syringe. Many styles of safety butterfly needles are available that have different types of safety shields that are activated at the conclusion of the draw. These are designed to meet Occupational Safety and Health Administration (OSHA) regulations and the Needle-Stick Safety and Prevention Act when manufacturer guidelines are followed.

Most butterfly needles are now designed to be used with an evacuated tube system. Those that are not can be fitted using a **Luer adapter**.

NEEDLE SAFETY

Accidental needle sticks are a major concern in health care. A recent study by the Centers for Disease

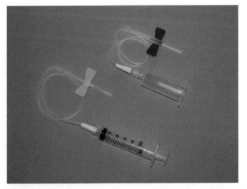

FIGURE 8-7 Winged infusion set attached to an evacuated tube holder with a Luer adapter.

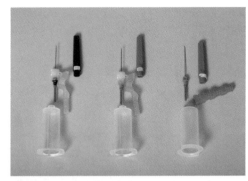

FIGURE 8-8 Needle safety devices. (Courtesy Zack Bent. From Garrels M, Oatis CS: *Laboratory testing for ambulatory settings: A guide for health care professionals*, Philadelphia, 2006, Saunders.)

Control and Prevention (CDC) estimated that approximately 1000 accidental needle sticks occur per day nationwide. Although most of these injuries are to nurses, phlebotomists are at risk too. To respond to this problem, the OSHA issued a directive in November 2000, stressing the use of safety devices to help reduce the number of sharps injuries. The Needlestick Safety and Prevention Act specified types of "engineering controls" mentioned in OSHA's Bloodborne Pathogens Standard to increase needle safety. Federal legislation enforces the use of safety devices, and many states have passed legislation related to safety devices.

Several standard strategies are used to increase needle safety. Self-capping needles have a plastic sheath that snaps shuts over the needle (Figure 8-8). Retractable technologies cause the needle to retract into the syringe, tube holder, or other device. The Vacutainer Push Button Blood Collection Set (winged collection set) manufactured by Becton, Dickinson and Company (BD) (Franklin Lakes, N.J.) has a button to push to retract the needle automatically from the vein and into the body of the needle device. This in-vein activation reduces the risk of needle sticks.

NEEDLE ADAPTERS

For most collections, you will use a multisample needle and an evacuated collection tube. To ensure a firm, stable connection between these two essential parts, a **needle adapter** (also called a **tube holder**) is used (Figure 8-9). A needle adapter is a translucent plastic cylinder. One end has a small opening that accepts the multisample needle. The other end has a wide opening that

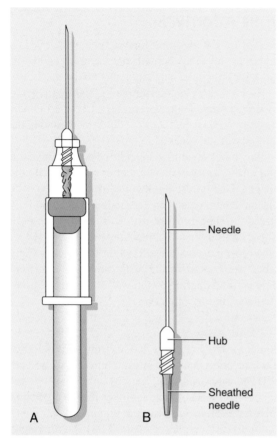

FIGURE 8-9 The evacuated tube system **(A)** and a multisample needle **(B)**.

accepts the collection tube. Adapters come in different sizes to fit tubes of different diameters, and it is important to choose an adapter that fits the tube you are using. Some manufacturers have standardized their tubes so that they all fit one adapter; others provide inserts that allow one adapter to fit a variety of tube sizes.

Adapters have a **tube advancement** mark indicating how far the tube can be pushed in without losing the vacuum.

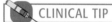

> **CLINICAL TIP**
>
> To prevent losing the vacuum, be careful not to push the tube past the tube advancement mark until you have inserted the needle in the vein.

Like a needle, an adapter is used only once, and it is discarded while still attached to the needle. According to OSHA regulations, reuse of an adapter is prohibited because of the risk of exposure to blood that may occur.

EVACUATED COLLECTION TUBES

Color-coded, evacuated collection tubes are at the center of modern phlebotomy. Tubes hold blood for later testing in the laboratory, and each type of tube may contain different sets of additives, which are chemicals designed to promote or prevent certain changes in the blood sample. Which tube to use depends on what tests have been ordered. A critical part of your training is learning and memorizing which tube to use for each test.

As shown in Figure 8-10, tube tops are either thick rubber stoppers or rubber stoppers with plastic tops (e.g., BD Vacutainer Hemogard system). The plastic top minimizes the chance of an aerosol spray forming when the stopper is removed. The tubes themselves are made of either glass or shatter-resistant plastic. Most tubes are plastic and thus are not only safer than glass for transportation, but also can withstand the extremely high forces inside a centrifuge. Unlike glass, plastic does not strongly activate platelets. Serum samples, which require platelet activation, are now usually collected in plastic tubes that contain a clot activator, although plain glass tubes are still being used in some circumstances or when the test is negatively affected by the presence of plastic.

Tubes are evacuated so that a measured amount of blood will flow in easily. They are available in a variety of sizes, from 2 to 15 mL. Be sure to match the needle gauge to the tube: A 23-gauge needle on a 15-mL tube will likely cause hemolysis, for instance. If you need a small needle, use two small tubes instead. "Partial-draw" tubes are also available. These have a smaller vacuum and pull a smaller volume of blood into the tube than would a fully evacuated tube.

The best tube size to use depends on several factors. Each test requires a particular minimum sample volume, which may range from less than 1 to 10 mL or more. Your laboratory's manual states the minimum

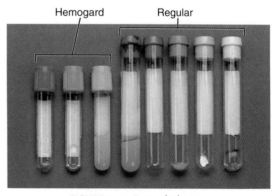

FIGURE 8-10 Types of tube tops.

volume required for each test. You may choose to draw a greater volume, however, perhaps because smaller tubes are more expensive or because testing equipment works better with a certain size of tube.

For example, for a basic metabolic panel, the minimum sample size is 0.5 mL of serum or plasma. As you learned in Chapter 7, whole blood is slightly more than half plasma. Routinely, you might use a 5-mL tube for convenience and cost. However, you could choose a 2.7-mL tube for a pediatric patient or for someone with small veins, knowing that the minimum test requirements would be met because this would give you about 1.5 mL of plasma.

Each tube carries an expiration date, and unused tubes must be discarded when they expire. Out-of-date tubes may have decreased vacuum, preventing a proper fill, or they may have additives that degrade with time. Use of an expired tube can cause inaccurate test results. When restocking supplies, tubes should be rotated by date so that the older tubes are up front and used first and the newer tubes are in the back. A computerized stock monitoring system may be available where you work, making the task easy. Even with such a system, however, it is ultimately the phlebotomist's duty to use only tubes with a valid date.

TYPES OF BLOOD SPECIMENS

Three types of blood specimens are used for analysis:
1. **Whole blood** is blood collected and mixed with an anticoagulant so that it will not clot. Whole blood is used for most hematology tests, including blood type and cell counts, and to determine the level of certain hormones and metals.
2. **Serum** is the fluid portion of blood that remains after clotting. No anticoagulant is used when collecting a serum sample. Complete clotting takes 30 to 60 minutes, depending on the presence of clot activators (discussed below). The sample can then be centrifuged to separate the serum. Serum is used for many laboratory tests, including most chemistry and immunology tests. Unlike plasma, serum does not contain fibrinogen or some other clotting factors (which are left behind or used up in forming the clot) and thus cannot be used for routine coagulation studies.
3. **Plasma** is the fluid portion of blood, including fibrinogen and other clotting factors. Plasma is obtained by collecting whole blood in a tube containing an anticoagulant and then centrifuging. Plasma is used for coagulation studies. It is also used for short turnaround time (stat) chemistry tests, when there is no time to wait for clotting to occur before centrifuging.

TUBE ADDITIVES

Except for the glass red-topped tube, which has no additives, all tubes contain one or more additives. Additives include anticoagulants to prevent clotting, clot activators to promote it, thixotropic gel to separate components, and preservatives and inhibitors of various cellular reactions to maintain the integrity of the specimen.

Any tube containing an additive must be inverted and mixed well immediately after removal from the adapter. Gently turning the tube over, and then back upright again, equals one inversion. You should *not* shake the tube because this will cause hemolysis. The exact number of inversions needed varies by tube type; most need five to eight inversions. Many tubes are coated inside with silicone to prevent blood from adhering to the wall of the tube and to slow the clotting process.

Anticoagulants

Anticoagulants prevent blood from clotting. Sodium or potassium ethylenediaminetetraacetic acid (EDTA) binds calcium, thereby inhibiting the coagulation cascade. Other additives that bind calcium include sodium citrate, potassium oxalate, and sodium polyanetholesulfonate (SPS). Another anticoagulant, heparin (linked with sodium, lithium, or ammonium), inhibits clotting by preventing the conversion of prothrombin to thrombin. Having the correct ratio of blood to anticoagulant is important, so you must take care to fill the tube completely. Anticoagulants must be mixed well by gently and repeatedly inverting the tube.

The choice of anticoagulant is determined by the tests to be done. EDTA preserves blood cell integrity well, prevents platelet clumping, and is compatible with blood staining, but it interferes with coagulation studies. Citrate is used for coagulation studies. SPS is used for blood cultures because it inhibits certain immune system components that could otherwise destroy blood-borne bacteria and neutralizes antibiotics that the patient may be taking. Heparin is preferred for plasma chemistry determinations and for blood gas determinations. Potassium oxalate, combined with sodium fluoride or iodoacetate, is used for glucose determination.

> **«‹¬ FLASHBACK**
> You learned about blood clotting in Chapter 7.

Sodium fluoride inhibits **glycolysis** and can be used for glucose determination. Glycolysis is a cellular

Tan

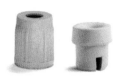

Tests: Lead analysis
Additives: Heparin
Specimen: Plasma
Note: The tube is formulated to contain less than 0.1 mcg/mL of lead.

Yellow, Nonsterile

Tests: Human leukocyte antigen (HLA) studies (paternity testing and tissue typing)
Additives: Acid citrate dextrose
Specimen: Whole blood
Notes: The dextrose nourishes and preserves RBCs, and the citrate is an anticoagulant.

Pink

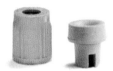

Tests: Blood bank compatibility test
Additives: K_2 EDTA
Specimen: Plasma or whole blood
Note: This tube is similar to the standard lavender-topped tube, but its closure and label meet the standards set by the American Association of Blood Banks.

 AVOID THAT ERROR!

It's the third day on the job for Maria Hernandez. She consults her requisition for the next patient, and sees that he needs a coagulation test. Maria assembles her materials, including tourniquet, swabs, bandage, and a lavender tube. She enters the patient's room, asks him to state his name, checks the wrist band, and proceeds with the draw. Afterward, she labels the tube, makes sure bleeding has stopped, and thanks the patient as she leaves. But as she closes the door, she stops, a look of panic on her face. What did she do wrong? And what should she do now?

ORDER OF DRAW

Patients often need to have more than one test performed and therefore more than one tube filled. Because the same multisample needle is used to fill all the tubes, material from an earlier tube could be transferred into a later tube if it contacts the needle.

Good technique can reduce this risk somewhat (discussed in more detail in the next chapter); however, it cannot eliminate it entirely. For this reason, the CLSI has developed a set of standards dictating the proper order of draw for a multitube draw (Figure 8-11). The order is the same for syringe samples as for direct filling from a multisample needle. The order-of-draw standards have undergone several revisions within the past decade, and not all institutions have adopted the most recent set of standards (termed H3-A6).

It is important for you to follow the order of draw used at your institution, even if it differs from the order given here.

1. Blood culture tubes (which are sterile) are drawn first. This prevents the transfer of unsterilized material from other tubes into the sterile tube.

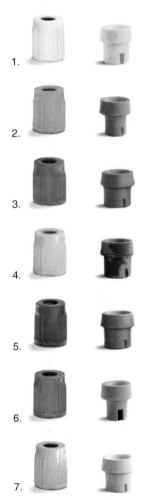

FIGURE 8-11 The order of draw, according to Standard H3-A6. *1,* Yellow, sterile. *2,* Light blue. *3,* Red. *4,* Gold, BD Hemogard Closure or red-gray. *5,* Green. *6,* Lavender. *7,* Gray. (Courtesy and © Becton, Dickinson and Company.)

FLASH FORWARD ↷≫

You will learn about blood culture collections and tubes in Chapter 14.

2. Light blue–topped tubes (for coagulation tests) are next. These tubes are always drawn before tubes containing other kinds of anticoagulants or clot activators because other additives could contaminate this tube and interfere with coagulation testing. If coagulation tests are the only tests ordered, you only need a light blue–topped tube. Your institution may have you draw a plain red-topped tube first and discard it (this may help prevent contamination by tissue fluids). The discard tube may be a plain red glass tube or a specially manufactured plastic tube without any additive. Also, if you are drawing with a butterfly, you must draw a discard tube to draw out the air in the tubing and prevent a short draw.

3. Glass red-topped tubes or plastic red-topped tubes may be drawn now.

4. Red-gray (gold BD Hemogard) tubes and plastic gold-topped tubes are next. These contain clot activators, which would interfere with many other samples if passed into other tubes.

5. Green tubes are drawn next. The heparin from the green tube is less likely to interfere with EDTA-containing tubes than vice versa.

6. Lavender-topped tubes are next. EDTA binds many metals, in addition to calcium, so it can cause problems with many test results, including giving falsely low calcium and falsely high potassium readings. For this reason, lavender tubes are drawn near the end.

7. The gray-topped tube is last. This tube contains potassium oxalate. The potassium would elevate the potassium levels measured in electrolyte analysis, and oxalate can damage cell membranes. Also, another additive, sodium fluoride, elevates sodium levels and inhibits many enzymes.

Other color tubes are typically drawn after these six, but you should check the instructions on the manufacturer's package insert and your laboratory's procedures manual for specific information. The glass red-topped tube (but not the plastic red-topped tube) may be drawn after the sterile tube if your institution allows it.

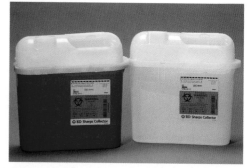

FIGURE 8-12 Needle disposal systems reduce the risk of accidental injury while removing the needle. (From Bonewit-West K: *Clinical procedures for medical assistants,* ed. 7, Philadelphia, 2008, Saunders.)

NEEDLE DISPOSAL CONTAINERS

Once you have withdrawn the needle from the patient's arm, it must be handled with extreme care to avoid an accidental needle stick. A used needle is considered biohazardous waste and must be treated as such. Dispose of the needle with the adapter still attached immediately after activating the needle safety device. Needles must be placed in a clearly marked, puncture-resistant biohazard disposal container (Figure 8-12). Containers must be closable or sealable, puncture resistant, leak-proof, and labeled with the correct biohazard symbol.

You must become familiar with the system in use at your workplace. Practice with a new system before you draw your first sample.

REVIEW FOR CERTIFICATION

The phlebotomist's tray includes tourniquets for locating veins; antiseptics and disinfectants for cleaning the puncture site; a variety of needles in different sizes, including multisample needles, syringe needles, and butterfly needles; needle adapters or tube holders; evacuated collection tubes; bandages; and a variety of other materials. The phlebotomist chooses the needle type and size to fit the characteristics of the patient and the test and then uses tubes that contain additives appropriate for the tests that have been ordered. A prescribed order of draw is used to minimize the effects of contamination among tubes.

BIBLIOGRAPHY

Calfee DP, Farr BM: Comparison of four antiseptic preparations for skin in the prevention of contamination of percutaneously drawn blood cultures: A randomized trial, *J Clin Microbiol* 40:1660–1665, 2002.

Chapman AK, Aucott SW, Milstone AM: Safety of chlorhexidine gluconate used for skin antisepsis in the preterm infant, *J Perinatol* 32(1):4–9, 2012.

CLSI: *Procedures for the collection of diagnostic blood specimens by venipuncture; Approved standard—sixth edition.* CSLI document GP41-A6 (formerly H03-A6). Wayne, Pa., 2007, Clinical and Laboratory Standards Institute.

CLSI: *Tubes and additives for venous and capillary blood specimen collection; Approved standard—Sixth edition.* CSLI document

GP39-A6. Wayne, Pa., 2010, Clinical and Laboratory Standards Institute.

College of American Pathologists (CAP). *So you're going to collect a blood specimen,* ed. 13, Northfield, Ill., 2010, CAP.

Lippi G, Salvagno GL, Montagnana M, et al: Phlebotomy issues and quality improvement in results of laboratory testing, *Clin Lab* 52:217–230, 2006.

Medical Safety Product Directory: *Advance for Medical Laboratory Professionals,* March 13, 2006.

OSHA: Disposal of Contaminated Needles and Blood Tube Holders Used for Phlebotomy. *Safety and Health Information Bulletin,* 2013. Retrieved from https://www.osha.gov/dts/shib/shib101503.html.

Winkelman J, Tanasijevic M: How RBCs move through thixotropic gels, *Lab Med* 30:476–477, 1999.

WHAT WOULD YOU DO?

You should not perform the draw. Although the vacuum might still be good, it might not, and using a defective tube could mean the patient must undergo a second draw, a potentially distressing and even harmful procedure. In the future, be sure to check the expiration on all the tubes when you stock your tray, and never arrive at the draw without extra tubes.

 AVOID THAT ERROR!

Maria's requisition called for a coagulation test, which should be drawn into a light blue–topped tube, which contains sodium citrate. But Maria used a lavender tube, which contains EDTA and is used for CBCs and sedimentation rate. Unfortunately, she has used the wrong tube and the sample is useless. She must ask the patient for permission to draw another sample.

STUDY QUESTIONS

See answers in Appendix F.

1. Explain the purpose of a tourniquet.

2. What does the gauge of a needle indicate?

3. Describe the consequences of using a needle with a large gauge number.

4. Explain the purpose of the rubber sleeve on the multisample needle.

5. Explain the advantages and disadvantages of the syringe method of drawing blood as opposed to the evacuated system.

6. Blood tubes are evacuated. Explain what this means.

7. Why must unused blood tubes be discarded when they expire?

8. Define SPS and explain what it is used for.

9. If a collection tube contains an anticoagulant, what must you do immediately after collection?

10. Explain the purpose of thixotropic gel in a collection tube.

11. Define glycolysis.

12. Name the three types of blood specimens used for analysis.

Match the collection tube top color to the type of test it is commonly used for:

13. Tan
14. Red or pink
15. Light blue
16. Lavender
17. Gray
18. Black
19. Gold BD Hemogard Closure
20. Green
21. Royal blue

a. blood bank
b. lead analysis
c. glucose tolerance test
d. chemistry testing
e. sedimentation rate
f. ABGs
g. CBC
h. trace metals
i. coagulation

22. Number the following in the correct order of draw using the evacuated method.

_____ light blue
_____ lavender
_____ green
_____ red, plastic tube
_____ yellow, sterile
_____ gray
_____ gold BD Hemogard Closure

CERTIFICATION EXAMINATION PREPARATION

See answers in Appendix F.

1. Which of the following is not an anticoagulant?
   a. Polymer gel
   b. Sodium heparin
   c. Sodium citrate
   d. EDTA

2. The most common antiseptic used in routine venipuncture is
   a. povidone–iodine solution.
   b. bleach.
   c. isopropyl alcohol.
   d. chlorhexidine gluconate.

3. How many times may a needle be used before discarding it?
   a. 1
   b. 2
   c. 3
   d. No limit

4. Which of the following indicates the largest-sized needle?
   a. 20 gauge
   b. 23 gauge
   c. 16 gauge
   d. 21 gauge

5. Complete clotting of a blood sample in a SST (gold or red-gray) tube takes _____ minutes at room temperature.
   a. 10
   b. 30
   c. 45
   d. 60

6. Serum contains
   a. fibrinogen.
   b. clotting factors.
   c. plasma.
   d. none of the above.

7. Which color-coded tube does not contain any additives?
   a. Red, plastic tube
   b. Red, glass tube
   c. Gold BD Hemogard Closure
   d. Royal blue

8. EDTA prevents coagulation in blood tubes by
   a. inactivating thrombin.
   b. binding calcium.
   c. inactivating thromboplastin.
   d. inhibiting glycolysis.

9. Tubes with gray tops are used for
   a. sedimentation rate tests.
   b. glucose tolerance tests.
   c. coagulation studies.
   d. CBC.

10. Tubes with green tops may contain
   a. sodium citrate.
   b. sodium heparin.
   c. sodium oxalate.
   d. sodium phosphate.

11. The smaller the gauge number, the
   a. larger the lumen diameter.
   b. longer the needle.
   c. shorter the needle.
   d. smaller the lumen diameter.

12. The syringe method of draw is useful because
   a. it allows for control of blood flow.
   b. it shows the appearance of blood at the hub.
   c. it allows for greater flexibility and less bulk.
   d. both a and b above.

13. The additive sodium citrate is used in blood collection to test for
    - a. blood alcohol.
    - b. prothrombin time.
    - c. lactic acid.
    - d. lead.

14. The most common gauge used for a routine venipuncture is
    - a. 16.
    - b. 21.
    - c. 25.
    - d. 23.

15. Blood banks use a _____ gauge needle to collect blood from donors for transfusions.
    - a. 16- to 18-
    - b. 20- to 22-
    - c. 22- or 23-
    - d. 23- to 25-

16. Blood collection tubes containing an anticoagulant should be
    - a. inverted gently and repeatedly after blood collection.
    - b. shaken aggressively after blood collection.
    - c. allowed to sit for 30 minutes before centrifugation.
    - d. centrifuged immediately.

17. Tubes containing the SPS anticoagulant are used for
    - a. antibody screen.
    - b. HLA studies.
    - c. nutritional analysis.
    - d. blood culture analysis.

18. Blood collected in lavender-topped tubes is used for which test?
    - a. FBS
    - b. CBC
    - c. Stat potassium
    - d. Stat chemistry

19. Blood collected in gray-topped tubes is used for which test?
    - a. FBS
    - b. CBC
    - c. Stat potassium
    - d. Stat chemistry

20. Blood collected in light blue–topped tubes is used for which test?
    - a. Sedimentation rate
    - b. Glucose tolerance
    - c. Toxicology
    - d. Coagulation

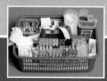

Routine venipuncture is the most common procedure a phlebotomist performs. The most important step in venipuncture is positive identification (ID) of the patient. This is done by matching the information on the requisition with, for inpatients, the information on the patient's ID band or, for outpatients, the information provided by the patient. Although most patients are suitable candidates for drawing blood with evacuated tubes, patients with fragile veins may be better candidates for wing-set ("butterfly") collection; the blood is transferred to evacuated tubes after the draw if a syringe is used.

OUTLINE

Requisitions
Advance Beneficiary Notice of Noncoverage
Patient Identification

Routine Venipuncture
Procedure 9-1: Routine Venipuncture

Routine Venipuncture With a Syringe
Procedure 9-2: Routine Venipuncture With a Syringe
Review for Certification

OBJECTIVES

After completing this chapter, you should be able to:

1. List the information that is commonly found on a patient's test requisition.
2. List, in order, the steps in a routine venipuncture.
3. Discuss the information that must be verified for inpatient identification (ID) before the blood collection procedure.
4. Explain how the ID of outpatients differs from that of inpatients.
5. Describe patient preparation and positioning.
6. Describe how to assemble the evacuated tube system.
7. Explain how to apply a tourniquet, and list three consequences of improper application.

8. List the veins that may be used for blood collection, and give the advantages and disadvantages of each.
9. Explain how to clean the venipuncture site.
10. Describe how to properly insert the needle into the vein.
11. Discuss how the needle should be removed when the last tube of blood has been collected.
12. List the information that must be included on the label of each tube.
13. Describe how venipuncture using a syringe differs from that using the evacuated tube system.

KEY TERMS

hematoma
hemoconcentration

hemolysis
palpation

petechiae
requisition

ABBREVIATIONS

ABN Advance Beneficiary Notice of Noncoverage
DOB date of birth
ICD-9-CM International Classification of Diseases, Ninth Revision, Clinical Modification

ICD-10-CM International Classification of Diseases, Tenth Revision, Clinical Modification
ID identification
stat short turnaround time

WHAT WOULD YOU DO?

It's midday at City Center Hospital, and your next draw is for Thomas Phelps in room 322. As you enter room 322, you see the patient sitting up in bed. You greet him. You ask his name, and he replies: "I'm Tommy Phelps." You then check the ID band on his wrist—the number matches the number on the requisition form. When you ask him to state his date of birth, he says, "June 14, 1985"—but the requisition gives the date of birth as July 14, 1985. Can you go ahead and draw?

REQUISITIONS

All blood collection procedures begin with a request for a test from the treating physician. A physician's request for tests can be presented on a prescription pad. The physician must provide the *International Classification of Diseases,* Ninth Revision, Clinical Modification (ICD-9-CM, or ICD-9) code for the requested tests (ICD-10 is scheduled to replace ICD-9 by October 1, 2015). The ICD-9-CM code is a billing code used to submit charges for services to insurance companies and other providers. For outpatients, the laboratory processes the physician's request and generates a **requisition**, a set of labels for the collection tubes, or both. Generally, procedures for inpatients arrive at the laboratory through the computer system, and no paper requisition is generated. Instead, only a set of labels is printed. Tests for outpatients may arrive via a paper requisition (Figure 9-1). The phlebotomist uses the requisition or labels (Figure 9-2) to determine what type of sample to collect from the patient.

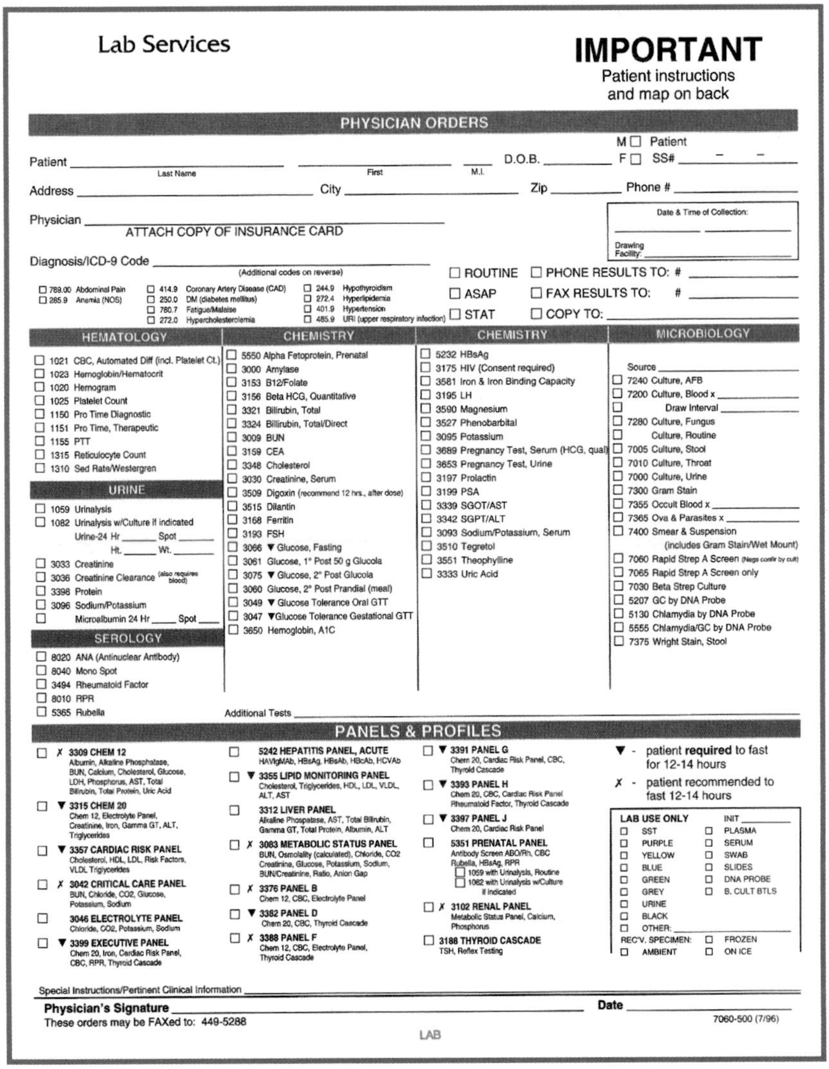

Lab Services

IMPORTANT
Patient instructions and map on back

PHYSICIAN ORDERS

Patient ____ (Last Name) ____ (First) ____ (M.I.) D.O.B. ____ M ☐ F ☐ Patient SS# ____ – ____ – ____
Address ____ City ____ Zip ____ Phone # ____
Physician ____
ATTACH COPY OF INSURANCE CARD
Date & Time of Collection: ____ ____
Drawing Facility: ____
Diagnosis/ICD-9 Code ____
(Additional codes on reverse)
☐ 789.00 Abdominal Pain
☐ 285.9 Anemia (NOS)
☐ 414.9 Coronary Artery Disease (CAD)
☐ 250.0 DM (diabetes mellitus)
☐ 780.7 Fatigue/Malaise
☐ 272.0 Hypercholesterolemia
☐ 244.9 Hypothyroidism
☐ 272.4 Hyperlipidemia
☐ 401.9 Hypertension
☐ 485.9 URI (upper respiratory infection)
☐ ROUTINE ☐ PHONE RESULTS TO: # ____
☐ ASAP ☐ FAX RESULTS TO: # ____
☐ STAT ☐ COPY TO: ____

HEMATOLOGY
☐ 1021 CBC, Automated Diff (incl. Platelet Ct.)
☐ 1023 Hemoglobin/Hematocrit
☐ 1020 Hemogram
☐ 1025 Platelet Count
☐ 1150 Pro Time Diagnostic
☐ 1151 Pro Time, Therapeutic
☐ 1155 PTT
☐ 1315 Reticulocyte Count
☐ 1310 Sed Rate/Westergren

URINE
☐ 1059 Urinalysis
☐ 1082 Urinalysis w/Culture if indicated
Urine-24 Hr ____ Spot ____
Ht. ____ Wt. ____
☐ 3033 Creatinine
☐ 3036 Creatinine Clearance (also requires blood)
☐ 3398 Protein
☐ 3096 Sodium/Potassium
☐ Microalbumin 24 Hr ____ Spot ____

SEROLOGY
☐ 8020 ANA (Antinuclear Antibody)
☐ 8040 Mono Spot
☐ 3494 Rheumatoid Factor
☐ 8010 RPR
☐ 5365 Rubella

CHEMISTRY
☐ 5550 Alpha Fetoprotein, Prenatal
☐ 3000 Amylase
☐ 3153 B12/Folate
☐ 3156 Beta HCG, Quantitative
☐ 3321 Bilirubin, Total
☐ 3324 Billirubin, Total/Direct
☐ 3009 BUN
☐ 3159 CEA
☐ 3348 Cholesterol
☐ 3030 Creatinine, Serum
☐ 3509 Digoxin (recommend 12 hrs., after dose)
☐ 3515 Dilantin
☐ 3168 Ferritin
☐ 3193 FSH
☐ 3066 ▼ Glucose, Fasting
☐ 3061 Glucose, 1° Post 50 g Glucola
☐ 3075 ▼ Glucose, 2° Post Glucola
☐ 3060 Glucose, 2° Post Prandial (meal)
☐ 3049 ▼ Glucose Tolerance Oral GTT
☐ 3047 ▼Glucose Tolerance Gestational GTT
☐ 3650 Hemoglobin, A1C

CHEMISTRY
☐ 5232 HBsAg
☐ 3175 HIV (Consent required)
☐ 3581 Iron & Iron Binding Capacity
☐ 3195 LH
☐ 3590 Magnesium
☐ 3527 Phenobarbital
☐ 3095 Potassium
☐ 3689 Pregnancy Test, Serum (HCG, qual)
☐ 3653 Pregnancy Test, Urine
☐ 3197 Prolactin
☐ 3199 PSA
☐ 3339 SGOT/AST
☐ 3342 SGPT/ALT
☐ 3093 Sodium/Potassium, Serum
☐ 3510 Tegretol
☐ 3551 Theophylline
☐ 3333 Uric Acid

MICROBIOLOGY
Source ____
☐ 7240 Culture, AFB
☐ 7200 Culture, Blood x ____
☐ Draw Interval ____
☐ 7280 Culture, Fungus
☐ Culture, Routine
☐ 7005 Culture, Stool
☐ 7010 Culture, Throat
☐ 7000 Culture, Urine
☐ 7300 Gram Stain
☐ 7355 Occult Blood x ____
☐ 7365 Ova & Parasites x ____
☐ 7400 Smear & Suspension (includes Gram Stain/Wet Mount)
☐ 7060 Rapid Strep A Screen (Negs confir by cult)
☐ 7065 Rapid Strep A Screen only
☐ 7030 Beta Strep Culture
☐ 5207 GC by DNA Probe
☐ 5130 Chlamydia by DNA Probe
☐ 5555 Chlamydia/GC by DNA Probe
☐ 7375 Wright Stain, Stool

Additional Tests ____

PANELS & PROFILES
☐ ✗ 3309 CHEM 12 — Albumin, Alkaline Phosphatase, BUN, Calcium, Cholesterol, Glucose, LDH, Phosphorus, AST, Total Bilirubin, Total Protein, Uric Acid
☐ ▼ 3315 CHEM 20 — Chem 12, Electrolyte Panel, Creatinine, Iron, Gamma GT, ALT, Triglycerides
☐ ▼ 3357 CARDIAC RISK PANEL — Cholesterol, HDL, LDL, Risk Factors, VLDL Triglycerides
☐ ✗ 3042 CRITICAL CARE PANEL — BUN, Chloride, CO2, Glucose, Potassium, Sodium
☐ 3046 ELECTROLYTE PANEL — Chloride, CO2, Potassium, Sodium
☐ ▼ 3399 EXECUTIVE PANEL — Chem 20, Iron, Cardiac Risk Panel, CBC, RPR, Thyroid Cascade
☐ 5242 HEPATITIS PANEL, ACUTE — HAVIgMAb, HBsAg, HBsAb, HBcAb, HCVAb
☐ ▼ 3355 LIPID MONITORING PANEL — Cholesterol, Triglycerides, HDL, LDL, VLDL, ALT, AST
☐ 3312 LIVER PANEL — Alkaline Phospatase, AST, Total Bilirubin, Gamma GT, Total Protein, Albumin, ALT
☐ ✗ 3083 METABOLIC STATUS PANEL — BUN, Osmolality (calculated), Chloride, CO2 Creatinine, Glucose, Potassium, Sodium, BUN/Creatinine, Ratio, Anion Gap
☐ ✗ 3376 PANEL B — Chem 12, CBC, Electrolyte Panel
☐ ▼ 3382 PANEL D — Chem 20, CBC, Thyroid Cascade
☐ ✗ 3388 PANEL F — Chem 12, CBC, Electrolyte Panel, Thyroid Cascade
☐ ▼ 3391 PANEL G — Chem 20, Cardiac Risk Panel, CBC, Thyroid Cascade
☐ ▼ 3393 PANEL H — Chem 20, CBC, Cardiac Risk Panel Rheumatoid Factor, Thyroid Cascade
☐ ▼ 3397 PANEL J — Chem 20, Cardiac Risk Panel
☐ 5351 PRENATAL PANEL — Antibody Screen ABO/Rh, CBC Rubella, HBsAg, RPR
☐ 1059 with Urinalysis, Routine
☐ 1082 with Urinalysis w/Culture if indicated
☐ ✗ 3102 RENAL PANEL — Metabolic Status Panel, Calcium, Phosphorus
☐ 3188 THYROID CASCADE — TSH, Reflex Testing

▼ - patient **required** to fast for 12-14 hours
✗ - patient recommended to fast 12-14 hours

LAB USE ONLY INIT ____
☐ SST ☐ PLASMA
☐ PURPLE ☐ SERUM
☐ YELLOW ☐ SWAB
☐ BLUE ☐ SLIDES
☐ GREEN ☐ DNA PROBE
☐ GREY ☐ B. CULT BTLS
☐ URINE
☐ BLACK
☐ OTHER: ____
REC'V. SPECIMEN: ☐ FROZEN
☐ AMBIENT ☐ ON ICE

Special Instructions/Pertinent Clinical Information ____
Physician's Signature ____ **Date** ____
These orders may be FAXed to: 449-5288
7060-500 (7/96)
LAB

FIGURE 9-1 Requisitions may be used for outpatients. The phlebotomist uses the requisition form to determine what type of sample to collect from the patient. The requisition may be computer generated or written by hand. (From Proctor DB, Adams AP: *Kinn's the medical assistant: An applied learning approach,* ed. 12, St. Louis, Saunders, 2014.)

FIGURE 9-2 Computer-printed label for specimen tube.

Requisitions or labels have the following information:
- Patient demographics, including full name, date of birth (DOB), sex, and race
- If an inpatient, hospital ID number and room and bed number
- Name or code of the physician making the request
- Test status (e.g., short turnaround time, or stat; timed; or fasting)

The number and type of tubes to collect may also be indicated. Test names may be abbreviated, so it is important to know the meaning of test abbreviations.

> **◀◀◀↰ FLASHBACK**
>
> Most common laboratory tests and their abbreviations were covered in Chapters 2, 6, and 7.

The information provided on the requisition or labels serves several purposes. First, it allows you to identify the patient correctly and may provide some helpful information about the patient. Second, it tells you what specimen should be collected. Third, it allows you to gather the necessary equipment for the collection before you encounter the patient. The requisition may not indicate any special handling procedures, and you may be required to consult laboratory resources to ensure both correct collection and

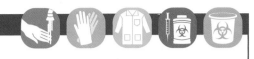

PROCEDURE 9-2–cont'd

Venipuncture With a Syringe

Holding the syringe upright, push the first tube up into the transfer device. Angle the tube slightly so blood flows slowly down the side of the tube, rather than dropping straight down, to prevent hemolysis. Allow the tube to fill without applying any pressure to the plunger. Pushing on the plunger causes hemolysis and increases the risk of causing an aerosol spray when the needle is removed. The evacuated tube will fill according to its vacuum capacity. If you need to fill a second tube, remove the first and insert the second tube just as you did the first.

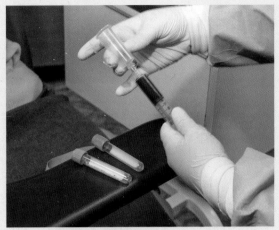

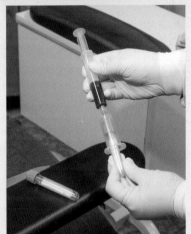

5. **Dispose of the syringe and transfer device together in the appropriate container.**

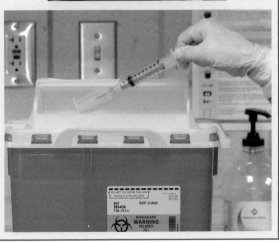

Continued

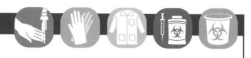

PROCEDURE 9-2–cont'd

Venipuncture With a Syringe

6. **Complete the procedure.**
   Finish the procedure as in steps 18 to 20 of
   Procedure 9-1.

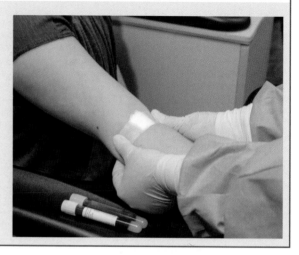

 AVOID THAT ERROR!

The waiting room at Consolidated Medical Services is filled, with seven outpatients still waiting for draws and more patients likely to arrive at any moment. Phlebotomist Tomas Sanchez knows the efficient functioning of the laboratory depends on him, and he is working quickly to clear the backlog. He seats his next patient, checks her ID against the requisition, prepares his tubes, applies the tourniquet, and swabs the site with alcohol. Moments later, he blows on the site to remove the last traces of liquid, then inserts the needle. The samples obtained, he finishes with the patient and labels the tubes. "Next!" What did he do wrong, and what should he have done?

WHAT WOULD YOU DO?

You must *not* draw blood from the patient. Drawing from the wrong patient can lead to incorrect diagnosis or treatment and may even lead to death of the patient. It can also get you fired and subject you to legal action. Although it seems likely the patient is the one you were expecting, there is a slight chance he is not—it is possible that two patients with the same name and similar dates of birth are both patients at the hospital and the ID numbers are in error. Find a nurse to determine where the error arose. You must resolve the discrepancy before you draw.

 AVOID THAT ERROR!

Ms. Campos has fainted, fortunately remaining on the bed rather than falling to the floor and risking severe injury. Sylvia should have insisted that the patient lie back in the bed, with enough support to prevent movement should she faint. Had Ms. Campos refused, Sylvia should have contacted the nurse. That is exactly what she must do now, to make sure the patient is safe and has not been injured during syncope.

AVOID THAT ERROR!

Tomas blew on the site, potentially contaminating it with bacteria or viruses from his mouth. Despite the need for rapid turnaround, he should have waited for the site to air-dry before proceeding with the draw.

STUDY QUESTIONS

See answers in Appendix F.

1. What is the most important aspect of any phlebotomy procedure?

2. Describe how to properly identify a patient.

3. What information is typically on a requisition form?

4. List the steps you should perform when requisitions are received.

5. Define hemoconcentration.

6. Name three veins in the antecubital area suitable for venipuncture.

7. Explain why the median cubital vein is the first choice for venipuncture.

8. Describe how veins, arteries, and tendons feel when palpating them.

9. What techniques can you use to help locate a vein?

10. Define hematoma.

11. Describe the correct position of the patient's arm after withdrawing the venipuncture needle.

12. Explain the correct procedure for labeling blood tubes.

13. List the information a phlebotomist must look for on a requisition slip.

14. Explain the reasoning behind preparing the patient before you wash your hands and put on gloves.

15. Describe the purpose of an ABN, and the phlebotomist's role in their use.

CERTIFICATION EXAMINATION PREPARATION

See answers in Appendix F.

1. Which is a purpose of the requisition?
   a. Identifying the patient
   b. Determining the specimens to be collected
   c. Allowing the equipment necessary for the collection to be gathered
   d. All of the above

2. Which vein is often the only one that can be palpated in an obese patient?
   a. Median
   b. Cephalic
   c. Basilic
   d. Iliac

3. Upon entering a patient's room, you should first
   a. assemble your equipment.
   b. put on your gloves.
   c. introduce yourself.
   d. identify the patient.

4. Which vein lies close to the brachial artery?
   a. Cephalic
   b. Median cubital
   c. Basilic
   d. Iliac

5. At what angle should a venipuncture needle penetrate the skin?
   a. 10 to 15 degrees
   b. 15 to 30 degree
   c. 30 to 40 degrees
   d. 45 degrees

6. Which information must match on the patient's ID band and the requisition?
   a. DOB
   b. ID number
   c. Patient's name
   d. All of the above

7. When should the tourniquet be removed from the arm in a venipuncture procedure?
   a. After the needle is withdrawn
   b. As the needle is withdrawn
   c. Before the needle is withdrawn
   d. The tourniquet should not be removed

8. Tourniquets should be placed _____ inches above the venipuncture site.
   a. 1 to 2
   b. 2 to 3
   c. 3 to 4
   d. 4 to 5

9. The following can occur if the tourniquet is left on the patient too long:
   a. nerve damage.
   b. hemoconcentration.
   c. occluded radial pulse.
   d. hematoma.

10. Hematomas can be caused by
    a. removing the tourniquet after removing the needle.
    b. withdrawing the needle before removing the last tube.
    c. withdrawing the needle too quickly.
    d. removing the tourniquet before removing the needle.

11. An increase in the ratio of formed elements to plasma is called
    a. hemolysis.
    b. petechiae.
    c. hemoconcentration.
    d. hematoma.

12. Small red spots on the skin are referred to as
    a. hemolysis.
    b. petechiae.
    c. hemoconcentration.
    d. hematoma.

13. If you are asked to perform a venipuncture on an inpatient who is not wearing an ID band, you should
    a. identify the patient by asking his or her name, and perform the venipuncture.
    b. ask the patient's nurse to attach a new ID band before proceeding.
    c. notify the physician.
    d. refuse to perform the venipuncture.

14. Which vein is the first choice for venipuncture?
    a. Basilic
    b. Median cubital
    c. Cephalic
    d. Iliac

15. During the venipuncture procedure, the tourniquet should stay on no longer than
    a. 30 seconds.
    b. 45 seconds.
    c. 1 minute.
    d. 2 minutes.

CHAPTER 10   Capillary Collection

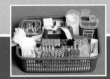

Capillary collection, also called dermal puncture or skin puncture, is the usual collection procedure for infants. In adults, it is an alternative collection procedure when minute amounts of blood are needed for testing, or for patients for whom venipuncture is inadvisable or impossible. In addition, it is typically used when collecting blood from infants and point-of-care testing. The depth of puncture must be carefully controlled to produce adequate flow while avoiding contact with underlying bone. Skin puncture devices deliver a precise incision, and microsample containers, sized to fit the desired sample, collect the blood from the puncture site.

OUTLINE

OBJECTIVES

After completing this chapter, you should be able to:

1. List situations in which a capillary collection might be preferred.
2. Explain why it is necessary to inform the physician when capillary blood is collected.
3. Describe the common skin puncture devices.
4. Discuss containers that may be used to collect capillary blood.
5. Explain how circulation may be increased at the puncture site.
6. Discuss proper capillary collection site selection.
7. Explain why it is important to control the depth of the puncture.
8. List, in order, the steps for capillary collection.
9. Describe how the cut should be made when a finger is used as the puncture site.
10. Explain why the first drop of blood is discarded.
11. List precautions to be observed when collecting capillary blood.
12. State the order of the draw in collecting capillary blood.
13. List, in order, the steps for performing a bleeding time (BT) test.

KEY TERMS

ancillary blood glucose test
bleeding time (BT) test
bilirubin, uric acid,
  phosphorus, and
  potassium (BURPP)
calcaneus
capillary tubes
Caraway or Natelson
  pipets
iatrogenic anemia
microcollection containers
microcollection
  tubes
microhematocrit
  tubes
osteochondritis
osteomyelitis
venous thrombosis

ABBREVIATIONS

ABG arterial blood gas
BT bleeding time
BURPP bilirubin, uric acid, phosphorus, and potassium
CBC complete blood count
CBG capillary blood gas

µL microliter
OSHA Occupational Safety and Health Administration
PFA platelet function assay

WHAT WOULD YOU DO?

You are working the morning shift at Bayview Walk-in Clinic. You call your next patient, Latisha Williams, from the waiting room. She hands you a requisition from her physician at the clinic, indicating she needs to have her serum glucose level checked. You ask her to sit down. As you collect your red-top tube and multisample needle, you notice she is looking a little nervous, so you try to calm her by chatting about the weather. As you begin to apply the tourniquet, she looks even more afraid. Suddenly she says, "Stop! Don't stick me with that needle! They never did that before!" What would you do?

REASONS FOR PERFORMING CAPILLARY COLLECTION

Although venipuncture is the most common way to obtain a blood sample, at times it is impossible or inadvisable to do so. In these situations, capillary collection (also called skin puncture or dermal puncture) offers a valuable alternative. Capillary collection is the preferred method for obtaining blood from newborns and infants for neonatal bilirubin, newborn screening, and point-of-care testing. Capillary collection is also used for **ancillary blood glucose testing**.

A requisition form generally does not state that a capillary collection should be performed, and it is up to the phlebotomist to choose the best collection method for the tests ordered. For this reason, you must be familiar with the advantages, limitations, and appropriate uses of capillary collection. Knowing how and when to perform a capillary collection is a vital skill for a phlebotomist.

Capillary collection is preferred in several situations and for several types of patients (Box 10-1). Adult patients undergoing frequent glucose monitoring are excellent candidates for capillary collection, because the test requires only a small amount of blood, which must be taken frequently. Access to venipuncture sites may be difficult with obese patients, whose veins are often hard to find, and with geriatric patients, who often have small or fragile veins that can make obtaining venous blood difficult. Venipuncture may be contraindicated for patients with burns or scars over venipuncture sites or for those at risk for **venous thrombosis** (caused when clots form within the veins), because

BOX 10-1	Patients for Whom Capillary Puncture May Be Considered

- Children, especially younger than age 2
- Geriatric patients
- Obese patients
- Patients at risk for serious complications associated with deep venous puncture
- Patients at risk for venous thrombosis
- Patients for whom only one blood test has been ordered for which a dermal puncture is appropriate
- Patients requiring frequent blood tests
- Patients undergoing frequent glucose monitoring
- Patients with burns or scars over venipuncture sites

venipuncture increases the risk of venous thrombosis. Other patients may be at risk for serious complications associated with deep venipuncture, including **iatrogenic anemia**, hemorrhage, infection, organ or tissue damage, arteriospasm, or cardiac arrest. Iatrogenic anemia is anemia caused by excessive blood draws.

Capillary collection is usually the preferred method of collection for newborns, infants, and children younger than 2 years. Young children's smaller veins and lower blood volume make venipuncture both difficult and potentially dangerous. Reducing blood volume through venipuncture is a concern for newborns and infants. It may lead to anemia and even cardiac arrest and death.

In addition to serving as a substitute for venipuncture, capillary blood gas (CBG) determination can be used as an alternative to arterial puncture for arterial blood gas (ABG) determination in infants.

FLASH FORWARD

Special considerations for collection from pediatric and geriatric patients are discussed in Chapter 12.

However, some tests cannot be performed on blood from a capillary collection. These include blood cultures and most routine coagulation tests. Capillary collection may not be appropriate for severely dehydrated patients, because test results may not be accurate. (This may also be a concern with venipuncture for such patients.) Capillary collection should not be used at sites that are swollen or where circulation or lymphatic drainage is compromised (such as a limb on the same side as a mastectomy).

DIFFERENCES BETWEEN VENOUS AND CAPILLARY BLOOD

A capillary puncture collects blood from capillaries. Because capillaries are the bridges between arteries and veins, blood collected by capillary puncture is a mixture of venous blood and arterial blood. The arterial proportion in the sample is increased when the collection site is warmed, as may be done to help increase blood flow before collection. Small amounts of tissue fluid from the puncture site may also be in the sample, especially in the first drop.

The levels of many substances are the same in both capillary and venous blood, but this is not the case for all substances, as indicated in Table 10-1. For instance, the normal potassium reading obtained by capillary collection is *lower* than that in a plasma sample obtained by venipuncture, but *higher* than that in a serum sample obtained by venipuncture. Because of these differences, results obtained by the two techniques cannot be compared. For this reason as well, it is important to record that the sample was obtained by capillary collection.

CLINICAL TIP

If a patient needs repeated determinations of potassium, calcium, total protein, hemoglobin, or glucose, you must use the same collection technique each time.

TABLE 10-1	Reference Values in Capillary and Venous Blood
Higher in Capillary Blood	Higher in Venous Blood
• Glucose	• Calcium
• Hemoglobin	• Total protein
• Potassium (serum sample)	• Potassium (plasma sample)

EQUIPMENT FOR CAPILLARY COLLECTION

Capillary collection equipment allows the phlebotomist to puncture the skin safely and collect the sample quickly and efficiently, with a minimum of discomfort for the patient.

Skin Puncture Devices

Skin puncture devices in the modern health care environment are designed with a retractable blade per Occupational Safety and Health Administration (OSHA) safety regulations. Some devices are contact activated, whereas others require the phlebotomist to depress a trigger to release the blade. Automatic puncture devices (Figure 10-1) deliver a swift puncture to a predetermined depth, which can be a significant advantage at sites where the bone is close to the skin (see "Site Selection"). The dimensions of the puncture are controlled by the width and

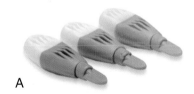

A

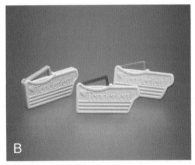

B

FIGURE 10-1 A, BD Microtainer Contact-Activated Lancet. **B,** Tenderlett Finger Incision Device. (**A** courtesy and © Becton, Dickinson and Company. **B** used with permission from International Technidyne Corporation [ITC] © 2010.)

depth of the point. Some automatic puncture devices have a platform that is positioned over the puncture site and color coded for different depths. (The automatic devices designed for home glucose testing make a cut that is too small for multiple tests or for filling several microsample containers and are not used in clinical practice.) Safety features include retractable blades and locks that keep a blade from being used a second time and prevent accidental sticks to the phlebotomist.

The Lasette laser lancing device is unique in that it uses a laser, rather than a sharp instrument, to pierce the skin, which causes less pain and bruising at the sample site. Cross-contamination between patients is avoided by disposing of the single-use lens cover between uses. The device is approved for patients 5 years and older.

Microsample Containers

Microsample containers come in different sizes to accommodate different volumes of blood.

Microcollection tubes (also called "bullets") hold up to 750 μL of blood. They are made of plastic and are available with a variety of anticoagulants and additives (Figure 10-2). The tubes are color coded by additive to match the coding of evacuated containers. Microcollection tubes are used for all types of dermal puncture collections and are the most common type of collection containers used for dermal puncture samples. They are also available with a plastic capillary tube that is fitted inside the container to aid in the collection of the sample.

> **FLASH FORWARD**
>
> See Appendix A to review metric symbols.

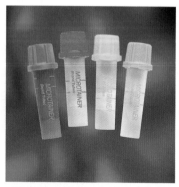

FIGURE 10-2 BD Microtainer Tubes with BD Microgard Closure. (Courtesy and © Becton, Dickinson and Company.)

Capillary tubes come in either plastic or glass, and in a range of sizes. These tubes are used primarily for the collection of samples for CBG determinations. **Caraway or Natelson pipets** are narrow glass tubes with capacities up to about 470 μL. The use of these tubes has declined in recent years because of heightened attention to sharps injury prevention, and OSHA recommends against using glass tubes of this sort. Plastic capillary tubes are increasingly being used instead.

Capillary tubes are available either plain, with a blue band, or heparin coated, with a red, yellow, or green band (colors may vary with the manufacturer). Once the sample is in the tube, one or both ends are sealed. Sealing used to be done by pushing the ends into soft clay. New, safer sealing methods are recommended that instead fit the ends with small plastic caps. Both ends must be sealed for a CBG determination. In the laboratory, the sample may be centrifuged to separate cells from plasma or serum. The sample can be removed with a syringe.

> **FLASH FORWARD**
>
> You will learn about collecting blood gas samples in Chapter 13.

Microhematocrit tubes are small tubes, either plastic or glass, with a volume up to 75 μL. These tubes are used infrequently and have been largely replaced by **microcollection containers**. However when a spun hematocrit is requested, a plastic capillary tube can be used.

Finally, capillary collection is also used in neonatal screening for a variety of inherited diseases. In this situation, no collection container is used. Instead, drops of blood are applied directly to specially prepared filter paper.

> **FLASH FORWARD**
>
> You will learn about neonatal screening collection in Chapter 12.

Additional Supplies

As in venipuncture, alcohol pads are used to prepare the site, and gauze pads are used to help stop the bleeding. A sharps disposal container is needed for the lancet.

Warming devices increase circulation. Simple towels or washcloths may be soaked in warm water and applied to the site. Be sure that the site is completely dry before puncture, however, as residual water will cause hemolysis and dilution of the specimen. Commercial warming packs are also available. The pack is first wrapped in a dry towel and then activated by squeezing. Such "heel warmers" are often used when blood must be collected from infants. The temperature of the device should not exceed 42° C, and it should be applied for 3 to 5 minutes. Glass slides are used to prepare blood smears for microscopic examination of blood cells.

FLASH FORWARD ⤳»

You will learn how to prepare a blood smear in Chapter 14.

SITE SELECTION
General Considerations

Capillary collection should be performed on warm, healthy skin that is free of scars, cuts, bruises, and rashes. The site must be easily accessible and have good capillary flow near the skin surface, but there must be enough clearance above the underlying bone to prevent the lancet from accidentally contacting it. Bone puncture can lead to **osteochondritis**, a painful inflammation of the bone or cartilage, or **osteomyelitis**, a potentially serious, sometimes fatal, bone infection.

You should also avoid skin that has been damaged or compromised in any way. Specific areas to avoid include skin that is callused, scarred, burned, infected, bruised, edematous, or bluish. Also avoid previous puncture sites as well as sites where circulation or lymphatic drainage is compromised.

Puncture Depth and Width

The depth of the puncture depends on the site and the patient (Table 10-2). To minimize the risk of inflammation and infection, the lancet should never penetrate more than 3.0 mm. For a heel puncture, the maximum depth is 2.0 mm, because the **calcaneus**, or heel bone, can lie very close to the surface. For premature babies, the recommended depth is 0.65 to 0.85 mm.

TABLE 10-2	Puncture Depth
Use	Depth
Finger stick	3.0 mm
Heel stick	2.0 mm
Heel stick (premature infants or neonates)	0.65–0.85 mm
Bleeding time	1.0 mm

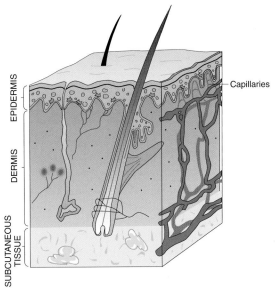

FIGURE 10-3 The proper sites for capillary collection are those that provide an adequate capillary bed and sufficient clearance from underlying bone. (From VanMeter KC, Hubert RJ: *Gould's pathophysiology for the health professions,* ed. 5, St. Louis, Saunders, 2015.)

Puncture width should not exceed 2.4 mm (Figure 10-3). At the right site, this achieves adequate blood flow but remains well above the bone. Puncture width is actually more important than depth in determining blood flow, because capillary beds may lie close to the skin, especially for newborns. A wider cut severs more capillaries and produces greater flow.

Capillary Collection Sites for Adults and Older Children

For adults and for children older than 1 year, dermal punctures are almost always performed on the fingertips of the nondominant hand. The best sites are the palmar surface of the distal segments of the third (middle) and fourth (ring) fingers (Figure 10-4). The thumb is likely to be callused, and the index finger's extra nerve endings make punctures more painful. The little finger (pinky) has too little tissue for safe puncture. If the fingers cannot be used, the big toe may be an option—check the policy at your workplace. Earlobes are never used for dermal puncture.

«« ↰   **FLASHBACK**

Anatomic terminology was discussed in Chapter 6.

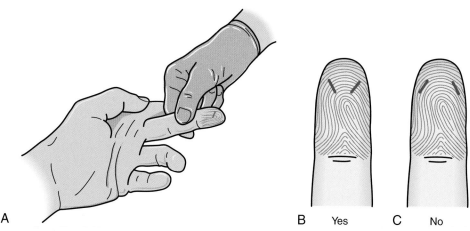

A   B   Yes   C   No

FIGURE 10-4 Dermal puncture in adults and children is performed on the third (middle) or fourth (ring) finger, on the palmar surface near the fleshy center of the distal segment.

The puncture should be made near the fleshy center of the chosen finger. Avoid the edge of the finger, as the underlying bone is too close to the surface. As indicated in Figure 10-4, the puncture should be made perpendicular to (across) the ridges of the fingerprint, which lessens the flow of blood into the grooves.

Capillary Collection Sites for Infants

For children younger than 1 year, there is too little tissue available in any of the fingers. For this reason, dermal puncture is performed in the heel (Figure 10-5). As shown in Figure 10-6, only the medial and lateral borders of the plantar (bottom) surface can be used. The center of the plantar surface is too close to the calcaneus, as is the posterior (back) surface. The arch is too close to nerves and tendons. For older infants, the big toe may be used if the heel is unacceptable. Be aware that the heel may be callused on young children who have begun to walk.

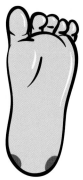

FIGURE 10-6 Dermal puncture in infants is performed on the heel, on the medial and lateral borders only.

> ⚠ **AVOID THAT ERROR!**
>
> When phlebotomist Brandon Mayhew entered the waiting room and saw his next draw, 1-month-old Derek Stevens, he knew he would need to be especially careful to make this dermal collection as smooth as possible for both the infant and the nervous mother. He greeted them warmly, smiled at Derek, and quickly cleansed the infant's big toe, which Brandon had chosen as the puncture site. Once it was dry, he collected the sample without delay, applied a bandage, labeled the tubes, and thanked the patient. Two weeks later, Derek was admitted to the hospital with a bone infection, and Brandon was named in a lawsuit for injuring Derek. What did Brandon do wrong? What should he have done? And what should he do now?

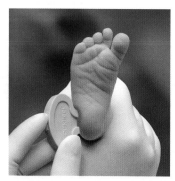

FIGURE 10-5 BD Microtainer Quikheel Lancet. (Courtesy and © Becton, Dickinson and Co.)

CAPILLARY COLLECTION

Procedure 10-1 outlines the steps for a capillary collection. In addition to these specific steps, you should always greet the patient, identify the patient, and obtain consent, as you would for a routine venipuncture.

PROCEDURE 10-1

Capillary Collection

1. **After documenting on the requisition that you are performing a capillary collection, sanitize your hands and put on gloves.**

   > **◄◄↰ FLASHBACK**
   >
   > Proper hand sanitation and gloving techniques were covered in Procedures 4-1 and 4-2.

2. **Assemble your equipment.**
   Use the patient's age and the tests ordered to determine which type of collection tube you will need, what type of skin puncture device to use, and whether to use a warming device.

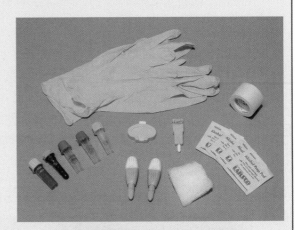

3. **Select and clean the site.**
   Warm the area first, if necessary. If the site feels cold, it should be warmed for at least 3 minutes at a temperature no greater than 42° C. If a wet washcloth is used, be sure to remove any residual water, as residual water will cause hemolysis and dilution of the specimen.

   Use 70% isopropyl alcohol to clean the site. Allow the site to dry completely. In addition to causing stinging, contamination, and hemolysis, residual alcohol interferes with the formation of rounded drops of blood on the skin surface. (Use of povidone–iodine is not recommended for dermal punctures, because it may elevate test results for **bilirubin, uric acid, phosphorus, and potassium.** Remember the acronym **BURPP** to help you learn this group of tests.)

   Massaging the finger proximal to the puncture site (closer to the palm) can help increase blood flow. To avoid hemolysis, massage gently, and do not squeeze.

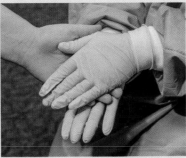

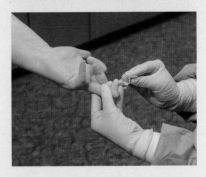

Continued

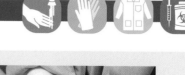

PROCEDURE 10-1—cont'd

Capillary Collection

4. **Position and hold the area.**

   Hold the finger or heel firmly. This prevents it from moving during the puncture and reassures the patient.

   Grasp the patient's finger with its palmar surface up, holding it between your thumb and index finger.

   To hold the patient's heel, place your thumb in the arch, wrap your hand over the top of the foot, and place your index finger behind the heel.

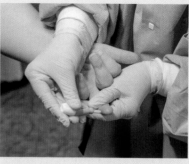

5. **Make the puncture, and dispose of the blade properly.**

   Align the device so the cut is made across the fingerprint ridges or heel lines. This allows the blood to flow out and make a rounded drop, rather than run into the grooves. Puncture the skin slightly lateral to the center of the finger (that is, slightly toward the pinky finger), so that the hand can be tilted for easier blood flow into the container. Do not lift the device immediately after the puncture is complete. Count to two before lifting the device to ensure that the blade has made the puncture to the full depth and then fully retracted. Scraping of the skin may occur if the blade is not retracted.

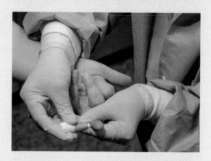

   Dispose of the used blade immediately in an appropriate collection container.

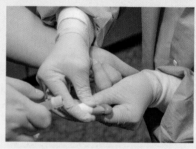

   Failure to obtain blood: If you are unable to obtain sufficient blood with the first puncture, the policy at most institutions is to attempt one more puncture. You must use a sterile lancet to make the new puncture. After two unsuccessful punctures, notify the nursing station and contact a different phlebotomist to complete the procedure.

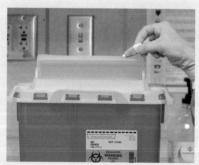

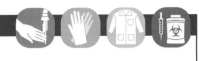

PROCEDURE 10-1—cont'd

Capillary Collection

6. **Prepare to collect the sample.**

   Wipe away the first drop of blood with a clean gauze pad to prevent contaminating the sample with tissue fluid.

   Keep the finger in a downward position to help encourage blood flow.

   You can alternate applying and releasing firm pressure proximal to the site to increase flow, but avoid *constant massaging,* as this will cut off flow, cause hemolysis, and introduce tissue fluid back into the sample.

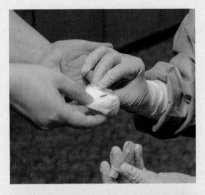

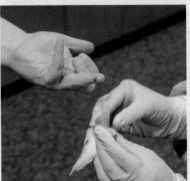

7. **Collect the sample.**

   Once blood is flowing freely, position the container for collection.

   Microcollection tubes should be slanted downward. Lightly touch the scoop of the tube to the blood drop, and allow the blood to run into the tube. Do not scrape the skin with the container. This causes hemolysis, activates platelets, and contaminates the sample with epithelial skin cells.

   Tap the container lightly to move blood to the bottom. Close the lid after the sample has been collected. Invert the tube 8 to 10 times after filling if additives are present. Be careful not to overfill the microcollection tube containing anticoagulant because the ratio of anticoagulant to blood will be exceeded and microclots will form. The collection will need to be repeated due to inaccurate test results.

   Order of collection: Platelet counts, complete blood counts (CBCs) and other hematology tests are collected first, followed by chemistry tests.

   Be mindful of specimens that require special handling before transport.

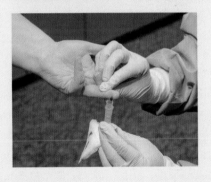

Continued

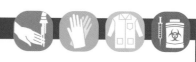

PROCEDURE 10-1—cont'd

Capillary Collection

8. Complete the procedure.

Apply pressure to the puncture site using a
clean gauze square. Once bleeding has
stopped, you can bandage the site for older
children and adults. Do not use a bandage
on children younger than age 2, as they may
remove the bandage and choke on it. When
drawing blood from children and infants,
be especially careful that all equipment has
been picked up and bed rails have been
placed back in position.

Label the microsample container, and place it in
a larger holder for transport to the laboratory.
As always, thank the patient.

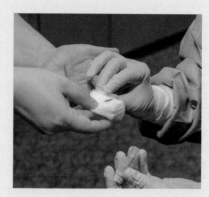

OTHER USES OF CAPILLARY PUNCTURE

Capillary puncture is used for bleeding time
tests and ancillary blood glucose testing (also
called bedside glucose testing). It can also be used
as an alternative to arterial puncture for ABG
determination.

Bleeding Time Test

A **bleeding time (BT) test** measures the length of
time required for bleeding to stop after an incision is
made. In the past, this test was used before surgery to
help assess the overall integrity of primary hemostasis. Inconsistencies in the test have led to its replacement by the platelet function assay (PFA) or other
tests. These are performed not on dermal puncture
samples but on venous blood. The procedure is
included here because you may be called upon to
perform it nonetheless. To perform a BT test, an automated incision device is used, with the depth set at
1 mm, and length at 5 mm. Some devices make one
incision; others make two incisions at the same time.
The steps of the BT test are shown in Procedure 10-2.

⟨⟨⟨↰   FLASHBACK
Hemostasis was discussed in Chapter 7.

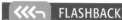

Results and Complications

Normal BT is 2 to 10 minutes and depends somewhat on the device used. Bleeding that does not stop

within 15 to 20 minutes means one of two things:
(1) either the patient has a condition that is interfering with normal platelet plug formation or (2) the
test was performed incorrectly—a capillary was
scratched, the incision was too deep, the filter paper
touched the incision site, or some technical error
was made. If only one incision was made, the test
may have to be repeated on the other arm. If two
incisions were made and the two BTs are within
several minutes of each other, it is unnecessary to
repeat the test. Be sure to learn the exact protocol
for your laboratory before this situation occurs.
Abnormally short BTs are probably caused by a test
error—for instance, the incision may have been too
shallow, the device may have been lifted too soon,
or there may have been hair at the incision site.

REVIEW FOR CERTIFICATION

Capillary collection is used for a variety of patients
with compromised or otherwise inaccessible veins,
including infants, or when only a small sample is
needed. A calibrated puncture device delivers a precise, carefully controlled puncture, avoiding contact
with the bone and reducing the risk of osteomyelitis
or osteochondritis. The size and purpose of the
sample dictate the collection container used,
although microcollection tubes are increasingly
used for most collections. The BT test assesses the
integrity of primary hemostasis by measuring the
time required to stop bleeding after a standard incision is made.

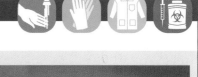

PROCEDURE 10-2

Bleeding Time Test

1. **Assemble your equipment.**
   You will need the following:
   - Antiseptic materials (alcohol pads)
   - Blood pressure cuff
   - Automated BT device
   - Stopwatch or timer with a second hand
   - Filter paper
   - Bandages

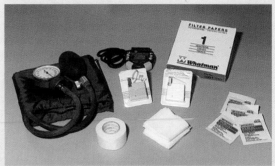

2. **Prepare the patient.**
   Explain the procedure to the patient. Be sure to
   explain that scarring may occur, especially in
   dark-skinned patients.

   Ask the patient about any medications he or
   she is taking or has taken recently, especially
   aspirin or other drugs that interfere with
   clotting. Salicylates, including aspirin,
   inhibit platelet function for 7 to 10 days
   after the last dose. Ibuprofen inhibits
   function for 24 hours. If the patient has
   taken such medications recently, follow
   the policy of your institution or consult
   with your supervisor about proceeding
   with the test.

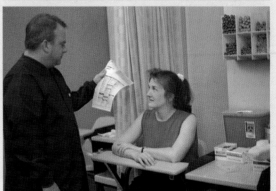

3. **Position the arm, select the site, and clean
   the site.**
   Place the arm on a flat, steady surface, with
   the palm facing up. Select a site 5 cm below
   the antecubital crease. The area must be
   free of veins, scars, hair, and bruises. For
   patients with very hairy arms, you may need
   to shave the site before cleaning it. Clean
   the site and allow it to dry, as you would
   for other dermal procedures.

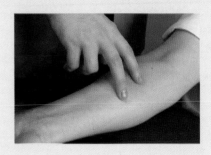

Continued

PROCEDURE 10-2—cont'd

Bleeding Time Test

4. **Apply the blood pressure cuff.**

   Place the cuff on the upper arm. Inflate it to 40 mm Hg. This pressure must be maintained throughout the procedure. Wait 30 to 60 seconds to ensure that the pressure is stable before making the incision.

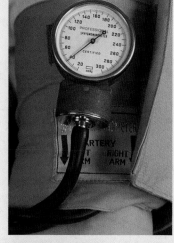

5. **Position the device.**

   The blade is placed perpendicular to the antecubital crease on the volar surface of the forearm.

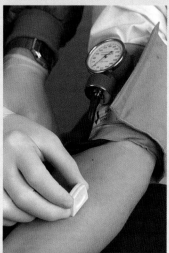

6. **Make the incision, and start timing.**

   Press the device on the arm without making an indentation.
   Press the trigger.
   Start timing as soon as the cut is made.
   Remove the device only after the blade has retracted.

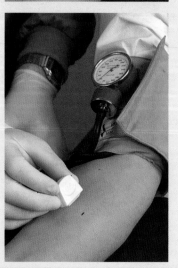

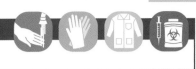

PROCEDURE 10-2—cont'd

Bleeding Time Test

7. **Wick the blood away every 30 seconds.**
   Use filter paper to absorb blood from the cut without touching the incision. Touch the edge of the filter paper to the surface of the blood drop without touching the skin or the incision. Wick until the drop disappears.

   Repeat every 30 seconds. Be careful not to touch the site between times, as this may disrupt the clot and alter the test results.

   If two incisions are made, follow this procedure for each incision independently.

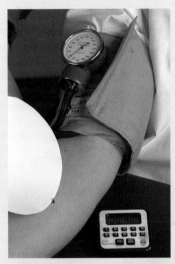

8. **Complete the test.**
   When blood is no longer absorbed by the filter paper, bleeding has stopped.
   Record the time.
   Remove the pressure cuff.

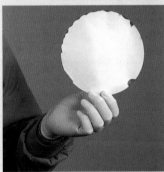

9. **Attend to the patient.**
   Clean the arm around the incision site with antiseptic wipe and apply a butterfly bandage. Be sure to pull the edges of the incision together when applying the butterfly bandage. Instruct the patient to keep the bandage in place for 24 hours to minimize scarring.

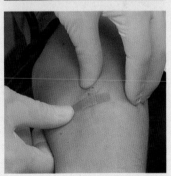

BIBLIOGRAPHY

Blumenfeld TA, Turi GK, Blanc WA: Recommended site and depth of newborn heel skin punctures based on anatomical measurements and histopathology, *Lancet* 313:230–233.

BD: *Vacutainer: LabNotes*, 2014. Retrieved from www.bd.com/vacutainer/labnotes/Volume17Number1/composition_differences.asp.

CLSI: *Performance of the bleeding time test; Approved Standard—Second edition.* CSLI Document H45-A2. Wayne, Pa., 2004, Clinical and Laboratory Standards Institute.

CLSI: *Procedures and devices for the collection of diagnostic capillary blood specimens; Approved standard—sixth edition.* CSLI document GP42-A6 (formerly H04-A6). Wayne, Pa., 2008, Clinical and Laboratory Standards Institute.

WHAT WOULD YOU DO?

Put away that needle and tube. Unless a patient gives consent, you may not proceed. And you do not need a whole tube of blood—when the only test a patient needs is glucose monitoring, a dermal puncture is sufficient. Thank your patient for reminding you of this, double-check the requisition to be sure a dermal puncture will suffice for the sample, and proceed with a dermal puncture.

 AVOID THAT ERROR!

Brandon chose an inappropriate site for dermal collection. In newborns, the bone in the toe is too close to the surface for safe dermal puncture. Brandon should have collected from the medial or lateral border of the plantar surface of the heel. Brandon also applied a bandage, which should not be used in children this young. At this point, Brandon will need to consult a lawyer to defend against the suit.

STUDY QUESTIONS

See answers in Appendix F.

1. Name two sites commonly used for adult capillary collection.

2. Explain why it is best to perform a capillary collection rather than a venipuncture on children.

3. List six types of patients, other than infants, for whom capillary collection may be advisable.

4. Explain why, in a capillary collection, the first drop of blood is wiped away with clean gauze.

5. Describe what microcollection containers are used for.

6. What can be used to stimulate blood flow to the capillaries?

7. List six specific areas of the skin to avoid when performing a capillary collection.

8. At what age are heel sticks preferred to finger sticks?

9. List four reasons alcohol must air-dry before a capillary stick.

10. Explain why povidone–iodine should not be used for capillary collection procedures.

11. Which fingers are acceptable to use for capillary collection?

12. Describe the order of collection for a capillary collection.

13. Explain the purpose of the BT test.

14. Why should bandages not be placed on young children following a dermal puncture?

CERTIFICATION EXAMINATION PREPARATION

See answers in Appendix F.

1. Capillary collections are performed on
   a. capillaries.
   b. veins.
   c. arteries.
   d. arterioles.

2. Which of the following has a higher value in a capillary sample as opposed to a venous serum sample?
   a. Potassium
   b. Calcium
   c. Total protein
   d. Hemoglobin

3. Good candidates for dermal collection include patients who
   a. require frequent collection.
   b. are obese.
   c. are severely dehydrated.
   d. All of the above
   e. a and b only

4. Capillary collection may be appropriate in geriatric patients because
   a. tourniquets are hard to place in this patient group.
   b. their veins tend to be small and fragile.
   c. most geriatric patients require only one blood test.
   d. they are likely to be obese.

5. An infant heel-warming device should be applied for approximately
   a. 1 to 2 minutes.
   b. 8 to 10 minutes.
   c. 30 seconds.
   d. 3 to 5 minutes.

6. The depth of a heel puncture should not be more than
   a. 3.0 mm.
   b. 2.0 mm.
   c. 2.0 cm.
   d. 1.5 cm.

7. Which finger is most widely used for capillary collection?
   a. Thumb (first digit)
   b. Index (second digit)
   c. Ring (fourth digit)
   d. Pinky (fifth digit)

8. In performing a dermal puncture, the puncture should be
   a. aligned with the whorls of the fingerprint.
   b. perpendicular to the whorls of the fingerprint.
   c. on the edge of the finger.
   d. on the tip of the finger.

9. The location for heel sticks is the
   a. center of the plantar surface.
   b. medial or lateral borders of the plantar surface.
   c. posterior surface.
   d. arch.

10. Which sample(s) is/are collected first in a capillary collection?
   a. Platelet counts
   b. Complete blood counts
   c. Chemistry tests
   d. All of the above
   e. a and b only

11. Which medication does not interfere with the BT test?
   a. Salicylates
   b. Ibuprofen
   c. Aspirin
   d. All of these interfere with the test

12. At what level does the blood pressure cuff remain during a BT test?
   a. 20 mm Hg
   b. 10 mm Hg
   c. 50 mm Hg
   d. 40 mm Hg

13. How frequently is the blood wicked during a BT test?
   a. Every 5 seconds
   b. Every 10 seconds
   c. Every 30 seconds
   d. Every 45 seconds

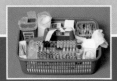
Although most venipuncture collections are routine and without problems, complications can arise. Many factors can interfere with the collection of blood, but most complications can be dealt with by knowing what to expect and planning ahead. Complications include problems with access to the patient, site selection, site cleaning, tourniquet application, sample collection, completion of the procedure, and sample integrity. In addition, patients may experience long-term health-related complications from venipuncture. Specimens may be rejected for a variety of reasons, requiring a re-draw. By learning the most common complications and the best approaches for avoiding or overcoming them, you will be better prepared in your work as a phlebotomist.

OUTLINE

OBJECTIVES

After completing this chapter, you should be able to:

1. Explain the procedure to be followed in these situations:
   a. The patient is not in his or her room.
   b. The patient has no identification band.
   c. The patient is sleeping, unconscious, or apprehensive.
   d. A member of the clergy or a physician is with the patient.
   e. Visitors are present.
   f. The patient cannot understand you.
   g. The patient refuses to have blood drawn.

2. List at least four sites that must be avoided when collecting blood, and explain why.
3. Describe techniques that can be used to help locate a vein.
4. Discuss limitations and precautions to be followed if a leg or hand vein is considered for venipuncture.
5. List at least two situations in which alcohol should not be used to clean the venipuncture site, and state at least one alternative.
6. Describe four potential problems associated with tourniquet application.

7. Define syncope, describe the signs of syncope, and explain what to do when a patient experiences this condition during the collection of blood.

8. Describe the actions to be taken if a patient has a seizure, complains of nausea, or vomits.

9. List three reasons that blood may not flow into a tube, and explain how to prevent or correct the problem.

10. Explain what should be done in the following situations:

   a. An artery is inadvertently punctured.
   b. No blood is collected on the first try.
   c. The patient requests something.
   d. There is prolonged bleeding from the puncture site.

11. List the causes of a hemolyzed sample, and name the test results that may be affected.

12. List tests that may be affected by a patient's position.

13. Describe five long-term complications associated with venipuncture, and explain how they can be avoided.

14. State the reasons a sample may be rejected by the laboratory.

KEY TERMS

compartment syndrome	hemolysis	occluded	sclerosed
emesis	lymphostasis	reflux	syncope

ABBREVIATIONS

BURPP bilirubin, uric acid, phosphorus, and potassium
CBC complete blood count
EDTA ethylenediaminetetraacetic acid
ER, ED emergency room, emergency department

ICU intensive care unit
ID identification
stat short turnaround time
WCS winged collection set

WHAT WOULD YOU DO?

You are preparing to draw samples from Cynthia Miller, an inpatient at Cedar Hills Hospital who is scheduled for surgery tomorrow. You have correctly identified her, studied the labels for and assembled the tubes you need, donned your personal protective equipment, applied the tourniquet, and found a good vein. Just as you are about to insert the needle, Cynthia's physician enters the room and says in a rather brusque tone, "I need to talk with Cynthia. Give us the room." Do you tell the physician you need to finish the draw, or do you pack up and leave? What would you do?

FACTORS THAT PREVENT ACCESS TO THE PATIENT

Locating the Patient

If the patient is not in his or her room, make every effort to locate the patient by checking with the nursing station. If the patient is in another department and the test is a short turnaround time (stat) or timed request, proceed to that area and draw the blood there.

Always let the nurse know if the request needs to be rescheduled.

Identifying the Patient

As you learned earlier in this book, positive identification (ID) of the patient is the most important procedure in phlebotomy.

Several situations can make ID difficult, including the following:

- Emergency requisitions
- Emergency room (ER) collections
- Orders telephoned in to the laboratory
- Requisitions picked up at the site

Despite the difficulties these situations may present, the information on the requisition must match exactly the information on the patient's ID band. *Any discrepancies must be resolved before collecting the specimen.* When the ID band is missing, contact the nursing station so that one can be attached by the nurse on duty. Even if an ID band is in the room, unless it is on the patient, you must not draw blood. Specific policies regarding the resolution of patient ID problems may vary from institution to institution. Be sure to follow the policy of your institution.

The American Association of Blood Banks requires special ID for patients receiving blood transfusions. Most institutions use a commercial ID system, in which the ID band comes with matching labels for the specimens. If you are collecting a blood bank specimen and your institution uses this system, be sure to have the appropriate labels.

BARRIERS TO COMMUNICATING WITH THE PATIENT

Sleeping or Unconscious Patients

If you encounter a sleeping patient, you should make one or two attempts to gently wake the patient, and give them time to become oriented, before you begin the draw. A sleeping patient cannot give informed consent or confirm their identity. Drawing from a patient without their consent may expose you to charges of assault. A patient who awakens during a draw may move suddenly, risking injury to himself or herself, or you. If the patient cannot be awakened, consult the nurse or your supervisor.

There are times when you must draw from a patient who is unconscious and cannot be awakened. Unconscious patients are most commonly encountered in the intensive care units (ICU), emergency department, and nursing home. The medical facility will have a protocol in place that needs to be followed for obtaining consent and ensuring the safety of the draw.

As a phlebotomist, you will often not know the reason a patient is unconscious. A patient may be recovering from a procedure, or experiencing the side effects of medications. Treat an unconscious patient just as you would a conscious one, including identifying yourself and describing the procedure. Unconscious patients may be able to hear you, even if they cannot respond.

Presence of Physicians or Clergy

If a physician or clergy member is in the room, return at another time for the procedure unless it is a stat or timed collection. In that case, you should respectfully interrupt and explain the reason for the interruption. If the physician enters while you are preparing to draw, leave the room until he or she is finished with the patient. If the physician enters after you have begun to draw blood, you may request a few minutes to complete the procedure.

Presence of Visitors

When you enter a room with visitors, greet them as you would the patient. Explain the purpose of your visit to the patient, and ask the visitors if they would mind stepping outside. Most visitors will exit to leave you to work without distraction. If the patient is a child, the presence of visitors or family members during the collection may be helpful.

> **FLASH FORWARD** →»
> Collecting blood from children is covered in Chapter 12.

Apprehensive Patients

Many patients have some apprehension about being stuck with a needle or having their blood drawn. Most patients can be easily calmed by engaging them in a little distracting conversation on neutral topics, such as the weather, traffic, or local news. If a patient is very nervous or you expect difficulty keeping the patient still or calm during the collection, it is helpful to request a nurse's assistance. This is especially true if the patient is a child.

Language Problems

When the patient cannot understand you, he or she cannot give informed consent. In this situation, you may need a translator. Alternatively, if you can effectively communicate with the patient by showing him or her what you will do, you may be able to obtain consent without a translator.

> **FLASH FORWARD** →»
> See Appendix B for useful Spanish phrases and vocabulary.

Patient Refusal

The patient always retains the right to refuse a blood collection. When a patient refuses to have his or her blood drawn, thank the patient and leave the room. Find the nurse and explain that the patient has refused the procedure. The nurse may ask you to return with him or her to the room. If the patient again refuses, document this on the request, along with the nurse's name, and notify the health care provider. Remember: never force a patient to have blood drawn.

FLASHBACK

Informed consent was discussed in Chapter 1.

PROBLEMS IN SITE SELECTION

The antecubital fossa is the most common site for routine venipuncture. However, the presence of certain conditions at the chosen site may alter the quality of a specimen or cause harm to the patient. In that case, another site must be chosen.

Occluded and Sclerosed Veins

Veins that are **occluded** (blocked) or **sclerosed** (hardened) feel hard or cordlike and lack resiliency. Occlusion and sclerosis can be caused by inflammation, disease, chemotherapy, prolonged IV therapy or repeated venipunctures. Such veins are susceptible to infection, and because the blood flow is impaired, the sample may produce erroneous test results.

Hematomas

Hematomas may be caused by the needle going through the vein, by having the bevel opening only partially in the vein, or by failing to apply enough pressure after withdrawal. Blood from a hematoma is no longer fresh from the vein, and the hematoma can obstruct the vein, slowing blood flow. Each of these factors can alter test results.

Edematous Tissue

The arm may appear swollen because of the accumulation of tissue fluid. Collection from edematous tissue alters tests results.

Burns, Scars, and Tattoos

Areas with burns, scars, or tattoos have impaired circulation, are susceptible to infection, and may be painful or difficult to penetrate.

Mastectomies

The removal of lymph tissue on the side of the mastectomy causes **lymphostasis**, or lack of lymph fluid movement. This can affect test results. The collection also may be painful to the patient, and the risk of infection may be increased. Your institution may require a physician's consent before drawing on the same side as the mastectomy.

IV Sites

Blood should not be drawn from an arm if there is an IV device in place. Use the other arm instead, or an alternative site. If no other sites are available, blood should be drawn from a site distal to (further away from), not proximal to, the IV.

FLASH FORWARD

Special considerations for vascular access devices are discussed in Chapter 12.

Other Situations

Any condition resulting in disruption of skin integrity means that the site should be avoided. Open or weeping lesions, skin rashes, recent tattoos, or incompletely healed stitches are examples of sites that should be avoided because of the increased risk of infection.

Difficulty Finding a Vein

When you cannot find a vein, several techniques can help.

Check the Other Arm

Examine the other arm for a suitable site. Ask the patient about sites of previous successful phlebotomy.

Enhance Vein Prominence

- Massage gently upward from the wrist to the elbow.
- Dangle the arm in a downward position to increase blood in the arm.
- Apply heat. Moist heat should be avoided if possible.
- Rotate the wrist to increase the prominence of the cephalic vein.

Use a Sphygmomanometer/Blood Pressure Cuff

A sphygmomanometer (blood pressure cuff) can be used instead of a tourniquet for hard-to-find veins. The blood pressure cuff should be placed 3 to 4 inches above the venipuncture site, and inflated to a pressure above the diastolic but below the systolic reading. If necessary, both arms should be checked to find a good vein. Check both arms for "good veins." The phlebotomist needs special training to use the blood pressure cuff in this way.

Use an Alternative Site

When a suitable vein cannot be found in the antecubital fossa, you will have to collect the blood from somewhere else—the hand, foot, or leg. The leg and foot are more susceptible to infections and clots, and they are not recommended sites for patients with diabetes or those on anticoagulant therapy (heparin or warfarin). Collection from the leg and foot usually requires the physician's permission.

The veins of the back of the hand (Figure 11-1) are small and fragile. For this reason, you should use a winged infusion set (WIS), or butterfly, with a smaller gauge needle and tube or a syringe. The steps in collecting blood from the back of the hand are similar to those for routine venipuncture, as described in Chapter 9. A butterfly is ideal for a hand draw, because the tubing allows for a lower angle of insertion than a standard needle and tube holder. A syringe allows you to control the suction to pull blood slowly from the veins, which is particularly important for elderly and pediatric patients. Procedure 11-1 outlines hand collection using a WIS.

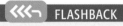

> **«« FLASHBACK**
> Butterflies were discussed in Chapter 8.

> **«« FLASHBACK**
> Syringe collection was discussed in Chapter 9.

PROBLEMS ASSOCIATED WITH CLEANING THE SITE

Alcohol cannot be used for site cleaning when drawing a blood alcohol test. It is also not a strong enough antiseptic for drawing blood cultures, blood gases, or blood donations. In these cases, povidone–iodine is used instead. For patients allergic to iodine, chlorhexidine gluconate is available. When you use an alternative antiseptic, note it on the requisition.

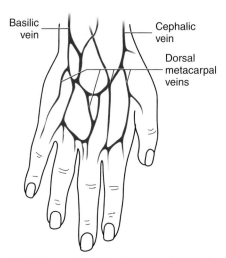

Basilic vein

Cephalic vein

Dorsal metacarpal veins

FIGURE 11-1 The veins of the back of the hand.

Povidone–iodine is not recommended for dermal punctures, because it may elevate test results for bilirubin, uric acid, phosphorus, and potassium (BURPP).

PROBLEMS ASSOCIATED WITH TOURNIQUET APPLICATION

Hemoconcentration

In Chapter 9, you learned that a tourniquet should not remain in place for more than 1 minute at a time. This is to prevent hemoconcentration, or alteration in the ratio of elements in the blood. When a tourniquet remains in place too long, the plasma portion of the blood filters into the tissue, causing an increase in the proportion of cells remaining in the vein. Primarily, this affects determinations of the large molecules, such as plasma proteins, enzymes, and lipids. It also increases red blood cell counts and iron and calcium levels. Prolonged tourniquet application can also alter potassium and lactic acid levels by a different mechanism. These problems can be avoided by releasing the tourniquet as soon as blood flow begins in the first tube. Hemoconcentration can also be caused by pumping of the fist, sclerosed or occluded veins, long-term intravenous therapy, or dehydration.

Formation of Petechiae

Petechiae are small, nonraised red spots that appear on the skin when the tourniquet is applied to a patient with a capillary wall or platelet disorder. The appearance of petechiae indicates that the site may bleed excessively after the procedure and requires longer application of pressure on the puncture site.

Tourniquet Applied Too Tightly

If there is no arterial pulse or the patient complains of pinching or numbing of the arm, the tourniquet is too tight. Loosen it slightly before proceeding.

Latex Allergy

Latex allergy is becoming increasingly common, and all patients must be asked whether they have a latex allergy. Nonlatex tourniquets and gloves are available and in wide use in hospitals, clinics, and nursing homes. Latex bandages should also be avoided for these patients.

> **«« FLASHBACK**
> You learned about latex allergy in Chapter 3.

PROCEDURE 11-1

Hand Collection Using a Winged Infusion Set

1. **Assemble your equipment.**

   Remove the WIS from the package.
   Straighten out the coiled tubing. Attach the
   WIS to the evacuated tube holder or the
   syringe.

   Insert the first tube. Lay this assembly next to
   the patient's hand. If using a syringe,
   loosen the plunger by pulling the barrel in
   and out.

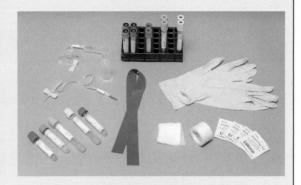

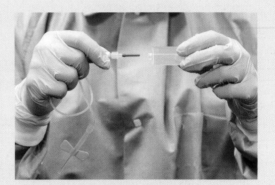

2. **Position the patient's hand, and apply the
   tourniquet.**

   Place the hand in an accessible position. Place
   a support (e.g., a towel) under the wrist,
   and ask the patient to gently curl his or her
   fingers under the hand. Tie the tourniquet
   in the usual manner around the wrist.

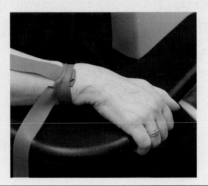

Continued

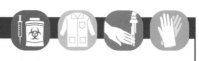

PROCEDURE 11-1—cont'd

Hand Collection Using a Winged Infusion Set

3. **Insert the needle.**

   Choose the largest and straightest vein, and clean the site in the usual manner.

   Anchor the vein firmly with your nondominant hand.

   Grasp the needle between the thumb and the index finger by folding the wings together in the middle.

   Insert the needle into the vein, bevel side up and lined up in the direction of the vein. The angle of insertion should be 10 to 15 degrees.

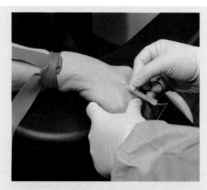

   Once the needle has entered the vein, a flash of blood should appear in the tubing. When using the syringe system, never pull the syringe plunger back if you do not see blood flash in the top of the syringe, as the suction may damage the tissue where the needle tip is positioned.

   Gently thread the needle up the lumen of the vein until the bevel is not visible, keeping the angle shallow.

   Hold the needle in place by one wing with the thumb of the opposite hand.

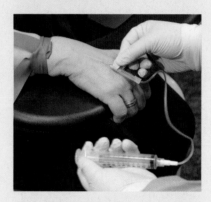

4. **Collect the sample.**

   If you are using evacuated tubes, push the collection tube into the adapter. Blood should appear in the tube. If you are using a syringe, pull the plunger back slowly, only matching the rate at which the blood is flowing into the syringe.

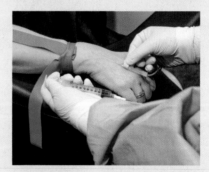

5. **Finish the collection.**

   When the tube is completely filled, release the tourniquet and remove the needle. Activate the needle safety device.

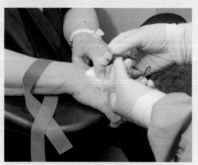

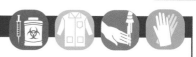

PROCEDURE 11-1—cont'd

Hand Collection Using a Winged Infusion Set

6. **Attend to the patient.**

   Apply pressure to the site, as you would for routine venipuncture.

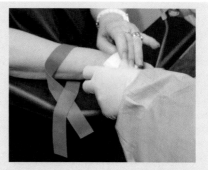

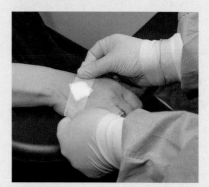

7. **Dispose of the WIS.**

   Special safety precautions must be observed when disposing of the WIS. The entire system should be gathered up in one hand. Leave nothing dangling that could get caught on something or cause an accidental needle-stick injury. Remove the tube from the adapter. Drop the tubing, needle, and the attached adapter into the sharps container.

   If using a syringe, discard the tubing and needle as for a WIS. Attach a needleless blood transfer device to the syringe to transfer the sample to the appropriate evacuated tubes, as outlined in Chapter 9.

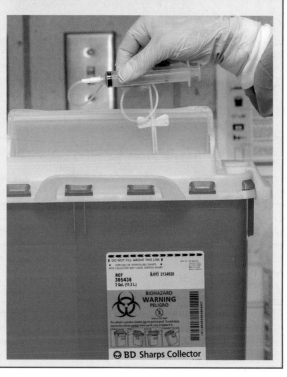

COMPLICATIONS DURING COLLECTION

Changes in Patient Status

In all of the following cases, be sure your patient is in a safe position before leaving the room.

Syncope

Syncope (pronounced "SIN-co-pee") is the medical term for fainting. Before syncope, the patient's skin often feels cold, damp, and clammy, beads of sweat may form on the forehead or upper lip; the patient may state that they are not feeling well, or will stop talking; their eyes may start to roll back, or their head could tilt either forward or backward.. If syncope occurs during the procedure, remove the tourniquet and needle immediately and apply pressure to the site. Fainting is more common with outpatients; inpatients lying in bed are less likely to faint. Outpatient draw areas should be equipped with pillows and blankets to properly respond to this emergency. It is also helpful to ask your patient before the draw if the patient has a history of fainting during a blood draw. Appropriate first aid must be applied. If the patient is conscious but woozy, have the patient lower his or her head between the knees, and apply a cold compress to the neck or forehead. Call a nurse to check the patient's blood pressure, or perform this yourself if you have been trained to do so. If the patient is unconscious, call the nurse immediately. The patient should be safely moved to a recumbent (lying down) position until he or she regains consciousness. All incidents of syncope must be documented.

Seizures

If a patient has a seizure during the procedure, remove the tourniquet and needle immediately and apply pressure to the site. Do not put anything in the patient's mouth; this is of no use during a seizure and can cause injury. Follow your institution procedures for patients having a seizure.

Nausea and Vomiting (Emesis)

When emesis (EM-eh-sis) occurs, reassure the patient and make him or her comfortable. Give the patient an emesis basin, and instruct him or her to breathe slowly and deeply. A wet washcloth for the head is often helpful.

Pain

To prevent the startle reflex, warn the patient before the needle stick that there may be a little poke, pinch, or sting.

Hematoma

When blood oozes from the vein into the surrounding tissue, a hematoma is formed. You can see the skin surrounding the puncture swell up and fill with blood. If this occurs during the procedure, remove the tourniquet and needle immediately and apply pressure to the site. A cool cloth or cold pack can slow swelling from blood and ease pain.

The following are the most common causes of hematoma are:

- Excessive probing to obtain blood
- Failure to insert the needle far enough into the vein
- The needle going through the vein
- Failure to remove the tourniquet before removing the needle
- Inadequate pressure on the site after removal of the needle
- Bending the elbow while applying pressure

> ### ⚠ AVOID THAT ERROR!
>
> For Kevin Masters, the draw for patient Richard Robinson was going great—easy access, great flow, no complaints. Kevin finished drawing the last tube, and placed a gauze pad over the puncture site. As he withdrew the needle, Mr. Robinson suddenly yelled out in pain. "You hurt me!" he said as he clutched his arm. Flustered, all Kevin could manage to reply was, "I do the best I can." He finished up without any more conversation. Five minutes later, Mr. Robinson returned to the outpatient laboratory with a swelling the size of a marble at the puncture site. What went wrong? What should Kevin have done and what should he do now?

Lack of Blood Flow

Lack of blood flow can be caused by a defective tube, an improperly positioned needle, or missing the vein. Intermittent or slow blood flow indicates improper needle position or a collapsed vein.

Defective Evacuated Tube

Occasionally, blood will not flow into a tube because the vacuum in the tube has been depleted. This may occur from a manufacturing defect, use of an expired tube, or a very fine crack (which may occur if the tube is dropped). If the tube has been pushed past the tube advancement mark on the holder before insertion in the vein, the vacuum has been depleted. Always take extra tubes to the bedside or the outpatient area to be prepared for defects or errors. If you find a defective tube, be sure to note the expiration date and lot number. Document this information, and then dispose of the defective tube in the appropriate sharps container immediately. Do not leave a defective tube lying around the draw area for someone else to use!

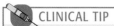 **CLINICAL TIP**

Be careful not to push the tube past the tube advancement mark before you insert the needle into the vein.

Improperly Positioned Needle

If the tube is not the problem, the needle may not be properly positioned in the vein, and you may need to adjust it. When the needle is not in the correct position with respect to the vein, blood flow may stop or may be intermittent. Any one of the following may have occurred:

- The bevel is stuck to the vein wall. Slightly rotate the needle (Figure 11-2).
- The needle has passed through both sides of the vein ("blowing" the vein). Slowly pull back on the needle (Figure 11-3).
- The needle is not advanced far enough into the vein. Slowly advance the needle (Figure 11-4).
- The vein was missed completely. Pull the needle out slightly, palpate to relocate the vein, and redirect the needle (Figure 11-5).
- The tube is too large for the vein, causing the excessive vacuum to pull the vein onto the bevel and block blood flow. Remove the tube, wait a few seconds, and then switch to a smaller-volume tube.

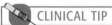 **CLINICAL TIP**

Probing causes pain and hematoma. Do not probe if the needle is positioned incorrectly or if the vein cannot be located by palpation. Instead, repeat the puncture with a new tube and needle.

Collapsed Vein

A collapsed vein is caused by too much vacuum on a small vein. When using the evacuated tube system, a collapsed vein becomes evident when the tube is pushed onto the inner needle. During a syringe collection, it may occur when the plunger is pulled too quickly. Using smaller tubes or pulling the syringe plunger more gently can help prevent collapsed veins. Once a vein collapses, remove the tourniquet, pull out the needle, and select a different vein, or switch to using a butterfly on a hand vein.

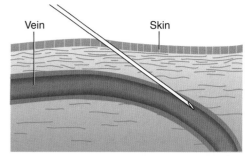

FIGURE 11-2 The bevel is stuck to the vein wall. Slightly rotate the needle.

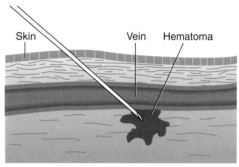

FIGURE 11-3 The needle has passed through both sides of the vein ("blowing" the vein). Slowly pull back on the needle.

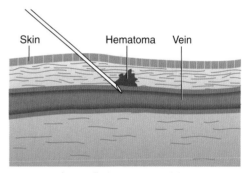

FIGURE 11-4 The needle is not advanced far enough into the vein. Slowly advance the needle.

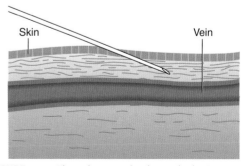

FIGURE 11-5 The vein was missed completely. Remove the tourniquet, pull the needle out slightly, palpate to relocate the vein, and redirect the needle.

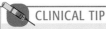

> **CLINICAL TIP**
>
> Moving the needle just a few millimeters up the vein minimizes collapsed veins and the likelihood of blowing the vein.

Inadvertent Puncture of the Artery

Puncture of the artery produces bright red blood and may cause spurting or pulsing of blood into the tube. A patient with a low blood oxygen level may have arterial blood that is darker in color, similar to venous blood. After sample collection and needle withdrawal, you should apply pressure for 10 minutes, and check the site before applying a bandage. The sample may not have to be redrawn, but because some values are different for arterial versus venous blood, label the specimen as an arterial sample. Notify the nurse if the artery was inadvertently punctured.

Failure to Collect on the First Try

The policy at most institutions is that a second try is acceptable. A new needle and tube must be used. For second tries, go below the previous site or use the other arm. After a second unsuccessful try, another phlebotomist should be found to draw blood from the patient.

> **AVOID THAT ERROR!**
>
> When Maria Lombard applied the tourniquet to Josie Burns, she was puzzled. There was no sign of the median cubital vein. She moved on to the cephalic vein, selecting a site and cleaning it. After it dried, she inserted her needle and blood dripped slowly into the tube; at this rate, the collection would take over 5 minutes and the sample would likely still be inadequate. She explained this to Ms. Burns, removed the needle, and inserted it again further up the vein. Still almost no flow. She reapplied the tourniquet, chose a site in the basilic vein, and tried again. This time there was no blood—she must have missed the vein. Well, if at first you don't succeed, she thought. "Hold it right there!" interrupted Ms. Burns. What did Maria do wrong? What should she do now?

PROBLEMS IN COMPLETING THE PROCEDURE

Patient Requests

Sometimes a patient may ask you for water or a change in bed position. Always check with the nurse on duty before you comply with any request.

Prolonged Bleeding

Normally, the site should stop bleeding within 5 minutes. However, aspirin or anticoagulant therapy can prolong bleeding times after the venipuncture

procedure. In all cases, you must continue to apply pressure until the bleeding has stopped. Inform the nurse if the patient has a prolonged bleeding time. Failure to apply adequate pressure, particularly with patients on excessive doses of warfarin (Coumadin) or with a coagulation disorder, can cause compartment syndrome (discussed later in this chapter). In these patients, it is important to apply pressure to the site beyond 5 minutes and ask the patient about any symptoms or significant pain.

FACTORS THAT AFFECT SAMPLE INTEGRITY

Hemolysis

Hemolysis is the destruction of blood cells, resulting in the release of hemoglobin and cellular contents into the plasma. Hemolysis can be caused by a range of factors, as indicated in Box 11-1. The serum or plasma is pinkish or red in a hemolyzed sample due to rupture of red blood cells. Hemolysis interferes with many test results, as shown in Box 11-2. The laboratory may request a redraw if the sample cannot give accurate results for the requested test.

Blood Drawn From a Hematoma

The blood in a hematoma is older than fresh venous blood, and use of such a sample can alter the results of some tests. The most frequent cause of hematoma is improper insertion or removal of the needle, causing blood to leak or be forced into the surrounding tissue.

Patient Position

The position of the patient during collection can affect some test results (Box 11-3) because body

Box 11-1	**Causes of Hemolysis**

- Blood frothing due to a needle improperly attached to a syringe
- Drawing blood too quickly into a syringe
- Excessively shaking or rotating the blood
- Failing to allow the blood to run down the side of the tube when using a syringe to fill the tube
- Forcing blood from a syringe into a vacuum tube
- Using too small a needle with respect to vein size
- Using a needle smaller than 23 gauge (usually, any smaller needle causes hemolysis)
- Using a small needle with a large vacuum tube
- Using a small needle to transfer blood from syringe to tube

Box 11-2	Chemistry and Hematology Tests Affected by Hemolysis

Seriously Affected
- Aspartate aminotransferase
- Potassium
- Lactate dehydrogenase

Moderately Affected
- Alanine aminotransferase
- Complete blood count (CBC)
- Serum iron
- Thyroxine

Slightly Affected
- Acid phosphatase
- Albumin
- Calcium
- Magnesium
- Phosphorus
- Total protein

Box 11-3	Tests Affected by Patient Position

- Albumin
- Bilirubin
- Calcium
- Cell counts
- Cholesterol
- Enzymes
- Hemoglobin or hematocrit
- High-density lipoprotein
- Iron
- Lipids
- Protein
- Triglycerides

fluids shift between the seated and supine positions. The standard position for drawing blood from an outpatient is with the patient seated. In very rare instances a physician may request that an outpatient lie down before specimen collection.

Reflux of Anticoagulant

Reflux is the flow of blood from the collection tube back into the needle and then into the patient's vein. This is rare, but it can occur when the tube contents come in contact with the stopper during the draw. Anticoagulant, as well as blood, may be drawn back into the patient's vein. This is a problem, because some patients have adverse reactions to anticoagulants (e.g., ethylenediaminetetraacetic acid, or EDTA), and loss of additive from the tube can alter test results. It may also result in the contamination

of the next tube with additive from the previous tube. To prevent reflux, keep the patient's arm angled downward so that the tube is always below the site, allowing it to fill from the bottom up. Also, after removing the tourniquet, disengage the tube from the needle before removing the needle from the patient's arm.

LONG-TERM COMPLICATIONS ASSOCIATED WITH VENIPUNCTURE

Iatrogenic Anemia

Iatrogenic anemia is anemia caused by excessive removal of blood at the request of a physician. Removal of as little as 3 or 4 mL of blood per day may result in the development of iron deficiency anemia in some patients. For this reason, it is important to minimize the amount of blood drawn and the frequency of collection. Your institution should have a procedure in place for documenting the total volume of blood drawn from a patient. If a single test is required, it may be appropriate to acquire blood with a dermal puncture instead of venipuncture.

Compartment Syndrome

For patients receiving excessive doses of anticoagulants such as warfarin, or who have a coagulation disorder, such as hemophilia, routine venipuncture may cause bleeding into the tissue surrounding the puncture site. A small amount of blood leads to a hematoma. Larger amounts may cause **compartment syndrome**, a condition in which pressure within the tissue prevents blood from flowing freely in the blood vessels. This causes swelling and pain, and it carries the risk of permanent damage to nerves and other tissues. Severe pain, burning, and numbness may be followed by paralysis distal to the puncture site. The patient should seek immediate medical attention if compartment syndrome is suspected.

Nerve Damage

Nerves in the antecubital area can be damaged if they are contacted with the needle during collection. The patient will experience a shooting pain or "electric shock" sensation down the arm, numbness, or tingling in the fingers. If the patient experiences this type of sensation, immediately remove the needle. The procedure should be performed at another site, preferably in the other arm. This incident should be documented according to your institution's protocol. To prevent nerve damage, avoid excessive or blind probing during venipuncture. *Avoid using the basilic vein whenever possible.*

‹‹↰ FLASHBACK
You learned about nerves in the antecubital area in Chapter 7.

Infection

Infection can be prevented by adhering to venipuncture protocol. Proper aseptic technique before and during collection must be followed. Do not touch the venipuncture site after it has been cleansed. Outpatients should be instructed to leave the bandage in place for at least 15 minutes.

SPECIMEN REJECTION

Specimens may be rejected by the laboratory for a variety of reasons (Box 11-4). Almost all of these can be avoided by proper care before, during, and after the procedure.

SPECIMEN RECOLLECTION

Sometimes, problems with the sample cannot be identified until after testing. In this case another

Box 11-4	**Reasons for Specimen Rejection**

- Clotted blood in an anticoagulated specimen
- Collection in the wrong tube
- Contaminated specimens and containers
- Defective tube
- Hemolysis
- Improper special handling
- Incompletely or inadequately filled tube
- No requisition form
- Unlabeled or mislabeled specimens

Box 11-5	**Reasons for Specimen Recollection**

- Clots in an anticoagulated specimen
- Contaminated specimens and containers
- Hemolysis
- Improper special handling
- Incomplete drying of antiseptic
- Quantity not sufficient (QNS)
- Unlabeled or mislabeled tube
- Use of the wrong antiseptic

sample will have to be collected. Some of the reasons for recollection are shown in Box 11-5.

REVIEW FOR CERTIFICATION

Complications of routine venipuncture may occur from a variety of causes. If the patient is not in the room, locate him or her if possible, especially if the collection is a stat request or for a timed test. Contact the nursing station for missing or improper ID bands. Apprehensive patients may need calming.

If the antecubital fossa is not appropriate due to scarring, burning, or other skin disruptions, use an alternative site such as the dorsal hand. Be aware of the potential for complications from improper tourniquet application. During the collection, remain aware of the patient's status, and be ready to cope with syncope, seizures, nausea, pain, and other responses to the procedure. Keep extra supplies handy in the event of defective tubes or needles. Specimen rejection, or redrawing and retesting, may be necessary due to improper collection, labeling, transport, or other errors.

BIBLIOGRAPHY

CLSI: *Procedures for the collection of diagnostic blood specimens by venipuncture; Approved standard—sixth edition*. CSLI document GP41-A6 (formerly H03-A6). Wayne, Pa., 2007, Clinical and Laboratory Standards Institute.

CLSI: *Procedures for the handling and processing of blood specimens for common laboratory tests; Approved guideline—fourth edition*. CSLI document GP44-A4 (formerly H18-A4). Wayne, Pa., 2010, Clinical and Laboratory Standards Institute.

Lusky K: Safety net: Juggling the gains, losses of phlebotomy routines. *CAP Today,* 2004.

Masoorli S: Caution: Nerve injuries during venipuncture, *Nurs Spectr,* 2006. Retrieved from ews.nurse.com/apps/pbcs.dll/article?AID=2005505010320.

Roberge RJ, McLane M: Compartment syndrome after simple venipuncture in an anticoagulated patient, *J Emer Med* 17: 647–649, 1999.

WHAT WOULD YOU DO?

When a physician enters a patient's room to consult with the patient, you should leave until they are done. The physician may be brusque or hurried, but he or she is in charge of the patient's care and the phlebotomist must comply with the request. If the needle is already in place, you may ask the physician for a few minutes to finish up because this will likely be more comfortable and safer for the patient than redrawing a second time. Even then, the physician may choose to have you leave and return later.

AVOID THAT ERROR!

Kevin likely damaged the vein while withdrawing the needle. This can happen if the needle is accidently pushed in at first, or if the tube is lifted away from the skin before the needle is completely removed. The damage causes pain and accumulation of blood, forming a hematoma. Kevin needed to pay as much attention to withdrawing the needle as he did to inserting it. Now, he should apologize, contact his supervisor, and make sure that Mr. Robinson gets treatment for the hematoma.

 AVOID THAT ERROR!

Maria may not have done anything wrong in her first two attempts—some patients are harder than others to draw from. But two attempts is the limit at most institutions; after that, she should have stopped and called her supervisor or a more experienced phlebotomist to complete the draw.

STUDY QUESTIONS

See answers in Appendix F.

1. What must be done if the patient is not in the room when you come to collect a specimen?

2. What hospital protocol is followed when you are supposed to draw blood from a patient who is not wearing an ID bracelet?

3. How is an unconscious patient approached for blood collection?

4. Name six potential barriers to communicating with a patient.

5. Define hemolysis.

6. Define occluded, and describe what occluded veins feel like.

7. Describe where the tourniquet is applied when performing a dorsal hand stick.

8. What antiseptic must be used when collecting for a blood alcohol test?

9. List four things that can cause hemoconcentration.

10. What symptoms might a patient exhibit immediately before syncope?

11. How can you correct the position of a needle whose bevel has stuck to the vein wall?

12. What can cause a vein to collapse during a blood draw?

13. How many venipuncture attempts by a phlebotomist are usually considered acceptable?

14. How can a phlebotomist prevent reflux of an additive during collection?

15. List five reasons specimens may be rejected.

CERTIFICATION EXAMINATION PREPARATION

See answers in Appendix F.

1. If a stat test is ordered and the patient is not in his or her room, you should
   a. wait in the patient's room until he or she returns.
   b. leave the request at the nurse's station for the nurse to perform the draw.
   c. locate the patient.
   d. postpone the collection.

2. Which laboratory department may require special patient ID?
   a. Microbiology
   b. Chemistry
   c. Hematology
   d. Blood bank

3. Collapsed veins can be caused by
  a. too large a needle for the vein.
  b. too much vacuum asserted on the vessel.
  c. the plunger being pulled too quickly.
  d. All of the above.

4. When an artery is inadvertently stuck during collection, which of the following statements is not true?
  a. The sample should be labeled as usual.
  b. The blood may be bright red.
  c. The blood may spurt or pulse into the tube.
  d. Pressure should be applied for 10 minutes.

5. Which of the following could be a cause of hemolysis?
  a. Vigorously mixing the tubes
  b. Allowing the blood to run down the side of a tube when using a syringe to fill the tube
  c. Drawing blood too slowly into a syringe
  d. Using a needle larger than 23 gauge

6. Reasons for specimen recollection include all of the following except:
  a. incomplete drying of the antiseptic.
  b. using the wrong antiseptic.
  c. prolonged bleeding after needle withdrawal.
  d. contamination by powder from gloves.

7. To avoid reflux of an anticoagulant, you should do all of the following except:
  a. keep the patient's arm elevated above the heart.
  b. allow the tube to fill from the bottom up.
  c. remove the last tube from the needle before removing the tourniquet.
  d. remove the last tube from the needle before removing the needle.

8. Conditions that may alter the quality of a specimen or cause harm to the patient during a blood draw include the following:
  a. edematous tissue.
  b. mastectomies.
  c. hematomas.
  d. All of the above

9. When performing a butterfly draw using a hand vein,
  a. place the tourniquet on the patient's arm above the antecubital fossa.
  b. place the tourniquet on the patient's arm below the antecubital fossa.
  c. place the tourniquet on the patient's wrist.
  d. a tourniquet is not required.

10. Povidone–iodine is not recommended for
  a. blood alcohol draws.
  b. dermal punctures.
  c. blood gas draws.
  d. blood cultures.

11. Hemolysis is
  a. the flow of blood from the collection tube back into the needle and the patient's vein.
  b. alteration in the ratio of elements in the blood.
  c. lack of lymph fluid movement.
  d. destruction of blood cells.

12. Which test result is not affected by patient position?
  a. Albumin
  b. Blood alcohol
  c. Cholesterol
  d. Enzymes

13. Lymphostasis is
  a. the flow of blood from the collection tube back into the needle and the patient's vein.
  b. alteration in the ratio of elements in the blood.
  c. lack of lymph fluid movement.
  d. destruction of blood cells.

14. To enhance vein prominence, you can
  a. elevate the arm in an upward position.
  b. tap the antecubital area with your index and middle finger.
  c. squeeze the patient's wrist.
  d. apply a cold pack.

15. Hemoconcentration is
  a. the flow of blood from the collection tube back into the needle and the patient's vein.
  b. alteration in the ratio of elements in the blood.
  c. lack of lymph fluid movement.
  d. destruction of blood cells.

Four special populations—pediatric patients, geriatric patients, patients requiring chronic blood draws, and patients in the emergency room/emergency department (ER/ED) or intensive care unit (ICU)—have special needs and require special knowledge and procedures to collect blood safely and considerately. In young children, loss of blood volume and the child's fear of the procedure are paramount concerns. In geriatric patients, skin changes and the possible presence of hearing loss or mental impairment are important considerations. Patients with certain diseases require regular blood tests for an extended or indefinite period, and the sites commonly used for drawing blood may become damaged from overuse. Patients in the ER or ICU may have vascular access devices or intravenous (IV) lines in place. Only specially trained personnel can draw blood from these devices on a physician's order, but the phlebotomist may be called on to assist in the draw or handle the samples during and after collection. Each of these special populations requires approaches and equipment beyond those needed for routine blood collection. By understanding these special requirements, you will gain the skills you need to collect blood from the widest possible patient population.

OUTLINE

OBJECTIVES

After completing this chapter, you should be able to:

1. Describe two physiologic differences between children and adults that should be considered when collecting blood from infants and children.
2. Describe steps that can be taken to help reduce a child's anxiety and make the venipuncture experience more pleasant.
3. Explain how blood collection supplies and the venipuncture procedure are modified for infants and children.
4. List the steps in dorsal hand venipuncture in children.
5. Define bilirubin, explain its significance, and describe precautions that must be observed when collecting blood for bilirubin testing.

6. Explain the usual procedure for collecting blood for neonatal screening tests, and list five tests that may be done.
7. Explain physical changes that may occur with aging that should be considered when collecting blood.
8. List conditions that may require blood draws for an extended period and alternative collection sites for patients with such conditions.
9. Define vascular access device, and describe eight types.
10. Describe how blood should be collected from a vascular access device.
11. List steps to be followed when collecting blood from a patient with an intravenous line in place.

KEY TERMS

arterial line	central venous line	homocystinuria	peripherally inserted
arteriovenous (AV) shunt	external arteriovenous	hypothyroidism	central catheter (PICC)
Bili light	(AV) shunt	implanted port	phenylketonuria (PKU)
bilirubin	fistula	internal arteriovenous	saline lock
biotinidase deficiency	galactosemia	(AV) shunt	sickle cell anemia
Broviac	Groshong	jaundice	triple lumen
central venous	heparin lock	kernicterus	vascular access
catheter (CVC)	Hickman	maple syrup disease	device (VAD)

ABBREVIATIONS

AV arteriovenous
CVC central venous catheter
EMLA eutectic mixture of local anesthetics
ER, ED emergency room, emergency department
HIV human immunodeficiency virus
ICU intensive care unit
ID identification
IV intravenous

LTC long-term care
PICC peripherally inserted central catheter
PKU phenylketonuria
RBCs red blood cells
stat short turnaround time
TLC tender loving care
VAD vascular access device
WBC white blood cell

WHAT WOULD YOU DO?

Even before you enter room 323 in the pediatric wing of Mount Sinai Hospital, you know your next draw may be a challenge. A young child is wailing and a parent is loudly telling the child to quiet down "or else." As you enter the room, you can see the child—your patient—is afraid and uncertain, but he has stopped crying for the moment, distracted by your entrance. The mother turns to you and says, "Look, I can't stay here—I can't stand the sight of blood." Should you proceed with the draw? Should you insist that the mother stay in the room? What would you do?

PEDIATRIC PATIENTS

Collecting blood from pediatric patients presents both technical and psychological challenges. Because greater technical expertise is required to perform phlebotomy on children than on adults, you should master your collection methods on adult patients first. Similarly, you should master collection in older children before moving on to young children and infants.

Special Physiologic Considerations

Children have a lower total blood volume than adults do. The younger (and smaller) the child, the lower the volume that can be safely withdrawn. For example, a 150-lb adult has about 5 L of blood, so a 10-mL sample represents about 0.2% of total blood volume. In contrast, that same sample from a 1-year-old represents 1% of total blood volume, and in a newborn about 3%. Removal of more than 10% of total blood volume can cause cardiac arrest.

Repeated withdrawal of even smaller amounts may cause iatrogenic anemia. Infants and children should not have more than 5% of their blood volume removed within a 24-hour period unless medically necessary. Removal of 3% or less is the preferred maximum. No more than 10% should be removed over a 1-month period unless medically necessary. Table 12-1 provides guidelines for determining safe volumes that may be withdrawn.

 CLINICAL TIP

When collecting blood from a child, log the time and the volume of blood taken to avoid blood depletion.

Dermal puncture requires a very small amount of blood and is the most common pediatric collection procedure. However, it cannot be used when a larger volume of blood is required, such as for blood

TABLE 12-1   Blood Volume and Safe Withdrawal Calculations in Newborns and Infants

Age	Approximate Blood Volume per Body Weight	Patient Weight	Maximum Safe Withdrawal (3%)		Safe Volume for Withdrawal in 24 hr
Premature neonate	95 mL/kg	_____	× 0.03	=	_____
Full-term neonate	85 mL/kg	_____	× 0.03	=	_____
Newborn	80 mL/kg	_____	× 0.03	=	_____
1- to 12-month-old	75 mL/kg	_____	× 0.03	=	_____
Example: 7-lb newborn	80 mL/kg	3.2 kg	× 0.03	=	7.68 mL

culture or cross-match testing or for coagulation testing. For blood culture in infants and small children, a sample of 1 to 5 mL is required. Consult with the laboratory's procedures manual for specific information on minimum draw volumes in infants.

Newborns also have a higher proportion of red blood cells (RBCs) than adults do (60% versus 45%) and a lower proportion of plasma (40% versus 55%), so more blood may be needed to obtain enough serum or plasma for testing.

Newborns and infants are also more susceptible to infection, because of the immaturity of their immune systems. Extra precautions should be taken to avoid exposing this group to potential sources of infection. Protective isolation procedures, discussed in Chapter 4, are often used.

Special Psychological Considerations

Children differ in their levels of understanding, ability to cooperate, and anxiety about medical procedures. For many children, needles represent pain, and their fear of pain often makes the collection procedure challenging for the phlebotomist. In addition to the fear of pain, children may be anxious about being in a hospital and away from home. Some children associate a white coat with all these fears, and seeing any stranger in a white coat enter the room can increase their anxiety level even before they see a needle.

As a phlebotomist, your goal is to make the collection as calm, comfortable, and painless as possible for the child (Figure 12-1). Keeping the child calm not only helps the child but also helps you carry out the procedure. Prolonged crying also affects the white blood cell (WBC) count and the pH level of the blood; therefore a calm experience ensures accurate test results.

Several strategies can be used to reduce the child's anxiety. Not all of them work for every child, and some are more appropriate for children of certain ages or dispositions. As you gain experience,

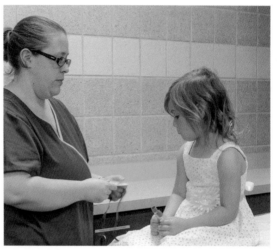

FIGURE 12-1 It is important that a phlebotomist use a calming approach with children.

you will be able to gauge how to best approach each child. You can do the following to minimize the child's anxiety:

- Prepare your equipment ahead of time, before you encounter the child. This means less time for the child's anxiety to build before the stick.
- If possible, perform the procedure in a room that is not the child's hospital room such as a procedure room. This allows the child to feel safe in his or her bed.
- Be friendly, cheerful, and empathetic. Use a soothing tone of voice.
- Explain what you will be doing in terms that are appropriate for the child's age. Even if the child will not or cannot respond, your explanation helps the child understand what is about to happen, lessening the fear of the unknown. Demonstrating on a toy can be helpful.
- Do not say that it will not hurt. Rather, explain that it will hurt a little bit and that it is okay to say "ouch" or even to yell or cry, but emphasize the need to keep the arm still.

- Give the child choices whenever possible to increase his or her feeling of control. You can ask the child which arm or finger to use or which type of bandage he or she prefers. This also keeps the child occupied, lessening anxiety.
- Use the shortest possible needle for the procedure, and keep it out of sight for as long as possible.
- Distract the child just before the actual stick so that he or she is looking away. If parents or siblings are in the room, they can be helpful here.
- During the draw, tell the child how much longer it will be ("just one more tube" or "a few more seconds"). This can help keep the child's anxiety from building during the procedure.
- Afterward, praise the child (even if he or she did not cooperate as well as you had hoped) and offer him or her a small reward, such as a sticker (for younger children) or a pencil (for older children).

Involvement of Parents and Siblings

Parents who are present during the procedure can help in several ways. Ask the parent whether the child has had blood drawn previously and, if so, what techniques helped ease the child's anxiety. Parents or siblings can help distract and comfort the child. Siblings should be offered small rewards as well.

Some parents may prefer not to remain with the child during the procedure because they are reluctant to see the child in pain or become queasy at the sight of blood. Respect their wishes. In some cases, parents can make the child more anxious through their words or reactions. If you feel that the parents cannot help the child, you can politely suggest that they might be more comfortable waiting outside. If the child needs restraining, check your employer's policy regarding the use of restraints.

Identification of Newborns

On their identification (ID) bracelets, newborns may be identified only by their last names, such as "Baby Boy (or Girl) Smith." As always, use the hospital ID number, not the name, as the ultimate proof of ID. Be especially careful with twins, who are likely to have similar names and ID numbers.

Supplies

When performing venipuncture, use shorter needles, if possible, and use the smallest gauge consistent with the requirements of the tests. Butterfly needles and smaller, partial-fill tubes should be used for pediatric draws.

You will need additional protective equipment in the premature nursery (and possibly in the full-term nursery) to reduce the risk of spreading infection. Check with the nursery supervisor regarding policy.

Take along a selection of rewards, such as stickers or small toys. Keep a stock of cartoon bandages as well. In a pinch, you can draw a smiley face on a regular bandage. Remember not to use these on infants younger than 2 years because of the danger of choking.

Anesthetics

Topical anesthetic cream may be useful for venipuncture procedures in pediatric patients. The most commonly used agent is EMLA (eutectic mixture of local anesthetics), a mixture of lidocaine and prilocaine. It must be applied 60 minutes before the draw, however, which means that the site must be chosen at that time. It is possible to numb more than one area if it is not practical to choose the site ahead of time. Anesthetic is not recommended for **phenylketonuria (PKU)** testing (described later). Some states and institutions do not allow phlebotomists to apply any medication—check with your institution first.

Immobilization of Infants and Children

Immobilizing pediatric patients may be necessary to ensure their safety during the draw. Wrapping newborns or very young infants in a receiving blanket is usually sufficient, as they are not strong enough to work themselves loose during the procedure. Older babies, toddlers, and young children need to be restrained. Know your employer's restraint policy. Older children may have the self-control to keep from moving, but a parent's care and attention can still be beneficial during the draw.

Pediatric draws are done with the patient either seated in the lap of a parent or other assistant or lying down, with the parent or assistant leaning over the child. For a seated child, the parent hugs the child's body, crosses his or her legs around the child's legs to prevent kicking and holds the arm not being used in the draw (Figure 12-2, *A*). For a child lying down, the parent or assistant leans over the child, holding the unused arm securely (Figure 12-2, *B*). The assistant may support the arm from behind, at the bend in the elbow, which helps immobilize the arm.

Pediatric Dermal Puncture

The procedures for dermal puncture were discussed in Chapter 10. As you learned in that chapter, heel

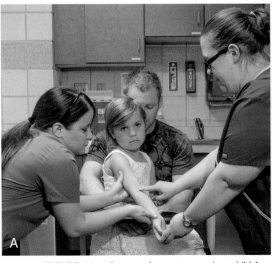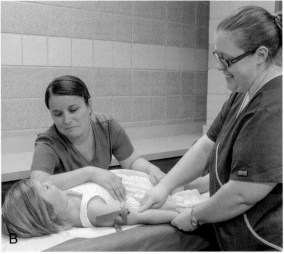

FIGURE 12-2 Suggested ways to restrain a child for phlebotomy. **A,** Hugging the child's body and holding the arm not being used in the draw. **B,** Obtaining a draw from a restrained child in a lying-down position.

puncture is preferred for children younger than 1 year, because the tissue overlying the finger bones is not thick enough for safe collection there. Safe areas for heel collection are diagrammed in Figure 10-6.

Special Considerations

Several special considerations apply when performing dermal punctures in newborns and young children:

- The ID band must be present on the infant. Be sure to match the ID number to the number on the requisition.
- Keep your equipment out of the patient's reach.
- Warm the heel for 3 to 5 minutes, using a heel-warmer packet. The packet contains sodium thiosulfate and glycerin, which undergo a chemical reaction when activated by squeezing. Wrap the packet in a towel before placing it against the skin.
- At the end of the procedure, be sure to remove all equipment from the crib and secure all bed rails in the up position.
- Avoid using adhesive bandages.
- Document the collection in the nursery log sheet. Record the date, time, and volume of blood collected.

Special Dermal Puncture Procedures
Neonatal Bilirubin

Bilirubin is a substance produced by the normal breakdown of RBCs. The liver is responsible for further processing of bilirubin so that it does not reach excessive levels in the blood. In newborns, the liver may not be developed enough to prevent bilirubin from accumulating in the blood. When this occurs, blood must be collected to assess the patient's clinical response to treatment to decrease bilirubin blood levels.

Excess bilirubin levels commonly occur when mother and child have mismatched blood groups and antibodies from the mother break down the infant's RBCs, increasing bilirubin levels beyond the infant's capacity to process it. Buildup of bilirubin causes **jaundice**, or yellowing of the skin, and can lead to brain damage if untreated, a condition called **kernicterus**.

When bilirubin is slightly above normal in a newborn, a **Bili light**, or ultraviolet light treatment, can be used. Higher levels, or levels that are rising rapidly, require blood transfusion.

Collection Precautions. Keep the following points in mind when collecting blood for bilirubin testing:

- Bilirubin is light sensitive. Bili lights should be turned off during collection. The specimen should be shielded from light using an amber-colored container, foil, or heavy paper to cover the container. Once the specimen is collected and shielded from the light, turn the Bili light back on.
- Hemolysis of the specimen falsely lowers the results, so precautions against hemolysis must be taken.
- Collection times must be recorded exactly to track the rate of bilirubin increase. Samples for

bilirubin testing are frequently collected as timed or short turnaround time (stat) specimens.

Neonatal Screening

Neonatal screening tests are required as a part of mandatory, state-based public health programs. The tests are used to detect inherited metabolic disorders that cause severe brain damage or other impairments, and allow for implementation of early intervention treatments. In 2006 the American College of Medical Genetics recommended standardization of 29 core conditions to be tested for in all infants. The 29 core conditions were adopted the same year by the U.S. Secretary of Health and Human Services. These tests include screening for **hypothyroidism** and PKU. Other diseases screened for include **galactosemia**, **homocystinuria**, **maple syrup disease**, and **biotinidase deficiency**. **Sickle cell anemia** is an inherited disorder of the hemoglobin molecule that may also be screened for in newborns from ethnic groups with the highest risk. Each state has the authority to determine what additional tests will be included with the 29 core conditions.

Specimen Collection. Blood for neonatal screening is collected by capillary heel stick on special filter paper. Recent studies have shown that the levels of phenylalanine are significantly different between capillary and venous samples. Reference values are based on capillary values.

The filter paper is supplied in a kit provided by the state agency responsible for screening tests (Figure 12-3, *A*). Both the ink and the paper are biologically inactive. When using the paper, do not touch or contaminate the area inside the circles, because this will alter the results.

To collect a sample for neonatal screening, first perform a routine heel stick. Wipe away the first drop of blood, and then apply one large drop of blood directly to the circle. The drop must be evenly spread (Figure 12-3, *B*). Do not touch the paper against the puncture site, and do not apply successive drops onto a single circle. Although applied to only one side of the filter paper, the blood should be visible from both sides. Air-dry the specimen on a dry, clean, flat, horizontal non-absorbent surface for a minimum of three hours. Keep it at room temperature and away from direct sunlight until it is delivered to the laboratory.

Causes for rejection include:
- Use of expired specimen collection card
- Collection date missing
- QNS (quantity not sufficient) blood submitted

- Blood not completely soaked through the filter paper
- Contaminated or discolored specimen
- Blood is caked, clotted, or layered on the filter paper circles
- Patient demographic information missing
- Form number does not match that of the blood circles
- Specimen is too old on receipt (received 14 or more days after collection)
- Requisition form received but no blood sample
- Specimen submitted on improper collection form
- Improper drying or collection resulting in serum separation
- Specimen torn or damaged during transit
- Laboratory accident

Venipuncture in Newborns

When a larger volume of blood is required, blood can be collected from newborns or children younger than 2 years by venipuncture of the dorsal hand veins. Special considerations include the following:
- No tourniquet is needed. Instead, clasp the infant's wrist between your middle finger and forefinger, and allow the infant to encircle your thumb with his or her fingers. Flex the wrist gently downward while you examine the dorsal surface of the hand.
- Using a 23-gauge needle, gently insert the needle 3 to 5 mm distal to the vein, slowly advancing until you see blood in the hub of the needle
- Once blood begins to flow, you can release your hold on the needle and use your free hand to pull gently on the syringe. An alternative to using a syringe and tubes is to let the blood freely flow in to appropriate microtainer tubes.
- After withdrawing the needle, apply firm pressure with sterile gauze until the bleeding stops. Do not apply a bandage because the child may remove it and put it in his or her mouth.
- Follow the procedure for using a blood transfer device to fill required tubes and dispose of used devices.
- Record volume of blood collected per your facility's protocol.

Scalp vein venipuncture can be used when other venipuncture sites are not accessible. The scalp vein is located by applying a large rubber-band tourniquet around the scalp at the level of the forehead and shaving the hair, if necessary. This procedure requires additional training and expertise.

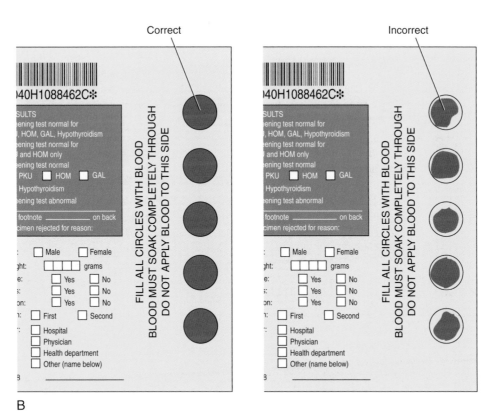

FIGURE 12-3 Neonatal screening tests. **A,** An example of filter paper used in neonatal screening. **B,** Correct and incorrect ways to fill in the circles. (Modified from Bonewit-West K: *Clinical procedures for medical assistants,* ed. 7, Philadelphia, 2008, Saunders.)

GERIATRIC PATIENTS

With the aging of the population, many of your patients are likely to be geriatric patients. As with infants, collection from geriatric patients presents both physical and psychological challenges. Working with geriatric patients also can bring considerable rewards for phlebotomists who take the time to get to know their patients as people.

You are likely to encounter geriatric patients in all types of facilities, from outpatient clinics to acute treatment hospital wards to long-term care (LTC) facilities, such as nursing homes, assisted living facilities, and rehabilitation settings. Geriatric patients are also the most likely clients in adult daycare settings and home care. Patients in LTC facilities are often coping with the special challenges that have led to the need for institutionalization. These challenges may include chronic illness, loss of mobility, or cognitive impairment or dementia. For some patients, institutionalization may engender feelings of anger, confusion, combativeness, or hopelessness. As a medical professional, your job includes adjusting to the challenges such patients may pose, with professionalism and compassion.

Geriatric patients may feel less in control of their medical situations than other patients do, and some may feel apprehensive about having you perform a collection. As you would with any patient, treat your geriatric patients with consideration for their special concerns and needs. A little extra tender loving care (TLC) goes a long way in this population (Figure 12-4). You can help ease their anxiety by being friendly, empathetic, and cheerful. Taking the time to listen to your patients and to talk with

them can make the experience not only easier for both of you but also more rewarding.

Physical Changes

As people age, their bodies undergo a number of changes that may have an impact on the safety and effectiveness of normal collection procedures. Skin changes are among the most important. The amount of collagen in the skin is reduced, so the skin becomes less elastic, and the layers of skin become thinner. Bruising is more likely, and it takes longer to replace cells, so longer healing times are needed.

> **CLINICAL TIP**
>
> Treat the skin of geriatric patients gently. Try massaging the site. Never slap the arm for a vein. A bandage may tear the skin when removed. Apply paper tape over the gauze instead.

Blood vessels, too, become less elastic and more fragile. Vessels may narrow because of atherosclerosis. Loss of supporting connective tissue leads to "loose skin," and loss of muscle tissue may allow veins to move from their usual locations, so the skin needs to be held very taut when anchoring the vein during venipuncture. Veins also are often closer to the skin; therefore, the penetration angle of the needle needs to be reduced.

Arteries are often closer to the surface in geriatric patients. Do not mistake an artery near the surface for a vein. Before sticking it, check your target "vein" to make sure it is not pulsing.

Common Disorders

Many conditions in geriatric patients may lead to the need for assistance in the draw, whether from other staff or from a family member.

Hearing loss is common among geriatric patients. Begin your encounter with a patient by speaking slowly and deliberately to be sure the patient understands. (However, do not continue using this style once the patient clearly indicates that he or she understands your normal speaking voice.)

Visual impairment is common, and may impair the patient's ability to comply quickly or easily with your requests. Such a patient may need guidance in finding the drawing chair, or returning to the hospital bed before a draw, for instance.

A number of conditions, including Parkinson's disease and stroke, can lead to unclear speech. Remember that difficulty speaking does not imply

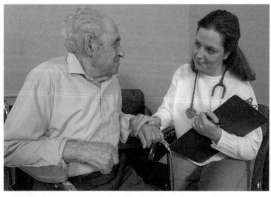

FIGURE 12-4 Phlebotomists should always be considerate to and respectful of geriatric patients.

difficulty understanding. Arthritis affects a large percentage of geriatric patients. Arthritis may prevent your patient from fully straightening his or her arm or fingers. Do not force a patient's arm flat; ask if the patient can do this or whether the action is uncomfortable. When the arm cannot be straightened, a butterfly may be useful in the antecubital area.

Many patients may be on anticoagulant therapy for previous heart attacks or strokes. Be aware of this possibility, especially because of the delay in clotting time it is likely to cause. These patients have an increased risk of hematoma.

Poor nutrition or chronic degenerative disease may lead to emaciation. Nutritional status can affect skin health, hemostasis, and ability to tolerate blood loss. Geriatric patients also may have increased susceptibility to infection due to disease or loss of immune function with age.

Tremor is common in advanced old age and may make it difficult for the patient to hold his or her arm steady during the blood collection process.

Mental Impairment

Forgetfulness, confusion, and dementia are more common among geriatric patients. These patients may have difficulty communicating and complying with requests and may also be combative. Assistance from a nurse or nursing assistant may be necessary, depending on the patient's mood and condition.

Use the wristband, not the patient's response, to confirm patient ID. Some patients may be in restraints to prevent them from hurting themselves or others. Be aware of your facility's policy for use of restraints. Always check with a nurse before loosening restraints.

Special Considerations for Blood Collection

Identifying the Patient

Be especially careful with patient ID. Rely on the ID bracelet if there is any doubt that the patient understands you.

Limiting Blood Loss and Bruising

Be aware of the frequency of blood draws because the risk for anemia is higher in geriatric patients. If possible, use a dermal puncture to reduce blood loss and bruising; however, poor circulation may make this inadvisable. Be especially gentle when applying pressure to the finger to avoid bruising.

Applying the Tourniquet

If you are performing venipuncture, you can apply the tourniquet over clothing to limit bruising. Do not apply the tourniquet as tightly as you would normally, because veins in geriatric patients collapse more easily, and release the tourniquet immediately after inserting the needle.

Locating the Vein

To improve access and comfort, place the arm on a pillow and have the patient grip a washcloth while the arm is supported on either side by rolled towels. Do not "slap" the arm to find a vein; rather, gently massage the area for several minutes to warm it and improve blood flow. The antecubital fossa may not be the best site. If it is not, look for veins in other locations.

Performing the Puncture

Anchor the vein firmly, as veins have a tendency to roll more easily in geriatric patients. Use a smaller needle or a butterfly and smaller tubes for more fragile veins. Do not probe to find the vein. After completing the venipuncture, apply pressure longer to ensure that bleeding has stopped.

PATIENTS REQUIRING BLOOD DRAWS FOR EXTENDED PERIODS

Patients with certain conditions require regular blood testing over an extended, possibly indefinite, period. Box 12-1 lists some of the most common conditions. Frequent blood drawing in these patients often causes the most commonly used sites to become damaged from overuse. The veins may become hardened and difficult to penetrate with the needle, and the skin may develop scar tissue. In some diseases, the trauma to the skin from

---

BOX 12-1	**Conditions Requiring Blood Draws for Extended Periods**

- Anticoagulant therapy
- Hepatitis C infection
- HIV infection
- IV drug use
- Leukemia
- Other chronic infections
- Sickle cell disease
- Terminal cancers

frequent needle puncture may cause it to become delicate and easily torn. Oncology patients present an added challenge since chemotherapy protocols are given by IV. These treatments cause additional trauma to the veins and skin, making venipuncture more difficult.

For these patients, try to minimize damage to the veins by frequently rotating the sites from which you draw and using the smallest needle consistent with the tests required. Consider alternative sites, such as on the forearm, on the underside of the arm, and on the wrist or fingers. If the antecubital vein has already been damaged from overuse, switch to these sites rather than attempting another draw from the damaged area.

SPECIAL EQUIPMENT USED IN THE INTENSIVE CARE UNIT AND EMERGENCY ROOM

Patients in the ICU or ER are likely to have some type of **vascular access device (VAD)** or indwelling line in place that may affect your collection. A VAD is a tube that is inserted into either a vein or an artery and is used to administer fluids or medications, monitor blood pressure, or draw blood.

Blood collection from a VAD is done only by trained personnel on the physician's order. The phlebotomist may be asked to assist with the collection or handle the sample after collection. Understanding the types of devices and the requirements they impose will improve your ability to work in these areas.

Types of Vascular Access Devices

The name of the VAD is based on the location of the tubing in the vascular system. A **central venous catheter (CVC)**, also called a **central venous line**, is the most common type of VAD. *Central* refers to the large veins emptying into the heart, into which the CVC is inserted. CVCs are most commonly inserted into the subclavian vein and then pushed into the superior vena cava, proximal to the right atrium (Figure 12-5). Access is gained through the several inches of tubing that sit outside the entry site. Types of CVCs include **Broviac**, **Groshong**, **Hickman**, and **triple lumen**.

An **implanted port** is a chamber located under the skin and connected to an indwelling line. This reduces the risk of infection. To access this device, a noncoring needle is inserted through the

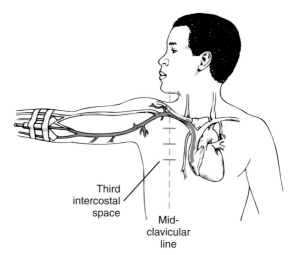

FIGURE 12-5 Central venous catheters are most commonly inserted into the subclavian vein and then pushed into the superior vena cava, proximal to the right atrium. (From Elkin MK, Perry AG, Potter PA: *Nursing interventions and clinical skills,* ed. 2, St. Louis, 2000, Mosby.)

skin into the chamber, through a self-sealing septum.

A **peripherally inserted central catheter (PICC)** is threaded into a central vein after insertion into a peripheral (noncentral) vein, usually the basilic or cephalic, accessed from the antecubital area. PICCs are most commonly used in angioplasty procedures, in which the lumen of an obstructed central vein is rewidened. They are not used for drawing blood, however, because the tubing collapses easily when aspirated.

An **arterial line** is placed in an artery for continuous monitoring of blood pressure or frequent collection of samples for blood gas testing. The radial artery is the most common site; the brachial, axillary, and femoral arteries are alternative sites.

A **heparin lock** or **saline lock** is a tube temporarily placed in a peripheral vein to administer medicine or draw blood. A winged infusion or IV catheter set connected to the tubing provides the venous access; the other end has a port with a rubber septum through which a needle can pass. These devices are most commonly inserted in the lower arm just above the wrist and may be left in place up to 48 hours (Figure 12-6). To prevent a clot from blocking the line, it is flushed with either saline or heparin just before and after the procedure. Saline is becoming the more frequent choice over heparin.

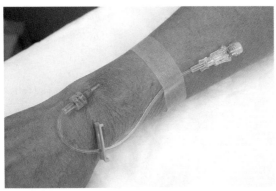

FIGURE 12-6 A heparin lock in place. (From Perry AG, Potter PA: *Clinical nursing skills and techniques,* ed. 7, St Louis, 2010, Mosby.)

An **arteriovenous (AV) shunt** is an artificial connection between an artery and a vein. AV shunts in the lower arm are used for dialysis patients to provide access for blood removal, purification, and return. Venipuncture should not be performed on an arm with an AV shunt. Nor should the arm be used for taking blood pressure or for any other procedure that would impair circulation.

An **external AV shunt** consists of a cannula with a rubber septum through which a needle may be inserted for drawing blood. An **internal AV shunt** consists of a **fistula**, or permanent internal connection between the artery and the vein, using the patient's tissue, a piece of bovine tissue, or a synthetic tube. An arm containing a fistula is used for phlebotomy procedures only with the physician's permission.

Drawing From a Vascular Access Device

As stated earlier, only specially trained personnel can draw blood from a VAD and usually only with the physician's order. Important considerations in the procedure include the following:

- Never use a syringe larger than 20 mL, because pulling on the plunger can create enough vacuum to collapse the line.
- VADs are often periodically flushed with heparin to keep the line open. For this reason, the first sample of blood collected through the line should not be used. The amount discarded depends on the dead-space volume in the line, the sample type, and the type of VAD. For noncoagulation specimens, discard twice the dead-space volume. For coagulation specimens, discard six times the dead-space volume, or 5 mL.

- The order of draw should be blood cultures, anticoagulated tubes, and then clotted tubes.

Working With Intravenous Lines

When a patient has an IV line in place in one arm, blood should be drawn from the other arm whenever possible. If this is impossible, or if there are lines in both arms, the following points should be kept in mind:

- Have the nurse turn off the IV drip before the draw for the appropriate amount of time for the IV to clear of medications. This may take from 2 to 15 minutes.
- Apply a tourniquet distal to the IV insertion site.
- Select a vein distal to the IV insertion site and different from the vein with the IV line.
- Discard the first 5 mL of blood, because it will be contaminated with the IV fluid.
- Note on the requisition that the specimen was drawn from an arm with an IV line, identify the IV solution, and note how long the drip was turned off.
- Once the draw is completed, notify the nurse so that the IV drip can be turned on.

REVIEW FOR CERTIFICATION

Special considerations apply when drawing blood from pediatric patients, geriatric patients, patients requiring chronic blood draws, and patients in the ER or ICU. Dermal puncture is the most common way to obtain samples from newborns and small children, as this minimizes blood loss. Dorsal hand or scalp venipuncture may be needed for larger blood volumes. Children's fears may be eased by a calm, soothing, and empathetic manner. Skin and vein changes are a prominent concern in geriatric patients, and careful technique is required to avoid bruising or collapsing the vein. The potential for hearing or vision loss or mental impairment should be considered, but do not assume that a geriatric patient is impaired without evidence. In patients requiring chronic draws, such as those with human immunodeficiency virus (HIV) or cancer, rotate collection sites to avoid damaging veins and tissue. ER and ICU patients are likely to have some type of VAD in place. Collection from a VAD is done only by specially trained personnel and on a physician's order. Venipuncture in such a patient takes place on the opposite arm whenever possible. If that is not possible, the puncture site should be distal to the IV site and in a different vein.

BIBLIOGRAPHY

American Congress of Obstetricians and Gynecologists: *Committee opinion: Newborn screening No. 481*, 2011. Retrieved from https://www.acog.org/Resources_And_Publications/Committee_Opinions/Committee_on_Genetics/Newborn_Screening.

Clagg ME: Venous sample collection from neonates using dorsal hand veins, *Lab Med* 20:248–250, 1989.

CLSI: *Blood collection on filter paper for newborn screening programs; Approved standard—sixth edition.* CLSI document NBS01-A6. Wayne, Pa., 2013, Clinical and Laboratory Standards Institute.

CLSI: *Collection, transport, and processing of blood specimens for testing plasma-based coagulation assays and molecular hemostasis assays; Approved standard—fifth edition.* CSLI document H21-A5. Wayne, Pa., 2008, Clinical and Laboratory Standards Institute.

CLSI: *Procedures and devices for the collection of diagnostic capillary blood specimens; Approved standard—sixth edition.* CSLI Document GP42-A6 (formerly H04-A6). Wayne, Pa., 2008, Clinical and Laboratory Standards Institute.

CLSI: *Procedures for the collection of diagnostic blood specimens by venipuncture; Approved standard—sixth edition.* CSLI document GP41-A6 (formerly H03-A6). Wayne, Pa., 2007, Clinical and Laboratory Standards Institute.

Faber V: *Communicating trust, empathy helps in collection,* Advance for Medical Laboratory Professionals, 1997.

Faber V: *Phlebotomy and the aging patient*, Advance for Medical Laboratory Professionals, 1998.

Garza D: *Tailoring phlebotomy to the patient,* Advance for Medical Laboratory Professionals, 1999.

Haraden L: *Pediatric phlebotomy: Great expectations,* 1997, Advance for Medical Laboratory Professionals.

Klosinski DD: Collecting specimens from the elderly patient, *Lab Med*, 1997.

Rogers TL, Ostrow CL: The use of EMLA cream to decrease venipuncture pain in children, *J Ped Nurs* 19:33–39, 2004.

Texas Department of State Health. (2014). *NBS Laboratory Services: Newborn Screening Tests. Causes for rejection.* Retrieved from www.dshs.state.tx.us/lab/mrs_nbs_tests_ns.htm.

Werner M, editor: *Microtechniques for the clinical laboratory: Concepts and applications*, New York, 1976, John Wiley & Sons.

WHAT WOULD YOU DO?

It can be difficult to know how to proceed with a pediatric draw when the parent seems to be part of the problem rather than the solution. At times like this, it is acceptable to ask the parent to wait outside. In this case, your choice is perhaps even clearer, since the mother does not want to stay. First, ask another phlebotomist or a nurse to assist you with the draw, as you will want someone to hold the child's arm, for instance. Then you may ask the mother to leave the room. As she does so, reassure the child that his mother will be right outside. Be calm and sincere, and proceed with the draw. Double-check the requisition because prolonged crying will affect test results for WBC count and pH. If these are called for, be sure to make a note that the child had been crying before the draw.

STUDY QUESTIONS

See answers in Appendix F.

1. List and explain five strategies you can use to help reduce a child's anxiety before a draw.

2. What type of needle may be used for pediatric patients younger than 2 years?

3. What is EMLA used for?

4. Name two safe ways that a child can be immobilized during a draw.

5. If an infant is under a Bili light, what must the phlebotomist do before collection?

6. How is a PKU sample collected?

7. Name four physical changes that geriatric patients undergo and the phlebotomist must consider when collecting blood.

8. Explain the procedure for drawing blood from a geriatric patient.

9. What is a VAD?

10. Explain the procedure for drawing blood from a patient who has an IV line.

11. List six types of VADs.

12. Name at least two psychological complications a child may experience during a phlebotomy procedure. List the actions you would take, as a phlebotomist, when drawing blood from a child.

13. List the special considerations to take when drawing blood from a newborn.

14. Name diseases that neonates may be screened for, besides PKU.

15. List at least two common disorders associated with geriatric patients and special considerations to take when drawing blood from such patients.

16. Why is it important to rotate the collection site in a patient with HIV infection?

CERTIFICATION EXAMINATION PREPARATION

See answers in Appendix F.

1. Which of the following is incorrect?
   a. Newborns have a higher proportion of RBCs than adults.
   b. More blood may be needed from newborns to provide enough serum or plasma for testing.
   c. Newborns have a higher proportion of plasma than adults.
   d. Newborns and infants are more susceptible to infection than adults.

2. Crying causes an increase in
   a. bilirubin.
   b. platelet count.
   c. WBC count.
   d. creatinine.

3. Which gauge needle is best to use for a draw on a child younger than 2 years?
   a. 18
   b. 21
   c. 23
   d. 28

4. Jaundice means
   a. yellowing of the skin.
   b. bruising of the skin.
   c. swelling of the skin.
   d. none of the above.

5. Which laboratory test assays jaundice?
   a. Glucose
   b. Electrolytes
   c. Bilirubin
   d. Complete blood count

6. Neonatal screening tests for which disorders are mandated by the United States?
   a. PKU and hyperthyroidism
   b. PKU and hypothyroidism
   c. PKU and sickle cell anemia
   d. PKU and vitamin D deficiency

7. Samples for PKU testing are typically collected
   a. in a microcollection container.
   b. in a collection tube.
   c. on special filter paper.
   d. in a micropipet.

8. Which of the following occurs as we grow older?
   a. The layers of the skin become more elastic.
   b. Hematomas are more likely.
   c. Arteries move farther from the surface of the skin.
   d. Blood vessels widen due to atherosclerosis.

9. Which of the following is not a VAD?
   a. CVC
   b. IV
   c. PICC
   d. EMLA

10. Blood should never be collected from the arm of a patient containing
    a. an AV shunt.
    b. an IV.
    c. an arterial line.
    d. a CVC.

11. Dermal punctures in pediatric patients are preferred for _____ testing.
    a. cross-match
    b. blood culture
    c. PKU
    d. serum

12. When warming an infant's heel for a dermal puncture, the heel should be warmed for
    a. 30 seconds.
    b. 1 to 2 minutes.
    c. 3 to 5 minutes.
    d. 6 to 8 minutes.

13. Which is not a type of CVC?
    a. Groshong
    b. Triple lumen
    c. Broviac
    d. Fistula

14. An arm containing _____ is never used for phlebotomy procedures.
    a. a heparin lock
    b. an arterial line
    c. a fistula
    d. an implanted port

15. Only specially trained personnel acting on a physician's order are allowed to collect specimens from
    a. geriatric patients.
    b. VADs.
    c. newborns.
    d. mentally impaired patients.

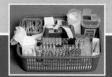

Arterial blood is collected to determine the level of oxygen and carbon dioxide in the blood and measure the pH. Arterial collection is more dangerous than venous collection to the patient, and it requires in-depth training beyond routine phlebotomy skills. It is usually performed by physicians, nurses, medical laboratory scientists (MLSs), medical laboratory technicians (MLTs), or respiratory therapists (RTs). Phlebotomists occasionally are asked to perform or assist with this procedure, and because of the ongoing changes in health care delivery, it is likely that at some point you will have to collect an arterial sample. However, you will not be permitted to participate in actual arterial collection before you receive specialized training at a health care institution. Only a qualified registered nurse, medical laboratory scientist (MLS), or RT may perform an arterial puncture. Arterial collection is most often performed in the radial artery, where collateral circulation from the ulnar artery can make up the loss to the supplied tissues. Arterial samples must be processed quickly after collection to minimize changes in analyte values.

OUTLINE

Composition of Arterial Blood
Arterial Blood Gas Testing
   Equipment for Arterial
    Puncture
   Site Selection
      Procedure 13-1: Modified
       Allen Test

Testing Collateral Circulation
Radial Artery Puncture
Arterial Puncture
   Complications
Sampling Errors
     Procedure 13-2: Radial
      Artery Puncture

Specimen Rejection
Capillary Blood Gas
  Testing
Review for
  Certification

OBJECTIVES

After completing this chapter, you should be able to:

1. Explain how arterial blood differs from venous blood.
2. Describe what is measured in arterial blood gas (ABG) testing, and explain the significance of abnormal results.
3. List the equipment needed to collect arterial blood, and discuss the differences from routine venipuncture equipment.
4. List the arteries that can be used for blood gas collection, and describe the advantages and disadvantages of each.
5. Explain the principle and procedure for testing collateral circulation.

6. Define respiratory steady state, and list the steps that should be taken to ensure that it exists when blood is collected.
7. Describe the steps in ABG collection.
8. Discuss at least five complications that may occur with arterial puncture.
9. List at least seven sample collection errors that may affect ABG testing.
10. Describe capillary blood gas testing, including uses, limitations, and procedure.

KEY TERMS

arterial blood gases (ABGs)
arteriospasm
brachial artery
capillary blood gas (CBGs)
collateral circulation

dorsalis pedis artery
embolism
femoral artery
flea
hyperventilation

modified Allen test
partial pressure of
  carbon dioxide (P_{CO_2})
partial pressure of
  oxygen (P_{O_2})

radial artery
respiratory steady state
scalp artery
thrombosis
umbilical artery

ABBREVIATIONS

ABGs arterial blood gases
CBGs capillary blood gases
COPD chronic obstructive pulmonary disease
EDTA ethylenediaminetetraacetic acid

Pco₂ partial pressure of carbon dioxide
Po₂ partial pressure of oxygen
RTs respiratory therapists

COMPOSITION OF ARTERIAL BLOOD

Arterial blood is rich in both oxygen and electrolytes; this is different from venous blood, in which the levels of these substances vary, depending on the metabolic activities of surrounding tissues. In addition, arterial blood is uniform in composition throughout the body. This makes arterial blood monitoring ideal for managing oxygen, electrolytes, and acid-base balance. Arterial collection is most often used for testing arterial blood gases (ABGs), ammonia, and lactic acid.

ARTERIAL BLOOD GAS TESTING

ABG testing determines the concentrations of oxygen and carbon dioxide dissolved in the blood and measures the pH. The absolute amount of oxygen is expressed as the **partial pressure of oxygen (P_{O_2})**. Similarly, the carbon dioxide level is expressed as the **partial pressure of carbon dioxide (P_{CO_2})**. Reference (normal) values for ABGs are shown in Table 13-1.

ABGs measure the gas-exchange ability of the lungs and the buffering capacity of the blood. A lower-than-normal P_{O_2} and a higher-than-normal P_{CO_2} indicate that gas exchange in the lungs is impaired. Abnormal values mean that the body's tissues are not getting adequate oxygen, a serious and potentially life-threatening situation. This may be caused by many conditions, including chronic obstructive pulmonary disease (COPD), lung cancer, diabetic coma, shock, cardiac or respiratory

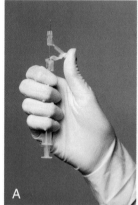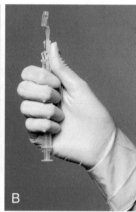

FIGURE   13-1 A, Arterial blood gas syringe with safety-engineered, syringe-hinged safety shield. **B,** Sliding shield syringe. (From Bonewit-West K: *Clinical procedures for medical assistants,* ed. 7, Philadelphia, Saunders, 2008.)

failure, and neuromuscular disease. Normal blood pH is 7.35 to 7.45. A lower pH indicates acidosis, and a higher pH indicates alkalosis. These also may be life threatening.

Equipment for Arterial Puncture

Figure 13-1 displays some of the special equipment needed for arterial collection. Also needed are bandages and a thermometer to take the patient's temperature.

Heparinized Syringe and Needle

Arterial blood is collected in a syringe that has been pretreated with heparin to prevent coagulation.

TABLE 13-1	Reference Values for Arterial Blood Gas Samples	
Parameter	Normal Range	Description
Hydrogen ion concentration (pH)	7.35–7.45	Measure of the acidity or alkalinity of the blood
Partial pressure of oxygen (P_{O_2})	80–100 mm Hg	Measure of the amount of oxygen dissolved in the blood
Partial pressure of carbon dioxide (P_{CO_2})	34–45 mm Hg	Measure of the amount of carbon dioxide in the blood
Bicarbonate ($HCO_3.$)	22–26 mEq/L	Measure of the amount of bicarbonate in the blood
Oxygen (O_2) saturation	97%–100%	Percentage of oxygen bound to hemoglobin

Syringes must be either glass or gas-impermeable plastic. The volume of blood required determines the syringe size; available syringe volumes range from 1 to 5 mL. Treated, prepackaged syringes are available. The choices of needle gauge and length are site dependent. The typical collection needle is usually 21 or 22 gauge, and 1 to 1½ inches long. The 1-inch needle is used for either the brachial or the radial artery. The 1½ inch needle is used for the femoral artery. Either the needle or the syringe should have a safety device to comply with federal safety regulations.

You may be required to prepare a heparinized syringe when no commercial prepackaged product is available. To do this, follow these steps:

1. Use a solution of sodium heparin with a concentration of 1000 U/mL.
2. Calculate the volume of heparin to draw up. Use 0.05 mL of heparin solution for each milliliter of blood to be drawn.
3. Attach a 20-gauge needle to the syringe, and draw up the heparin by slowly pulling back on the plunger.
4. Rotate the liquid in the syringe to coat the barrel.
5. Remove the 20-gauge needle and replace it with the needle you will use for collection.
6. Expel the excess heparin and any air by depressing the plunger fully with the needle pointed down.

Antiseptic

The risk of serious infection is greater with arterial puncture than with venipuncture. For this reason, both alcohol and povidone–iodine or chlorhexidine are used to clean the site.

Lidocaine Anesthetic

Arterial collection can be painful. To lessen pain, 0.5 mL of lidocaine, a local anesthetic, may be injected subcutaneously, using a 25- to 26-gauge needle on a 1-mL syringe. Note that not all hospitals use lidocaine before the puncture.

Safety Equipment

Arterial blood is under pressure and may spray out of the puncture. You need a fluid-resistant gown, face protection, and gloves. You also need a puncture-resistant container for sharps.

Luer Tip

This plastic tip covers the syringe top after you have removed the needle. This keeps air from reaching the specimen and altering gas concentrations.

Other Equipment

Other equipment needed for arterial puncture includes the following:

- Crushed ice
- Ice and water
- Gauze pads
- Pressure bandages
- Thermometer (to take the patient's temperature)
- Transport container

No tourniquet is needed because arterial blood is under pressure.

Site Selection

The artery used for collection must be located near the skin surface and be large enough to accept at least a 23-gauge needle. In addition, the region distal to the collection site should have **collateral circulation**, meaning that it receives blood from more than one artery. This allows the tissue to remain fully oxygenated during the collection procedure. Collateral circulation is tested using the modified Allen test (Procedure 13-1). Finally, the site should not be inflamed, irritated, edematous, or proximal to a wound.

Arteries Used for Arterial Puncture

The arteries used for arterial puncture are shown in Figure 13-2. Phlebotomists collect only from the radial or brachial arteries; other collections require a physician or other specially trained professional. Other arteries that can be used include the femoral and dorsalis pedis.

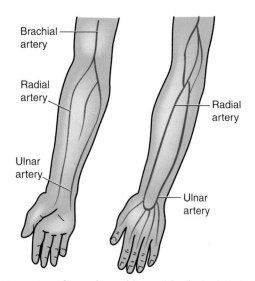

FIGURE 13-2 The arteries used for arterial collection include the radial, brachial, and femoral.

PROCEDURE 13-1

Modified Allen Test

1. **Extend the patient's wrist over a towel, and have the patient make a fist.**

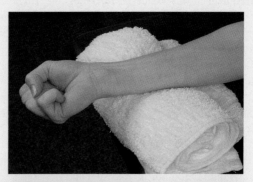

2. **Locate pulses of both the ulnar and the radial arteries, and compress both arteries.**

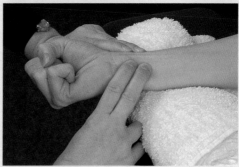

3. **Have the patient open and close the fist repeatedly.**
   This squeezes blood out of the hand. The patient's palm should blanch (become lighter).

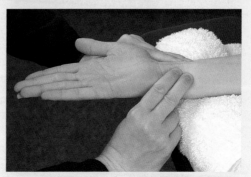

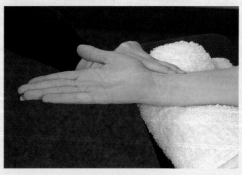

4. **Release the pressure from the ulnar artery.**
   Observe the color of the patient's palm within 5 to 10 seconds.

5. **Interpret the results.**
   Negative result: If no color appears during the 5 to 10 seconds, there is inadequate collateral circulation and the artery should not be used.
   Positive result: If color appears within 5 to 10 seconds, there is adequate collateral circulation and you may proceed with the radial puncture.

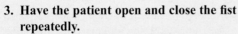

The radial artery, supplying the hand, is the artery of choice. Although it is smaller than either the brachial or the femoral artery, it has good collateral circulation and is easily accessible along the thumb side of the wrist. The ulnar artery provides collateral circulation to the hand. The radial artery can be compressed between the ligaments and the bones, allowing easy application of pressure after puncture and reducing the chance of hematoma. Its small size is a disadvantage in patients with low cardiac output because it is hard to locate.

The brachial artery is large; therefore, it is easy to palpate and puncture. It is located in the antecubital fossa, below the basilic vein and near the insertion of the biceps muscle. It has adequate collateral circulation, although not as much as the radial artery. Nevertheless, the brachial artery has important disadvantages. It is deep and is close to the median nerve. Puncturing the median nerve is a significant risk in brachial artery collection. Also, unlike the radial artery, the brachial artery lies in soft tissue and therefore is more difficult to compress, increasing the risk of hematoma and bleeding into the puncture site.

The femoral artery is the largest artery used. It is located in the groin area above the thigh, lateral to the pubic bone. The femoral is used when the previously mentioned sites are not available for puncture. Its large size and high volume make it useful when cardiac output is low. However, it has poor collateral circulation. In addition, it is a difficult site to keep aseptic, increasing the risk of infection, and the puncture itself may dislodge accumulated plaque from the arterial walls. Only personnel with advanced training can perform femoral artery puncture.

Alternative sites in adults include the dorsalis pedis artery in the foot. In infants, the umbilical artery and scalp artery are used. When puncturing the dorsalis pedis, the posterior tibial must be checked for an adequate pulse. These punctures are performed only by qualified and trained personnel.

In newborns who have difficulty breathing, blood may be collected from both the umbilical artery and the umbilical vein. These samples are tested separately and the results compared.

Testing Collateral Circulation

The modified Allen test is the most common method used to assess the adequacy of collateral circulation in the radial artery. Procedure 13-1 illustrates how to perform this test.

Radial Artery Puncture

Procedure 13-2 illustrates how to perform a radial artery puncture.

Arterial Puncture Complications

Complications from arterial puncture may include the following:
- Arteriospasm, the spontaneous constriction of an artery in response to pain. Arteriospasm may close the artery, preventing oxygen from reaching tissue.
- Embolism, or blood vessel obstruction, due to an air bubble or dislodged clot in the artery. This can cause arterial occlusion (blockage), leading to loss of blood flow.
- Hematoma, resulting from inadequate pressure on the site. This is more likely in elderly patients, whose artery walls are not as elastic and thus not as likely to close spontaneously.
- Hemorrhage. This is more likely in patients who have coagulation disorders or are receiving anticoagulant therapy (heparin or warfarin).
- Infection, from skin contaminants. Contaminants are easily carried to the rest of the body without encountering the immune system.
- Lightheadedness, nausea, or fainting.
- Nerve damage, caused by inadvertent contact with a nerve. This is more likely during arterial puncture than venipuncture because the needle passes more deeply into tissue.
- Severe pain.
- Thrombosis, or clot formation, within the artery.

Sampling Errors

Arterial collections are particularly prone to technical errors that affect the values determined in the laboratory. The most significant source of error is failure to deliver the sample to the laboratory immediately or to properly store the sample on ice if delivery will be delayed. Blood cells continue to respire after collection, and this may cause considerable changes in the analyte values, including PO_2, PCO_2, and pH. Samples collected in a plastic syringe are not iced, and must be analyzed within 30 minutes of collection. Samples collected in a glass syringe may be iced if they are not to be delivered to the laboratory within 5 to 10 minutes. Iced samples must be delivered within 1 hour. Ice should not be used if the sample is being tested for potassium because lower temperatures affect those levels.

Other sources of error include:
- Allowing air bubbles to enter the syringe, decreasing the carbon dioxide reading.

PROCEDURE 13-2

Radial Artery Puncture

1. **Prepare the patient, and examine and complete the requisition form.**

   Take the patient's temperature and respiration rate and record them on the requisition form if required by your facility's protocol. Also document the oxygen received by the patient and the device used to deliver the oxygen (e.g., "95% oxygen through nasal cannula" or "patient is on room air").

   The patient should be in a **respiratory steady state**, meaning that he or she has received the specified amount of oxygen and has refrained from exercise for at least 30 minutes. It is important to maintain this steady state during collection. Keep the patient calm, and make sure that he or she is not experiencing **hyperventilation**, because this changes the arterial oxygen and carbon dioxide levels. Pediatric patients should not be crying or holding their breath. Reassurance and distraction help keep the patient from becoming agitated.

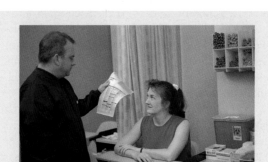

2. **Choose and prepare the site.**

   Perform the modified Allen test to assess collateral circulation in the hand. If the result is positive, proceed. Position the patient comfortably. Fully extend the arm, with the anterior surface facing upward. Palpate for the artery with either the middle or the index finger to locate the greatest maximum pulsation.

   Clean the site with the antiseptic required by your institution.

   Inject the local anesthetic. Wait 1 to 2 minutes for the anesthetic to begin working.

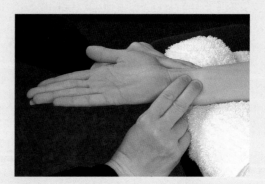

PROCEDURE 13-2—cont'd

Radial Artery Puncture

3. **Perform the puncture.**

    Cleanse the fingers of your nondominant hand and place them over the area where the needle should enter the artery, using the index finger and middle finger of your nondominant hand to stabilize the artery.

    Hold the syringe like a dart with your dominant hand, with the needle tip pointed bevel up toward the upper arm. The syringe plunger should be pushed all the way in toward the hub. Insert the needle 5 to 10 mm distal to the finger you placed on the artery. Insert it at an angle 45 to 60 degrees above the plane of the skin.

    As the needle is inserted into the artery, blood should appear in the hub. It should be bright red and move with the pulse. Do not withdraw the syringe plunger. Blood pressure should push the blood into the syringe without any assistance.

4. **Withdraw the needle, apply pressure, and ice the syringe.**

    Withdraw the needle with your dominant hand.

    With your nondominant hand, apply direct pressure to the site with a folded gauze square. Hold it for at least 5 minutes. You, not the patient, must continue to apply pressure until the bleeding stops. If the patient is on anticoagulant therapy, apply pressure for at least 15 minutes, and longer if necessary, until bleeding stops.

    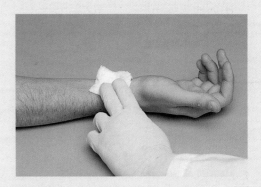

    Meanwhile, with the hand holding the syringe, depress the plunger slightly, if necessary, to expel any air that may have entered the needle. Engage the safety device for the needle. Cap off the syringe with the Luer tip cap. To mix the blood with heparin, roll the syringe between your thumb and fingers for 5 seconds, followed by gentle inversion for 5 seconds. Place the syringe in the ice.

Continued

PROCEDURE 13-2–cont'd

Radial Artery Puncture

5. **Examine the puncture site.**

   After 5 minutes (or 15 minutes for patients on anticoagulant therapy), check the site to ensure that the bleeding has stopped. A number of medications increase bleeding times, including anticoagulants (e.g., heparin and warfarin) and thrombolytics (e.g., tissue plasminogen activator, streptokinase, and urokinase). Once the bleeding has stopped, clean the site with alcohol to remove the iodine, and apply a bandage.

   Check for a pulse distal to the site. If the pulse is absent or weak, contact the nurse immediately.

6. **Label and ice the specimen.**

   Dispose of the needle in the sharps container.

   Label the specimen with a waterproof pen, and return the syringe to the ice.

   Deliver the specimen to the laboratory immediately. Ice the specimen if you are unable to deliver to the lab within 30 minutes.

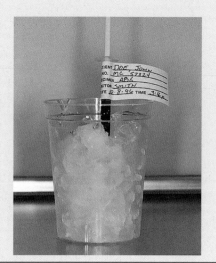

- Exposing the specimen to the atmosphere after collection, which is prevented by using a Luer tip to cover the syringe after you remove the needle.
- Mixing insufficiently, causing the specimen to clot.
- Puncturing a vein instead of an artery.
- Using an improper anticoagulant, as pH is altered by ethylenediaminetetraacetic acid (EDTA), oxalates, and citrates.
- Using an improper plastic syringe, which allows atmospheric gas to diffuse in and specimen gases to diffuse out through the plastic.
- Using too little heparin, causing the specimen to clot.
- Using too much heparin, which lowers the pH value.

Specimen Rejection

Specimens may be rejected by the laboratory for a variety of reasons, including:
- Air bubbles in the specimen
- Clotting
- Failure to ice the specimen
- Improper or absent labeling
- Inadequate volume of specimen for the test
- Too long a delay in delivering the specimen to the laboratory
- Use of the wrong syringe

CAPILLARY BLOOD GAS TESTING

Capillary blood gas (CBG) testing is an alternative to ABG testing when arterial collection is not possible or is not recommended. Capillary blood is not as desirable a specimen for blood gas testing because it is a mixture of blood from the capillaries, venules, and arterioles and is mixed with tissue fluid. In addition, this method of collection is open to the air, and the specimen may exchange gases with room air before it is sealed.

Capillary blood gas testing is most commonly performed on pediatric patients, as they generally should not be subjected to the deep punctures required for ABG testing.

The collection is done using a normal heel-stick procedure. Important points in the procedure are as follows.

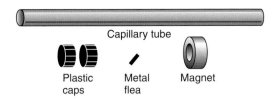

Capillary tube

Plastic caps   Metal flea   Magnet

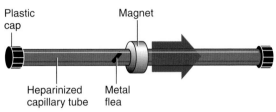

Plastic cap   Magnet

Heparinized capillary tube   Metal flea

FIGURE 13-3 A metal filing, called a flea, is inserted into the capillary tube before collection. A magnet is used to stir the sample after collection.

1. Warm the site to 40° C to 42° C for 5 to 10 minutes before the stick to maximize the arterial character of the capillary blood.
2. Clean the site with the appropriate antiseptic swab, using the antiseptic required by your institution. Allow the site to dry for the appropriate time.
3. Collect the sample in a heparinized glass pipet. Before collection, insert a metal filing, called a flea, into the tube. After collection, a magnet is used to draw the flea back and forth across the length of the tube to mix the contents with the heparin (Figure 13-3).
4. Fill the tube completely with blood so that no air bubbles remain.
5. Seal both ends of the tube with clay or plastic caps to prevent air contamination.
6. Mix well using the magnet and flea, and transport the specimen to the laboratory on ice.

REVIEW FOR CERTIFICATION

Because of the increased danger of arterial blood collection, special training is required beyond that needed for routine venipuncture. Arterial blood monitoring is ideal for managing oxygen, electrolytes, and acid-base balance. ABGs measure the gas exchange ability of the lungs and the buffering capacity of the blood. Arterial blood is collected in a syringe pretreated with heparin to prevent coagulation. The site is cleansed with both alcohol and chlorhexidine to minimize the serious risk of infection. Lidocaine is used as an anesthetic. The site is selected after testing the adequacy of collateral circulation using the modified Allen test. A rapid return of color indicates that the site has adequate collateral circulation and may be used for collection. In adults, the radial artery is the preferred site. The patient must be in a respiratory steady state and should be kept calm during the procedure. The specimen should be delivered immediately or kept on ice if a delay of more than 5 to 10 minutes is expected. Complications include arteriospasm, nerve damage, hematoma, hemorrhage, thrombosis, and infection. Sampling errors affecting test values may be introduced from improper cooling, delay in delivery, too much or too little heparin, insufficient mixing, exposure of the sample to air, and improper collection technique. Capillary blood gas testing is an alternative to ABG testing when arterial collection is not possible or recommended. A metal flea and magnet are used to mix the contents with the heparin.

BIBLIOGRAPHY

Bishop ML, Fody EP, Schoeff LE: *Clinical chemistry: Principles, procedures, and correlations,* ed. 7, Philadelphia, 2013, Lippincott.

Burton GG, Hodgkin JE, Ward JJ: *Respiratory care: A guide to clinical practice,* ed 4, Philadelphia, 1997, Lippincott.

CLSI: *Procedures for the collection of arterial blood specimens; Approved standard—fourth edition.* CSLI document GP43-A4 (formerly H11-A4). Wayne, Pa., 2004, Clinical and Laboratory Standards Institute.

Conover K: *Blood gases: Not as complicated as they seem,* Version 1.8, 2010. Retrieved from www.pitt.edu/~mercyres/Abg-ref.pdf.

Lockshin MBL: *Arterial blood gas,* 2010. Retrieved from www.wisc-online.com/objects/ViewObject.aspx?ID=NUR202.

Shapiro BA: *Clinical application of blood gases,* ed. 5, St. Louis, 1994, Mosby.

STUDY QUESTIONS

See answers in Appendix F.

1. Arterial collection is most often used for what type of testing?

2. List four conditions that produce abnormal ABG values.

3. What is a normal blood pH?

4. What is the difference between acidosis and alkalosis?

5. Describe the difference between a syringe used for venipuncture and a syringe used for ABG collection.

6. Besides alcohol, which other antiseptic must be used for arterial puncture?

7. What local anesthetic may be used to numb the site?

8. What safety precautions must be taken by the phlebotomist when collecting blood from an artery?

9. What gauge needle is most often used for blood gas collection?

10. Define collateral circulation, and state which test is used to determine whether this is present.

11. For an arterial collection, at what angle is the needle inserted into the artery?

12. How long must pressure be applied to the puncture site after an arterial collection?

13. Define arteriospasm.

14. List five ABG sampling errors.

15. Name five reasons that ABG specimens may be rejected.

16. In which population is capillary blood gas testing most commonly performed, and on what part of the body is this procedure usually done?

17. Why is capillary blood not as desirable as arterial blood for testing blood gases?

CERTIFICATION EXAMINATION PREPARATION

See answers in Appendix F.

1. Arterial blood collection monitors all of the following except
   a. ammonia.
   b. glucose.
   c. lactic acid.
   d. blood gases.

2. A normal blood pH is
   a. 7.35.
   b. 7.00.
   c. 7.60.
   d. 7.75.

3. The ABG syringe is coated with
   a. sodium citrate.
   b. sodium fluoride.
   c. EDTA.
   d. heparin.

4. A typical needle gauge for ABG collection is
   a. 16.
   b. 20.
   c. 22.
   d. 18.

5. Which artery is most frequently used for ABG collection?
   a. Brachial
   b. Femoral
   c. Dorsalis pedis
   d. Radial

6. Which of the following is not an ABG sampling error?
   a. Delivery of an un-iced sample to the laboratory 15 minutes after collection
   b. Use of the anticoagulant EDTA
   c. Air bubbles in the syringe
   d. Use of a gas-impermeable plastic syringe

7. The modified Allen test determines
   a. P_{O_2}.
   b. P_{CO_2}.
   c. collateral circulation.
   d. pH.

8. In an arterial collection, the needle should be inserted at a _____ degree angle.
   a. 90
   b. 45
   c. 30
   d. 70

9. If lidocaine is injected before an arterial blood collection, wait _____ minutes for the anesthetic to begin working.
   a. 1 to 2
   b. 2 to 3
   c. 3 to 4
   d. 4 to 5

10. The modified Allen test is performed on the _____ and _____ arteries.
   a. ulnar, brachial
   b. brachial, radial
   c. ulnar, radial
   d. radial, femoral

11. Which of the following is not a complication of ABG collection?
   a. Petechiae
   b. Arteriospasm
   c. Thrombosis
   d. Hematoma

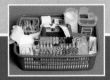

CHAPTER 14   Special Collections and Procedures

Although routine venipuncture is the most common procedure you will perform as a phlebotomist, special collecting or handling procedures are needed in many situations for samples that involve one or more special circumstances. Fasting specimens, timed specimens, blood cultures, and blood donor specimens all require collection procedures specific to the sample being collected. A variety of samples require special handling, which may involve keeping the sample warm, cool, or away from light, or providing immediate delivery or legal documentation. In this chapter, you will learn when and why these special procedures are needed and the details of how to perform them.

OUTLINE

OBJECTIVES

After completing this chapter, you should be able to:

1. Define basal state.
2. Define and explain the uses of:
   a. Fasting specimens
   b. Timed specimens
   c. 2-hour postprandial specimens
3. Describe the procedure for performing the various tolerance tests.
4. Define diurnal variation, and list the blood constituents that may be affected by it.
5. Define therapeutic drug monitoring (TDM), describe the differences among a random level and peak and trough levels, and explain how TDM samples are collected.
6. Describe the reasons and procedures for collecting blood for culture.
7. Explain the steps in collecting blood from donors for transfusion.

8. Define and explain the uses of autologous donation and therapeutic phlebotomy.
9. Explain how samples to be tested for or suspected of containing cold agglutinins, cryofibrinogen, or cryoglobulin should be handled.
10. List samples that should be chilled until tested.
11. List samples that are light sensitive, and explain how they should be handled.
12. Describe the precautions to be taken when collecting legal or forensic specimens.
13. List samples that are time sensitive, and explain how they should be handled.
14. Explain how to prepare blood smears, describe features of unacceptable smears, and list the possible causes.
15. Explain how to prepare smears to be examined for malaria.

KEY TERMS

aerobic bacteria	differential count (diff)	half-life	sepsis
agglutination	diurnal variation	hemochromatosis	sodium polyanethole
anaerobic bacteria	epinephrine tolerance test	hyperglycemia	sulfonate (SPS)
bacteremia	fasting specimen	hypoglycemia	therapeutic drug
basal state	feathered edge	lactose tolerance	monitoring (TDM)
blood culture (BC)	fever of unknown	test (LTT)	therapeutic phlebotomy
chain of custody (COC)	origin (FUO)	oral glucose tolerance	trough level
cold agglutinins	gestational diabetes	test (OGTT)	2-hour postprandial test
cryofibrinogen	glucagon tolerance test	peak level	
cryoglobulin	glucose tolerance test (GTT)	polycythemia	

ABBREVIATIONS

AABB American Association of Blood Banks
ACTH adrenocorticotropic hormone
BC blood culture
COC chain of custody
DNA deoxyribonucleic acid
FDA Food and Drug Administration
FUO fever of unknown origin
GTT glucose tolerance test

HIV human immunodeficiency virus
LTT lactose tolerance test
NIDA National Institute on Drug Abuse
OGTT oral glucose tolerance test
RBCs red blood cells
SPS sodium polyanethole sulfonate
stat short turnaround time
TDM therapeutic drug monitoring

WHAT WOULD YOU DO?

After you have had 2 months on the job at City General Hospital, your supervisor is ready to let you collect blood culture specimens. She asks your coworker, Tom, to go along with you in case you have any problems. You perform your first draw flawlessly, although it took longer than expected, and Tom has started looking at his watch. You begin prepping your second patient, hoping to do this one a bit faster, but as you are about to insert the needle, your gloved finger grazes the site. Oh no! Is the site contaminated? Do you need to start all over again? You look at Tom. "Don't worry," he says. "You can just go ahead and draw. It'll be fine. The lab is OK with that kind of thing." What would you do?

FASTING SPECIMENS AND THE BASAL STATE

As detailed in Box 14-1, many factors influence the composition of blood. **Diurnal variation** refers to the normal daily fluctuations in body chemistry related to hormonal cycles, sleep–wake cycles, and other regular patterns of change.

FLASH FORWARD

In Chapter 18, you will learn more about factors that affect test results and how to avoid making errors in your collection and transport.

To minimize the variations introduced by normal fluctuations in blood composition, reference ranges

BOX 14-1	Factors That Influence Blood Composition

- Age
- Altitude
- Body position
- Dehydration
- Diet
- Diurnal variation
- Drugs
- Environment
- Exercise
- Gender
- Pregnancy
- Smoking
- Stress

for blood tests are based on healthy patients in what is known as the **basal state**. The basal state is defined as the body's state after 8 to 12 hours of fasting and abstention from strenuous exercise. Routine phlebotomy rounds are scheduled for the early morning, because most patients are in the basal state at that time.

Some test results are more affected than others when a patient has not been scrupulously fasting for 12 hours. Glucose and triglycerides are especially affected. For this reason, a **fasting specimen** may be requested that is drawn after a 12-hour complete fast. Caffeine and nicotine are also prohibited during the fasting period, as these are metabolic stimulants. If a fasting specimen is requested, the phlebotomist must ask the patient if he or she has had anything to eat or drink other than water, or has had any caffeine or nicotine, within the past 12 hours. It is better to ask the question in this form than to ask, "Have you been fasting for 12 hours?" because some patients may not consider an evening snack or morning juice to be a violation of their fast. If the patient has violated the fast, you can still draw the sample, but make a note on the requisition. You may also contact your supervisor to see whether the physician should be notified before the draw. Often, the physician will reschedule the lab work, particularly if a lipid profile is ordered.

Timed Specimens

Timed specimens are taken to determine changes in the level of some substance of interest over time. Timed specimens are most often used to monitor:

- Medication levels (e.g., digoxin for heart disease or levodopa for Parkinson disease).
- Changes in the patient's condition (e.g., a decrease in hemoglobin level).
- Normal diurnal variation in blood levels at different times of the day (e.g., cortisol or other hormones).
- Cardiac enzymes, used to diagnose or rule out myocardial infarction (heart attack); these are tested at admission and then twice more at 8-hour intervals.

2-Hour Postprandial Test

The **2-hour postprandial test** is used to test for diabetes mellitus. It compares the fasting glucose level with the level 2 hours after consuming glucose, either by eating a meal or by ingesting a measured amount of glucose (*postprandial* means "after a meal"). In patients with diabetes mellitus, the glucose level will be higher than normal, whereas the level in normal patients will have returned to the fasting level. After the phlebotomist has obtained a fasting specimen, the patient is instructed to eat a full meal and then return to the lab 2 hours after eating for collection of the second specimen.

Glucose Tolerance Test

The **glucose tolerance test (GTT)**, also called the **oral glucose tolerance test (OGTT)**, tests for both diabetes mellitus and other disorders of carbohydrate metabolism. **Hyperglycemia**, or abnormally elevated blood sugar, is most commonly caused by diabetes; **hypoglycemia**, or abnormally lowered blood sugar, may be due to one of several endocrine disorders or other metabolic disruptions. Hyperglycemia is detected with a 3-hour GTT, and hypoglycemia is detected with a 5-hour GTT. Longer testing periods are sometimes used as well to identify a variety of metabolic disorders. The GTT has fallen out of general use for the diagnosis of diabetes mellitus, and has been replaced by either a fasting glucose sample (at least 8 hours without caloric intake) or a random glucose sample.

Glucose tolerance testing is still widely used in pregnant women, to diagnose **gestational diabetes**. Gestational diabetes is insulin-resistant diabetes that develops in almost 20% of women late in pregnancy. The initial screen is a 1-hour GTT, performed without fasting. The patient drinks an intensely sweetened liquid, and a sample is taken 1 hour later. Elevated glucose in the sample indicates potential gestational diabetes. That finding usually prompts the physician to order a fasting GTT.

Patients will be instructed by their physicians regarding pretest preparation, which includes eating high-carbohydrate meals for several days and then fasting for 12 hours immediately before the test.

Testing begins between 0700 (pronounced "oh-seven-hundred") and 0900 (7 AM to 9 AM), with the collection of a fasting blood specimen and sometimes a urine specimen. These specimens should be tested before the GTT proceeds. In the event that the glucose level is severely elevated, the physician may decide not to proceed with the test.

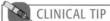

CLINICAL TIP

Times are given in military time. To get clock time, subtract 1200 for times of 1300 or later. Example: 1430 = 2:30 PM.

The patient then drinks a standardized amount of glucose solution within 5 minutes. Timing for the rest of the procedure begins after the drink is fin-ished. The phlebotomist makes a collection sched-ule. The first collection is 1 hour after glucose ingestion. The second collection is 2 hours after glucose ingestion, and so on, for the number of hours the physician has indicated. Note that some procedures may call for collection of the first sample at 30 minutes after ingestion of the glucose solution, followed by another collection 30 minutes later at the 1 hour mark, and then hourly samples after that. Follow the protocol of your facility. The phle-botomist gives the patient the collection schedule and instructs the patient to return to the collection station at the appropriate times (Table 14-1). Patients also should be instructed to continue to fast and drink plenty of water so that they remain adequately hydrated throughout the test.

Some patients do not tolerate the test well. Any vomiting should be reported to the physician ordering the test. If the patient vomits shortly after the test begins, the procedure will have to be started again.

All collections should be made on time and using the same collection method (i.e., venipuncture or dermal puncture) and anticoagulant for each sam-ple. A urine specimen may be collected at the same time. Samples should be labeled with the time from test commencement (1 hour, 2 hours, and so forth).

> **FLASH FORWARD** ↱≫
> Urine specimen collection is covered in Chapter 15.

Other Tolerance Tests

Similar procedures are used for other tolerance tests. The epinephrine tolerance test determines the patient's ability to mobilize glycogen from the liver. In response to a dose of the hormone epineph-rine, glycogen is converted to glucose and released into the bloodstream. The test begins with a fasting specimen, followed by the epinephrine injection administered by the physician. Specimen collection begins 30 minutes later. The glucagon tolerance test is identical in purpose and procedure, except that the hormone glucagon is injected instead of epinephrine.

The lactose tolerance test (LTT) determines whether the lactose-digesting enzyme lactase is present in the gut. A 3-hour GTT is performed first to produce a baseline glucose uptake graph. The following day a lactose tolerance test is performed. The procedure is identical to the GTT except that lactose is consumed and a tourniquet may not be used. Be sure to follow the protocol for your facil-ity. Because lactose is broken down into glucose and galactose, the timed samples should produce an identical glucose uptake graph. Lower glucose lev-els indicate a problem with lactose metabolism.

Lactose intolerance can also be determined using the hydrogen breath test, which does not require a blood sample. In this test, the patient drinks a lactose solution and then exhales into a collection bag. Hydrogen in the breath is a sign of undigested lactose in the gut.

A stool acidity test may be ordered for patients and children who are unable to undergo the other tests. Lactic acid and other acids from undigested lactose can be detected in a stool, or fecal, sample.

> **FLASH FORWARD** ↱≫
> You will learn about fecal samples in Chapter 15.

Diurnal Variation

Many substances in the blood (especially hormones) show diurnal variation, or regular changes through-out the day (Box 14-2). Cortisol, for instance, is usually twice as high in the morning as in the late afternoon. The time for the draw is usually

TABLE 14-1	Collection Schedule for Oral Glucose Tolerance Tests
Test	Schedule
2-Hr glucose tolerance test (GTT)	Fasting, 1 hr, and 2 hr
3-Hr GTT	Fasting, 1 hr, 2 hr, and 3 hr
5-Hr GTT	Fasting, 1 hr, 2 hr, 3 hr, 4 hr, and 5 hr

BOX 14-2	Representative Blood Constituents That Show Marked Diurnal Variation

- Cortisol
- Estradiol
- Glucose
- Hormones
- Progesterone
- Serum iron
- Testosterone
- White blood cells (eosinophils show especially pronounced variation)

scheduled for the diurnal peak or trough. Cortisol is usually drawn at 1000 or 1600, for instance.

Therapeutic Drug Monitoring

Patients differ greatly in the rate at which they metabolize or excrete medications. In addition, the "margin of safety," or the difference between the level at which a drug is therapeutic and the level at which it becomes toxic, may be narrow. To maintain constant therapeutic plasma drug levels and ensure that the drug does not reach toxic levels, a patient may require timed specimens to measure the levels of the medication. This is known as **therapeutic drug monitoring (TDM)**. Results of TDM are used by the pharmacy to adjust drug dosing. Table 14-2 lists some commonly monitored drugs. The rate of metabolism is often given in terms of the drug's **half-life**, the time for half of the drug to be metabolized. Drugs with long half-lives, including digoxin, often require only one timed specimen. Drugs with short half-lives, such as the aminoglycoside antibiotics (including gentamicin, tobramycin, and vancomycin) require the most careful monitoring. Monitoring for these rapidly metabolized antibiotics is done with a pair of specimens, known as a peak and a trough.

Collection is usually timed to coincide with either the trough or the peak serum level. The **trough level** is the lowest serum level and occurs immediately before the next dose of medicine is given. The requisition will specify the actual collection time, which is usually 30 minutes before the dose. The **peak level**, or highest serum level, occurs sometime after the dose is given; exactly when depends on the characteristics of the drug, the patient's own metabolism, and the method of administration. The tube should be labeled with the draw time in all cases. Careful attention to the correct timing of draw, and accurate labeling, is vital to the patient's health. TDM results are needed promptly, because the pharmacy is usually waiting for the results to determine both the timing and the concentration of the next dose of drug. By properly timing the administration of medications, the doctor can have the maximum beneficial effect with the fewest side effects. Most drugs need to be collected in a red top tube because the gel in a serum separator tube interferes with the analysis of the drugs.

> ⚠️ **AVOID THAT ERROR!**
>
> When phlebotomist Thomas Jordan picks up the stack of requisitions waiting for him in the laboratory at City General Hospital, he notices that the one for Leonard Brisco, in room 311, calls for a chem panel as well as a peak-level test for valproic acid, an epilepsy drug, to be drawn at 11 AM. Thomas arrives at 10:55 AM, prepares the patient, and begins the draw precisely at 11, filling a gold-top Hemogard tube, inverting it five times after the draw. He thanks the patient, labels the tube, and heads off to his next patient. What did he do wrong? What should he have done, and what should he do now?

BLOOD CULTURES

A **blood culture (BC)** is ordered to test for the presence of microorganisms in the blood, a potentially life-threatening situation. Such microorganisms include bacteria, fungi, and protozoa. **Bacteremia** refers specifically to the presence of bacteria in the blood. Bacteria occasionally enter the bloodstream, for instance through the gut or from excessively vigorous toothbrushing, which breaks capillaries. These rarely cause illness. Septicemia is a life-threatening infection caused by rapid multiplication of pathogens in the bloodstream. When microorganisms in the blood trigger a systemic inflammatory response, it is called **sepsis**. Patients with symptoms of chills and fever, or **fever of unknown origin (FUO)**, may require a BC. BCs are ordered as short turnaround time (stat) or timed specimens.

Isolating pathogenic organisms from blood is difficult because the number of organisms may be low (leading to false-negative results) and the potential for sample contamination is high (leading to false-positive results). To increase the likelihood of finding pathogens and decrease the number of false positives, collection is performed at timed intervals and from multiple sites. Aseptic collection technique is critical for meaningful results. Drawing the correct volume is also critical, because the ratio of blood to culture media depends on the system used. Always check your institution's guidelines.

TABLE 14-2	Commonly Monitored Therapeutic Drugs
Drug Name	Therapeutic Purpose
Dilantin and valproic acid	Anticonvulsant
Gentamicin	Antibiotic
Procainamide and digoxin	Heart medication
Theophylline	Antiasthmatic
Tobramycin	Antibiotic
Vancomycin	Antibiotic

Volumes for pediatric patients differ from those for adults.

Types of Collection Containers

There are three basic types of containers for collecting BCs:
1. A long-necked bottle, which accepts a BD Vacutainer needle and tube holder.
2. A shorter bottle, which accepts a winged infusion device, such as a BD Bactec, using a special adapter.
3. A standard evacuated tube with sodium polyanethole sulfonate (SPS) anticoagulant.

Figure 14-1 shows these three types of collection containers.

Timing

The number of organisms in the bloodstream is often highest just before a spike in the patient's temperature. By frequently recording the temperature, these spikes can often be predicted and collection scheduled accordingly. In other situations, collection may be timed at regular intervals, often hourly or just before antibiotic administration.

Multiple Sites

Contamination of the sample by skin bacteria is a frequent complication of BC collection. However, distinguishing contaminants from true pathogens can be difficult because some contaminants can grow on indwelling devices, causing infection in the patient. To reduce errors caused by this contamination, a known skin contaminant must be cultured from at least two different sites to be considered a

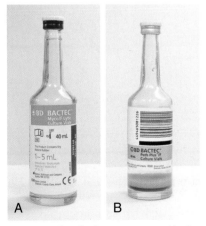

FIGURE 14-1 Examples of culture systems used in the collection of blood cultures (BCs). **A,** Adult blood culture collection container. **B,** Pediatric blood culture collection container.

blood pathogen. It is even better to collect two pairs of samples from two different sites. This helps detect contamination of samples by skin bacteria. The physician should be consulted about the exact sites and timing of the two sets.

Sample Collection

Procedure 14-1 outlines the steps in BC collection. As noted earlier, samples are collected either directly into a bottle containing culture media or indirectly into a sterile anticoagulated tube for later transfer to culture media in the laboratory. The ratio of blood to culture media is crucial to the culture, so be sure to collect the sample size indicated on the bottle. In addition to culture media, some tubes contain activated charcoal, which absorbs antibiotics from the patient's blood so that they do not inhibit growth of the bacteria in the culture tube. Also, some bacteria, called anaerobic bacteria, cannot tolerate oxygen, while others, called aerobic bacteria, use it. Some samples you collect will exclude oxygen and will be used to grow anaerobic bacteria. Other samples you collect will include oxygen and will be used to grow aerobic bacteria.

For direct collection into culture media, two samples, one aerobic and one anaerobic, are collected from each site. When using a syringe, collect the anaerobic sample first and the aerobic sample second, since the second sample will be more likely to have been exposed to air. The transfer must be performed with the appropriate transfer safety device. When using a butterfly, the opposite order is used: Collect the aerobic sample first, since there is air inside the butterfly tube, and then collect the anaerobic sample. Be sure to label the samples to reflect their order of collection.

For anticoagulated tube collections, only one tube is collected per site. At the laboratory, the specimen is cultured onto the appropriate media.

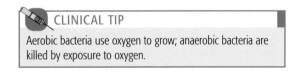

CLINICAL TIP

Aerobic bacteria use oxygen to grow; anaerobic bacteria are killed by exposure to oxygen.

BLOOD DONOR COLLECTION

Blood donation is a vital link in the health care system, and the phlebotomist plays a central role in the collection of donated blood. Blood banks collect and store donated blood for use in both emergency and scheduled transfusions. Guidelines for uniform collection procedures and safeguards have been

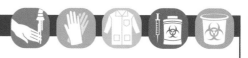

PROCEDURE 14-1

Blood Culture Collection

1. Prepare the site.

Proper site preparation is critical to obtain a valid blood culture (BC) specimen. After identifying the site, scrub it vigorously with alcohol to clean 1½ to 2 inches beyond the intended puncture site.

Scrub vigorously with 2% iodine or a povidone–iodine swab stick. Using a new swab stick, clean the site, moving outward in a concentric circle. An alternative is to use a one-step Medi-flex ChloraPrep applicator instead of the two steps outlined here.

Allow the site to dry for 1 minute. This ensures enough time for the iodine to kill surface bacteria.

Avoid touching the site once it has been cleaned. If you must touch it, reclean the site afterward.

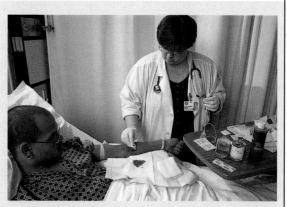

2. Prepare your collection equipment.

Clean the tops of collection bottles with iodine or alcohol, depending on your institution's protocol (rubber tops are usually cleaned with alcohol). Place a clean alcohol pad on top of each bottle until it is inoculated. Immediately before inoculation, wipe the top with the pad to prevent iodine contamination of the sample. Be sure not to touch the bottle tops directly.

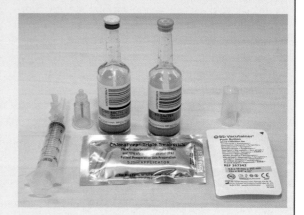

3. Collect the sample.

Reapply the tourniquet, and perform the venipuncture. Collect two samples. Label one "anaerobic" and the other "aerobic," and indicate the site of the puncture. (Remember that for a syringe collection the first sample is anaerobic and the second is aerobic. For a butterfly collection, the first sample is aerobic and the second is anaerobic.)

4. Attend to the patient.

After collection, remove the iodine from the patient's arm with alcohol. Do not touch the puncture site because this could cause stinging for the patient at that site.

Check the puncture site to be sure bleeding has stopped.

Apply a bandage, using a fresh adhesive bandage or placing adhesive tape over the gauze square.

Raise the bed rail if you lowered it.

Dispose of all contaminated materials in a biohazard container.

established by the American Association of Blood Banks (AABB) and the U.S. Food and Drug Administration (FDA).

Potential donors must be screened to ensure that the donation is not harmful to the donor or the recipient. Donors must be at least 17 years old (16 years in some states), weigh a minimum of 110 pounds, and not have donated blood in the past 8 weeks. Donor screening is usually done by the phlebotomist. All information provided during the screening is confidential. The screening process is performed every time a person donates blood. Screening involves the following:

- *Registration.* The donor must provide his or her name, date of birth, address, other identifying information, and written consent. All information must be kept on file for at least 10 years.
- *Interview and medical history.* This is done in private by a trained interviewer. All responses are kept confidential. Potential donors may be rejected for a variety of reasons, including exposure to human immunodeficiency virus (HIV) or viral hepatitis, current drug use, or cardiovascular conditions.
- *Physical examination.* The donor's weight, temperature, blood pressure, pulse, and hemoglobin level are determined. Hemoglobin is usually measured with a drop of whole blood from a dermal puncture. A hematocrit may be substituted for the hemoglobin determination.

Collection Procedure

Blood is collected by the *unit,* whose volume is 400 to 500 mL, or approximately 0.5 liter (Figure 14-2). It is collected directly into a sterile plastic bag, which

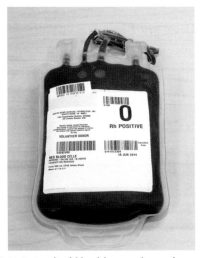

FIGURE 14-2 A unit of blood has a volume of approximately 400 to 500 mL.

hangs below the collection site and fills by gravity. The weight of the filled bag triggers a clamp that stops the collection. A 16- to 18-gauge needle is used for collection. This large needle speeds the collection and prevents hemolysis.

A large vein in the antecubital area is used for donor collection. The site is cleaned first with soap and water and then with iodine. After the puncture, the needle is secured to the arm with tape to prevent motion during the collection. The donor is instructed to pump his or her fist to increase flow. (Hemoconcentration may result from this action, but this is not a concern with blood collected for transfusion.) The phlebotomist stays with the donor during the collection and observes for any signs of distress, anxiety, or pale skin. After needle removal, the phlebotomist instructs the patient to apply firm pressure to the site and bandages the site when the bleeding has stopped.

Autologous Donation

An autologous donation is blood donated by a patient for his or her own use later. Patients planning surgery often make autologous donations before the procedure. This may reduce the likelihood of complications and may be especially useful for patients with rare blood types. Because multiple units might be needed during surgery, patients may need to donate several times. A patient can donate as often as every 72 hours, assuming that his or her health is good. Hemoglobin is checked during the donation series and should not fall below 11 g/dL.

Therapeutic Phlebotomy

Therapeutic phlebotomy is the removal of blood from a patient's system as part of the treatment for a disorder. The principal disorders treated by therapeutic phlebotomy are **polycythemia**, a disease characterized by excessive production of red blood cells (RBCs), and **hemochromatosis**, an excess of iron in the blood. In both cases, periodic removal of a unit of blood may be part of the treatment program. Because such a large volume must be removed, therapeutic phlebotomy is performed in the donor center, although a special area may be set aside for this purpose. This blood cannot be used for transfusion in most instances.

SPECIAL SPECIMEN HANDLING
Cold Agglutinins

Cold agglutinins are antibodies often formed in response to infection with *Mycoplasma pneumoniae,* a cause of atypical pneumonia. The antibodies created by the immune system during the infection may also react with RBCs at temperatures below body temperature, causing them to stick together, hence *cold agglutinins* (**agglutination** is the process of sticking together). Because the agglutinins attach to RBCs at cold temperatures, the specimen must be kept warm until the serum is separated from the cells to avoid falsely lowering the agglutinin levels. A patient with cold agglutinins is sometimes asymptomatic, but the presence of the antibodies can cause problems if the patient's body temperature falls. This may occur when a patient undergoes cardiopulmonary bypass, for example, which requires cooling the patient to slow the metabolic activity of the heart. If the patient has undetected cold agglutinins, this hypothermia will cause dangerous agglutination of red blood cells. A presurgical screening is therefore sometimes required to detect these cold agglutinins.

To collect a cold agglutinin sample, prewarm a plain red-topped tube (containing no gel) in a 37° C incubator for 30 minutes. To keep the specimen warm, it can be wrapped in an activated heel-warmer pack or placed in the incubator. Deliver the specimen as quickly as possible to the laboratory.

Cryofibrinogen and Cryoglobulin

Warm collection and storage are required for two other types of samples: **cryofibrinogen** (an abnormal type of fibrinogen) and **cryoglobulin** (an abnormal serum protein). Both precipitate when cold and redissolve when warmed. These samples should be collected and handled in the same manner as a cold agglutinin sample.

Chilled Specimens

A number of tests require that the specimen be chilled immediately after collection (Box 14-3). Chilling is used to prevent chemical changes that would alter test results. The sample should be placed in crushed ice or in an ice and water mixture and immediately delivered to the laboratory. The temperature should be 1° C to 5° C, and the sample should be transported to the laboratory for testing within 5 minutes of collection (Figure 14-3). A lactic acid sample should also be collected without a tourniquet, and without the patient making a fist, since both of these can raise lactic acid.

Light-Sensitive Specimens

Exposure to light can break down or alter certain blood constituents (Box 14-4). Specimens to be tested for these constituents must be protected from light after collection. This is done by wrapping the tube in aluminum foil immediately after collection (Figure 14-4). An amber-colored microtube can be used for dermal collection (e.g., of bilirubin samples).

Time-Sensitive Specimens

Some analytes are unstable or volatile. Because of this, the tests must be performed rapidly after the sample is taken. Box 14-5 lists analytes that are time sensitive.

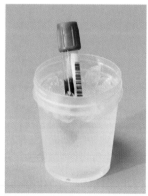

FIGURE 14-3 Samples that must be kept cold should be placed in crushed ice or in an ice and water mixture with a temperature of 1° to 5° C.

BOX 14-3	Tests Requiring Chilled Specimens

- Adrenocorticotropic hormone
- Ammonia
- Arterial blood gases
- Glucagon
- Gastrin
- Homocysteine
- Lactic acid
- Parathyroid hormone
- Pyruvate

BOX 14-4	Blood Constituents That are Light Sensitive

- Beta-carotene
- Bilirubin
- Porphyrins
- Vitamin A
- Vitamin B$_6$

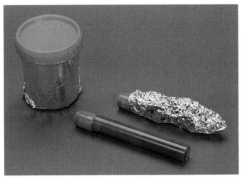

FIGURE 14-4 Samples that must be protected from light should be wrapped in aluminum foil immediately after collection. Amber-colored tubes also can be used.

BOX 14-5	**Time-Sensitive Blood Constituents**

- Adrenocorticotropic hormone (ACTH)
- Ammonia
- Brain natriuretic peptide
- Lactate
- Platelet aggregation
- Prostatic acid phosphatase

Legal and Forensic Specimens

Blood specimens may be collected for use as evidence in legal proceedings, including alcohol and drug testing, deoxyribonucleic acid (DNA) analysis, or paternity or parentage testing. Such samples must be handled with special procedures designed to prevent tampering, misidentification, or interference with the test results.

The most important concept in handling forensic specimens is the **chain of custody (COC)**, a protocol that ensures that the sample is always in the custody of a person legally entrusted to be in control of it. The chain begins with patient identification and continues through every step of the collection and testing process. COC documentation includes special containers, seals, and forms, as well as the date, time, and identification of the handler (Figure 14-5).

The National Institute on Drug Abuse (NIDA) has established requirements for patient preparation and specimen handling in COC samples. These requirements include the following:
- The purpose and procedure of the test must be explained to the patient.
- The patient must sign a consent form.
- The patient must present picture identification.

- The specimen must be labeled appropriately to establish a COC.
- The specimen must be sealed in such a way that any tampering can be identified.
- The specimen must be placed in a locked container before transport to the testing site.
- The recipient must sign for delivery of the specimen.

Legal Alcohol Collection

Collection for alcohol testing is most common in emergency departments. This collection requires special handling to prevent alteration of the test results. Important features of alcohol testing include the following:
- The site must not be cleaned with alcohol, as this would falsely elevate the result. Instead, use soap, water, and sterile gauze or another nonalcoholic antiseptic solution.
- Tubes must be filled as full as the vacuum allows to minimize the escape of alcohol from the specimen into the space above.
- Note on the requisition form that the site was cleansed with soap and water or another a nonalcoholic solution.

BLOOD SMEARS

Blood smears are made to allow microscopic examination of the blood cells. The blood smear is used for determining the proportion of the various blood cell types, called a **differential count**; counting reticulocytes; and performing special staining procedures.

> **⟪⟨↵ FLASHBACK**
> You learned about blood cell types in Chapter 7.

Blood Smear Preparation

Blood smears are usually prepared following dermal puncture. Slides are made in pairs. Figure 14-6 illustrates a good smear, as well as several examples of unacceptable smears. Procedure 14-2 outlines how to prepare blood smears.

Malaria Smears

Malaria is caused by blood-borne protozoa of the genus *Plasmodium.* A patient with malaria has cycles of fever and chills that coincide with the life cycle of the parasite in the bloodstream. Malaria is diagnosed with a blood smear, drawn as a stat or timed collection just before the onset

TOXICOLOGY LABORATORY

Chain of Evidence Form

SUBJECT NAME _____   SUBJECT SOCIAL SEC. # _____

DATE/TIME OF COLLECTION _____   COLLECTED BY _____

NUMBER OF SPECIMENS _____   TYPE OF SPECIMEN: _____ BLOOD _____ SERUM _____ URINE

WITNESS _____

Sent by Name/Date/Time	Received by Name/Date/Time	Condition of Seals
1.		
2.		
3.		
4.		
5.		

Specimen Opened for Testing Name/Date/Time	Witnessed by Name/Date/Time	Condition of Seals
A. Outside Package 6.		
B. Specimen 7.		

LABORATORY ACCESSION NUMBER:

This form must remain with the specimen until line #7 is completed. At that time the form should be turned over to the laboratory supervisor or the designate for filling.

FIGURE 14-5 Chain of custody documentation includes special containers, seals, and forms, as well as the date, time, and identification of the handler. (From Kaplan LA, Pesce AJ: *Clinical chemistry: Theory, analysis, correlation,* ed. 5, St. Louis, 2010, Mosby.)

of fever or chills. The test requires two to three regular smears, plus a thick smear. To make the thick smear, use a larger drop of blood, and spread it out to only about the size of a dime (Figure 14-7). The sample must be allowed to dry for at least 2 hours; it is then stained to reveal the parasites.

REVIEW FOR CERTIFICATION

Routine phlebotomy specimens are often collected in the early morning for inpatients and nursing home patients because most patients are in the basal state at that time. A 12-hour complete fast may be required for some tests, especially glucose and

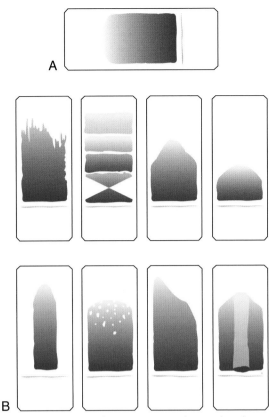

FIGURE 14-6 Blood smear slides. **A,** A good smear. **B,** Several examples of unacceptable smears. (From Rodak BF, Fritsma GA, Keohane E: *Hematology: Clinical principles and applications,* ed. 4, St. Louis, 2012, Saunders.)

triglycerides. The phlebotomist must ensure that the patient has complied with the fast and note any irregularities on the requisition. Timed specimens include the 2-hour postprandial test for diabetes mellitus and the GTT for diabetes mellitus, gestational diabetes, hyperglycemia, and hypoglycemia. TDM tests are timed to coincide with the peak or trough of serum drug levels. Testing for the presence of microorganisms in the blood requires a BC, with collection at timed intervals from multiple sites, using aseptic collection of the proper volume. Units of blood may be collected for donation to the blood bank or for use by the patient during later surgery. Therapeutic phlebotomy removes blood from the patient, most often to treat polycythemia or hemochromatosis. Samples to test for cold agglutinins,

antibodies formed against *Mycoplasma pneumoniae,* must be kept warm after collection, as must those for cryofibrinogen and cryoglobulin. Other specimens may require chilling or protection from light.

Legal or forensic samples require documentation of the COC, a protocol that ensures that the sample is always in the custody of a person legally entrusted to be in control of it. Alcohol specimens must be handled carefully to avoid contamination of the sample with alcohol and prevent escape of alcohol from the blood.

Blood smears are used for differential counts, counting reticulocytes, and special staining procedures. An acceptable smear must have a feathered edge, prepared by careful drawing of the blood drop across the slide using another slide.

PROCEDURE 14-2

Blood Smear Preparation

1. **Prepare the smears.**
   Place one drop of blood on a clean slide, ½ to 1 inch from the end, centered between the two sides.

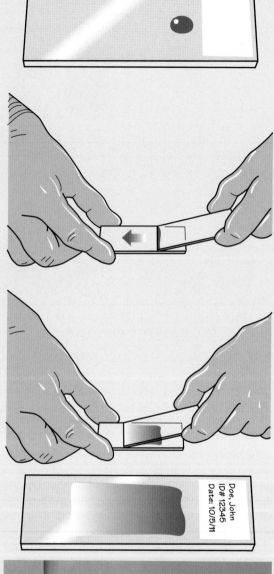

   Place the edge of a second slide, the "spreader," onto the first slide in front of the blood at a 25- to 30-degree angle, and draw it back to just contact the drop.

   Move the spreader slide forward, away from the drop, in one continuous movement to the end of the slide. The blood will be drawn along over the slide.

   To make the second slide, place a drop of blood onto the spreader slide. Using the first slide as the spreader, repeat the procedure.

   Dry and label the slides. Use pencil on the frosted end; do not use pen, as ink may run when the slide is stained.

   Doe, John
   ID# 12345
   Date: 10/5/11

2. **Examine the smears.**
   An acceptable smear must have a **feathered edge**, meaning that the cells appear to thin out farther from the original drop. At the far end, you should see a very thin transparent layer. This is the area from which the differential count is made. See Figure 14-6 for examples of blood smears. Table 14-3 describes common problems with smears and their likely causes.

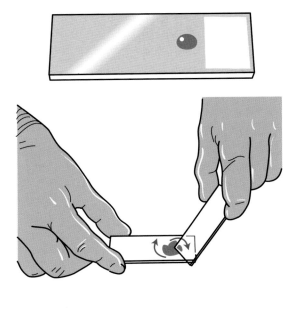

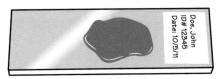

FIGURE 14-7 The thick smear for a malaria sample. This blood smear uses a larger drop of blood and is spread out only to about the size of a dime.

TABLE 14-3	Unacceptable Smears and Their Causes
Result	Cause
Holes in the smear	Dirty slide
No feathered edge	Drop that is too large
	Drop that is not placed close enough to the far edge of the slide
	Spreader slide that is lifted before it reaches the end of the sample slide
Smear that is too thick and long	Drop of blood that is too big
	Angle of the spreader slide >30 degrees
Smear that is too thin and short	Drop of blood that is too small
	Angle of the spreader slide <25 degrees
Streaks in the feathered edge	Chipped or dirty spreader slide
	Spreader slide that is not placed flush against smear slide
	Drop of blood that is in front of the spreader slide
Uneven distribution of blood	Uneven pressure on the spreader slide
	Uneven movement of the spreader slide

BIBLIOGRAPHY

American Diabetes Association: Standards of medical care in diabetes, *Diabetes Care* 32:S13–S61, 2009.

Black JG: *Microbiology principles and procedures,* ed. 8, Hoboken, N.J., 2012, John Wiley & Sons.

Blaney KD, Howard PR: *Basic and applied concepts of blood banking and transfusion practices,* ed. 3, St. Louis, 2013, Mosby.

Burtis CA, Bruns DE: *Tietz fundamentals of clinical chemistry and molecular diagnostics*, ed. 7, St. Louis, 2015, Saunders.

CLSI: *Principles and procedures for blood cultures; Approved guideline.* CSLI document M47-A. Wayne, Pa., 2008, Clinical and Laboratory Standards Institute.

CLSI: *Procedures for the collection of diagnostic blood specimens by venipuncture; Approved standard—sixth edition.* CSLI Document GP41-A6 (formerly H03-A6). Wayne, Pa., 2007, Clinical and Laboratory Standards Institute.

Ernst DJ: Controlling blood culture contamination rates, *Med Lab Observer,* May 2000.

Mayo Clinic Staff. *Lactose intolerance,* 2014. Retrieved from www.mayoclinic.org/diseases-conditions/lactose-intolerance/basics/tests-diagnosis/con-20027906.

Rodak BF, Fritsma GA, Keohane E: *Hematology: Clinical principles and applications,* ed. 4, St. Louis, 2012, Saunders.

Tille PM: *Bailey & Scott's diagnostic microbiology,* ed. 13, St. Louis, 2014, Mosby.

WHAT WOULD YOU DO?

You should not perform the draw without recleansing the site, even though it will take more time. The potential for contaminating the sample is significant because your gloves are almost certain to be carrying some bacteria. No matter what your coworker may say, the laboratory will not be able to perform the proper tests with a contaminated sample. Take your time and do it right—that is the essence of good patient care.

 AVOID THAT ERROR!

Mr. Brisco needed a therapeutic drug monitoring sample. In general, these samples should not be drawn into tubes with gel because the gel can absorb the drug. Instead, a red-topped glass tube should have been used. Before redrawing, Thomas should check with the ordering physician to determine whether the gel will interfere with the specific drug being tested.

STUDY QUESTIONS

See answers in Appendix F.

1. Define basal state.

2. List 10 factors that influence blood composition.

3. What three things are timed specimens most often used to monitor?

4. What is a GTT?

5. What is TDM, and why would this be ordered?

6. Why are BCs ordered?

7. What collection technique is critical for meaningful BC results?

8. Describe the screening process a potential blood donor goes through.

9. What special handling procedure is necessary for cold agglutinin samples?

10. List five tests that require transport on ice.

11. Explain COC.

12. Describe the important features of blood alcohol testing.

13. Explain the procedure for preparing a blood smear.

14. Describe the procedure for preparing a thick smear to test for malaria.

15. List the disorders for which therapeutic phlebotomy is used. Define the diseases based on the word roots, prefixes, suffixes, or a combination of these.

CERTIFICATION EXAMINATION PREPARATION

See answers in Appendix F.

1. Timed specimens are most frequently collected to monitor
    a. bilirubin.
    b. medication levels.
    c. cold agglutinins.
    d. cryoglobulins.

2. A 2-hour postprandial test is used to test for
    a. blood alcohol.
    b. medication levels.
    c. malaria.
    d. diabetes mellitus.

3. Hyperglycemia means
    a. decreased glucose.
    b. decreased hemoglobin.
    c. increased glucose.
    d. increased hemoglobin.

4. For a 3-hour GTT, how many blood samples will be collected?
    a. 3
    b. 4
    c. 5
    d. None of the above

5. Within what time period should a patient drink the glucose solution required for a GTT?
    a. 5 minutes
    b. 10 minutes
    c. 15 minutes
    d. 20 minutes

6. The epinephrine tolerance test determines the patient's ability to
    a. mobilize glycogen from the liver.
    b. digest lactose.
    c. metabolize carbohydrates.
    d. metabolize medications.

7. BC collection involves
    a. a peak and a trough sample.
    b. an aerobic and an anaerobic sample.
    c. a chilled sample.
    d. an accompanying urine sample.

8. Therapeutic phlebotomies are commonly performed on patients with
    a. hemochromatosis.
    b. leukemia.
    c. polycythemia.
    d. a and c.

9. To collect a cold agglutinin sample,
    a. warm the sample tube for 30 minutes before collection.
    b. pack the sample tube in ice before collection.
    c. wrap the sample in aluminum foil after collection.
    d. pack the sample tube in ice after collection.

10. Which specimen requires chilling during transfer to the laboratory?
    a. Cryofibrinogen
    b. Cryoglobulin
    c. Ammonia
    d. Cold agglutinins

11. When making smears for malaria,
    a. prepare two regular smears only.
    b. prepare two to three regular smears and one thick smear.
    c. prepare one thick smear only.
    d. prepare one regular smear and one thick smear.

12. It is necessary for a patient to fast for 12 hours before
    a. blood donation.
    b. BC.
    c. GTT.
    d. therapeutic phlebotomy.

13. Factors influencing blood composition include all of the following except:
    a. altitude.
    b. gender.
    c. age.
    d. weight.

14. Which of the following specimens is not sensitive to light?
    a. Vitamin A
    b. Lactic acid
    c. Beta-carotene
    d. Bilirubin

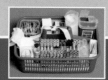

CHAPTER 15   Special Nonblood Collection Procedures

A phlebotomist is rarely just a phlebotomist today. In addition to collecting blood, you may be called on to collect nonblood specimens, assist the nurse or physician in doing so, or instruct patients regarding the procedures for collecting or handling such specimens. Nonblood specimens can provide valuable information about a patient's health or disease state. Each of the specimen types discussed in this chapter is collected to provide specific information about the physiologic processes occurring in the body or about the presence of infection or foreign substances. Strict adherence to collection protocols is as important for these procedures as it is for blood collection. Nonblood specimens include urine, feces, semen, and other body fluids. Special handling procedures are needed for some specimens to maintain sterility, preserve specimen integrity, or ensure chain of custody (COC).

OUTLINE

OBJECTIVES

After completing this chapter, you should be able to:

1. Describe six kinds of urine samples, explain how each is collected, and state one use for each.
2. Instruct a patient how to collect a midstream clean-catch urine specimen.
3. Explain how a urine sample can be collected from an infant, and state at least one limitation.
4. Discuss why a fecal sample may be requested, list three types of samples, and describe collection methods.
5. Discuss how and why semen samples may be collected.
6. Explain the proper procedure for collecting a throat sample and a nasopharyngeal sample.

7. Explain the reason and the procedure for collecting a sweat electrolyte/chloride sample.
8. Describe how cerebrospinal fluid is collected, and explain how the tubes collected should be distributed.
9. Define each of the following terms, and list at least one reason for collecting each fluid:
  a. pericardial fluid
  b. peritoneal (ascitic) fluid
  c. pleural fluid
  d. synovial fluid
10. Explain how amniotic fluid is formed, and describe three reasons for testing it.

KEY TERMS

amniocentesis	iontophoresis	nasopharyngeal (NP)	72-hour stool specimen
catheterized urine sample	iontophoretic	culture	suprapubic aspiration
8-hour specimen	pilocarpine test	occult blood specimens	sweat electrolytes (SE)
first morning specimen	midstream clean catch	random specimen	timed specimens

ABBREVIATIONS

C&S culture and sensitivity
COC chain of custody
CSF cerebrospinal fluid
hCG human chorionic gonadotropin
NP nasopharyngeal

O&P ova and parasites
RSV respiratory syncytial virus
SEs sweat electrolytes
stat short turnaround time

WHAT WOULD YOU DO?

Looking over your morning collection route for inpatients at Union Hospital, you notice your first collection is a first morning urine specimen on the eighth floor of the far wing, about as far away from the laboratory as you could be. You realize that the urine specimen needs to reach the laboratory within an hour of collection or else be refrigerated. You've got 3 hours' worth of other samples to collect, and if you go straight to the laboratory after the urine collection, you may not have time to do your other collections afterward. But you have no idea where you might find a refrigerator to hold the sample. What should you do?

URINE SPECIMENS

Why Collect a Urine Specimen?

Urine is created by the kidneys as they filter the blood. Urine contains excess salts, waste products, and small amounts of the many types of molecules that naturally circulate in the bloodstream. For this reason, urine provides a valuable snapshot of the inner workings of the body. As with blood, normal values and ranges have been established for the various substances expected to be found in urine. These values are different from those for blood, and the normal ranges are often wider because concentrations are significantly affected by fluid intake. Urine samples should be delivered to the laboratory within 1 hour of collection to prevent the breakdown of unstable compounds. When this is not possible, refrigeration of the specimen is an appropriate means of preserving the integrity of the urine's constituents. **Timed specimens**, which are specimens collected at specific times, are the exception, as discussed later.

> **‹‹‹↰ FLASHBACK**
>
> You learned about the kidney's role in urine formation in Chapter 6.

Types of Urine Specimens

Random Specimen

A **random specimen** can be collected at any time. It is used to screen for obvious metabolic abnormalities by measuring the presence of protein, glucose, blood, and other significant constituents of urine. One disadvantage of a random specimen is that it may be too dilute for accurate testing for all analytes, such as a urine pregnancy, or human chorionic gonadotropin (hCG), test.

First Morning Specimen

A **first morning specimen**, also called an **8-hour specimen**, is collected immediately after the patient awakens. It is a concentrated specimen that ensures the detection of chemicals or pathogens that may not be found in a more dilute, random sample.

Among other tests, this specimen is used for pregnancy testing, as the concentration of the pregnancy hormone, hCG, is greater in a first morning specimen. This sample should be delivered to the laboratory within 1 hour of collection to prevent breakdown of unstable compounds.

Timed Specimen

This is a series of samples often collected over 24 hours and combined to provide a single, large specimen (Figure 15-1). It is used to measure the amounts of protein, creatinine, and hormones. Creatinine is used to assess the ability of the kidney to clear waste products from the blood. In addition, some compounds are excreted in varying amounts over the course of a day, so a timed specimen is used to determine an average value.

The typical procedure is to have the patient void and discard the first morning sample, and then collect and combine all urine for the next 24 hours, ending at the same time as the patient started the test the previous day. Exact timing and collection of samples are critical. If delivery of the urine sample will not be made within 1 hour, the patient may need to refrigerate it until it can be delivered to the laboratory the following day depending on the test that is ordered. Some samples need a preservative added to them. This is usually done by the laboratory personnel. Specific instructions for each test should be given in the laboratory manual at your health care facility.

Collection Procedures for Urine Specimens

The most common procedure for collecting many types of urine specimens is known as the midstream

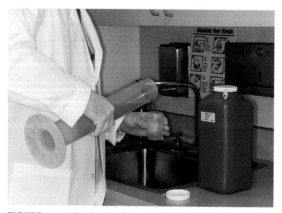

FIGURE 15-1 The timed urine specimens are often combined to provide a single, large specimen. (From Stepp CA, Woods MA: *Laboratory procedures for medical office personnel*, Philadelphia, 1998, Saunders.)

clean catch. It is collected after the patient has passed several milliliters of urine. This allows microorganisms from the urethra to be flushed out and not collected in the sample. When properly collected, the specimen is sterile or nearly so, unless the patient has a urinary tract infection. This sample can be used for urine culture, as well as for chemical and microscopic analysis. Procedure 15-1 outlines the steps for collecting a midstream urine specimen. In many cases, the patient can perform the collection himself or herself. The procedure instructions can be adapted to the situation you encounter. Other types of procedures may be more appropriate for special populations.

Pediatric Collection

Pediatric specimens for routine urinalysis can be collected using a soft, clear plastic bag with an adhesive that fits over the genital area of the child (Figure 15-2). This is not a sterile collection.

Catheter Collection

A catheterized urine sample is collected by a physician, nurse, or medical assistant. A catheter (narrow plastic tube) is inserted through the urethra into the bladder. This technique may be used for a culture and sensitivity (C&S) test when a urinary tract infection is suspected and obtaining a normal clean-catch specimen is not possible. It may also be used if the patient is unable to collect a sample independently. The phlebotomist may assist in processing the sample after collection.

Suprapubic Aspiration

A suprapubic aspiration sample is collected by a physician. A needle is inserted through the abdominal wall into the bladder for collection of a sample. The specimen is used for bacterial culture of anaerobes (bacteria that do not grow in the presence of oxygen) and for cytologic (cell) examination in cases of suspected bladder cancer. The phlebotomist may be involved in transport of the specimen to the laboratory.

Urine Samples for Drug Testing

Urinalysis can reveal the presence of many types of drugs and metabolites in the bloodstream. Drug testing is becoming increasingly common in outpatient settings, driven by the concern for a drug-free workplace. In addition, drug testing may be performed on athletes to monitor the use of performance-enhancing drugs, such as anabolic steroids, or on patients to determine whether prescription drugs have been misused.

PROCEDURE 15-1

Midstream Clean Catch

1. Clean the genitalia.

For women, use sterile soap to cleanse the area surrounding the urethra. The labia should be separated to improve access. Begin at the urethra and work outward.

For men, use towelettes with benzalkonium and alcohol. For uncircumcised men, retract the foreskin for cleaning. Begin at the urethra and work outward. Avoid using strong bactericidal agents such as povidone–iodine (Betadine) or hexachlorophene.

2. Collect the sample.

Specific procedures for sample collection may differ between institutions. At some, the patient is instructed to begin voiding into the toilet. He or she should then stop the flow of urine and move the cup into position before resuming flow. At others, the patient is instructed to begin voiding into the toilet and then, *without* stopping the flow, move the cup into the urine stream for collection. The cup should be held a few inches from the urethra, and the patient should urinate until the cup is about half full. He or she may then finish voiding into the toilet bowl. Be sure to follow the protocol for your institution.

3. Finish the collection.

Cap the container. Refrigerate or add preservatives if necessary. Label the specimen with the patient's name and the date and time of collection.

Samples for drug testing are collected in a chemically clean container, usually as a random sample via a clean catch. The collection of the sample is usually performed by the patient alone, but in a room without running water to prevent alteration of the specimen. The collection container also has a temperature-sensitive strip on the outside. A freshly collected sample will have a temperature similar to body temperature. Thus you should read the temperature strip immediately after collection. Collection and handling procedures must follow COC guidelines because the sample may be used in a legal proceeding or in decision making regarding employment or athletic participation. The COC is documented with special forms, seals, and containers.

> ### ◀◀◀⤶ FLASHBACK
> You learned about chain of custody in Chapter 14.

FECAL SPECIMENS

Why Collect a Fecal Specimen?

The two most common reasons for ordering a fecal sample are to look for intestinal infection and to

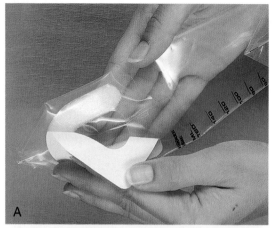

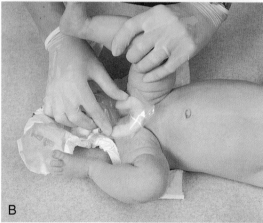

FIGURE 15-2 Pediatric specimens for routine urinalysis can be collected using a soft, clear plastic bag with an adhesive **(A)** that fits over the genital area of the child **(B).** (From Bonewit-West K: *Clinical procedures for medical assistants,* ed. 9, St. Louis, 2015, Saunders.)

screen for colorectal cancer. Microscopic examination of feces reveals the presence of intestinal ova and parasites (O&P) from organisms such as *Giardia* and tapeworm. Feces can be cultured to look for diarrhea-causing bacterial diseases such as cholera or salmonella. Cancer of the colon or rectum causes bleeding, and this blood, called occult blood, can be detected chemically. Feces also can be chemically analyzed to reveal digestive abnormalities such as excess fat and undigested meat fibers, which may indicate a gallbladder disorder or other digestion abnormalities.

Types of Fecal Specimens

Random Specimen

A random specimen is used for most determinations, including bacterial cultures, O&P, and fats and fibers.

Occult Blood Specimen

Occult blood specimens are collected after 3 days of a meat-free diet. Patients are instructed to avoid aspirin and vitamin C as well, as these can interfere with test results. Several types of special test cards are available, which may be prepared by the patient at home and sent in (Figure 15-3).

Seventy-two–Hour Stool Specimen

A 72-hour stool specimen is used for quantitative fecal fat determination. A special large container is provided for collection. This specimen is rarely called for and is ordered when a random specimen is positive for excess fat.

Collection Procedure for Fecal Specimens

Patients should be given the appropriate collection container and instructed to defecate into it, not the toilet, which would contaminate the sample with cleaning compounds. Patients should also be instructed to avoid contamination of the specimen with urine. Containers resemble a gallon-sized paint can and are typically plastic or wax-coated cardboard. The container should be tightly sealed and then wrapped in a plastic bag for transport. Specimens should be kept at room temperature until delivery to the laboratory. If the sample cannot be analyzed immediately, it may be necessary to transfer a portion of the stool to vials containing a preservative. This is especially important when it is to be examined for O&P. Kits with such vials are available commercially, or they may be prepared locally. They can be given directly to the patient, who is responsible for adding the appropriate amount of stool. O&P containers use

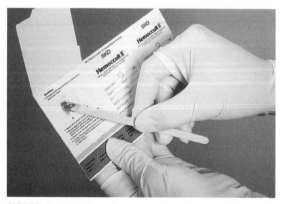

FIGURE 15-3 Fecal specimens are collected on special test cards, which may be prepared by the patient at home and sent in. (From Bonewit-West K: *Clinical procedures for medical assistants,* ed. 7, St. Louis, 2008, Saunders.)

formalin as a preservative, which is a carcinogen, and should not be sent home with the patient. Instead, the patient delivers the sample to the laboratory soon after collection, where it is transferred to the vials according to the laboratory's instructions.

SEMEN SPECIMENS

Why Collect a Semen Specimen?

Semen specimens are used to determine whether viable sperm are present in the semen, either for fertility testing or to assess the success of a vasectomy. Semen may also be collected as a forensic specimen from a rape victim, but this is collected with a special kit by trained personnel and handled with COC.

Collection Procedure for Semen Specimens

The patient should be instructed to avoid ejaculation for 3 days before the collection. The sample should be ejaculated into a sterile plastic container. A condom containing spermicide is an unacceptable collection container. The time of the collection should be recorded because sperm die quickly, and viability analysis is based on the time elapsed since collection. For fertility testing, the volume of semen is also important, so the patient should report whether the sample collected is complete or partial. The sample should be kept close to body temperature and delivered directly to the laboratory department responsible for testing within 30 minutes of collection. It is best if the sample is collected in a private room in the health care facility and delivered to the laboratory immediately.

THROAT SPECIMENS

Why Collect a Throat Specimen?

A throat culture sample (throat swab) is used to diagnose a throat infection. In particular, the sample is used to determine whether the infection is caused by group A *Streptococcus* bacteria, for which antibiotics are an effective treatment. Diagnosis is performed with either a standard bacterial culture or a rapid strep test.

Collection Procedure for Throat Specimens

Procedure 15-2 outlines the procedure for collecting a throat culture.

NASOPHARYNGEAL SPECIMENS

Why Collect a Nasopharyngeal Specimen?

The nasal passages and pharynx host many types of infectious organisms, particularly in children. A **nasopharyngeal (NP) culture** is used to diagnose whooping cough, croup, pneumonia, respiratory syncytial virus (RSV), and other upper respiratory tract infections.

Collection Procedure for Nasopharyngeal Specimens

The sample is collected using a cotton- or Dacron-tipped sterile wire (Figure 15-4). This swab is passed carefully through the nostril to reach the back of the nasopharynx. It is rotated gently to collect a mucus sample and then removed. The swab is placed in either transport media or growth media, depending on the test to be performed.

SWEAT ELECTROLYTE/CHLORIDE SPECIMENS

Why Collect a Sweat Electrolyte/Chloride Specimen?

Sweat electrolytes (SEs) are the salts, including chloride, present in normal sweat. The sweat electrolyte/chloride test is performed as part of the diagnosis for cystic fibrosis. A person with cystic fibrosis has elevated levels of chloride and sodium in the sweat.

Collection Procedure for Sweat Electrolyte/Chloride Specimens

Sweat electrolyte/chloride specimens are subjected to the **iontophoretic pilocarpine test**, which requires special training. Sweating is induced by applying a weak electrical current (known as **iontophoresis**) and the drug pilocarpine to the test area. Pilocarpine increases sweating. Sweat is collected on a piece of sterile filter paper, which is then weighed and analyzed for the amount of chloride.

BODY FLUID SPECIMENS

Fluid from various body cavities may be withdrawn for analysis or therapy. Table 15-1 lists the most common collection sites and the fluid removed. These collections are always performed by physicians. Fluid is collected in a sterile container, labeled, and transported to the laboratory for analysis as a stat specimen. The phlebotomist may be responsible for transport.

PROCEDURE 15-2

Throat Swab

1. Assemble your equipment.
You will need a tongue depressor, flashlight, sterile collection swab, transport tube with transport media (as shown in the photo), and mask and gloves.

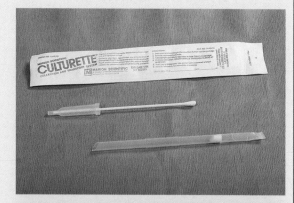

2. Collect the sample.
The patient is usually sitting upright. Ask the patient to tilt his or her head back with the mouth opened wide.

Gently depress the tongue with the tongue depressor. Inspect the back of the throat with the flashlight to locate the areas of inflammation.

Touch the tip of the swab quickly to the tonsils and any other inflamed area. Speed is essential because the patient may gag involuntarily and touch the swab with the tongue. Be careful not to touch the inside of the cheek, the tongue, or the lips because this will contaminate the sample and necessitate another collection with a new swab.

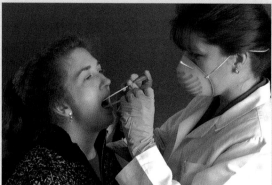

3. Process the sample.
Return the swab to the holder. Use care replacing the swab in the holder. Touching the outside or top of the holder can contaminate the swab.

Crush the ampule (containing a preservative) at the bottom of the holder containing the transport media, allowing the media to soak into the pledget, or barrier pad that separates the media and swab. Label the sample and deliver it to the laboratory.

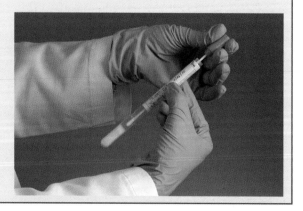

Cerebrospinal Fluid Specimens

Why Collect a Cerebrospinal Fluid Specimen?

Cerebrospinal fluid (CSF) circulates in the brain and spinal cord where it provides nourishment and removes wastes from the central nervous system. It is most commonly collected by lumbar puncture (spinal tap), in which a needle is inserted between the vertebrae at the base of the spine. CSF is used most commonly to diagnose meningitis or other central nervous system infections.

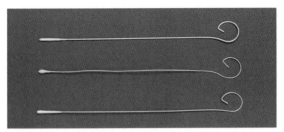

FIGURE 15-4 A nasopharyngeal (NP) culture specimen is collected using a cotton- or Dacron-tipped sterile wire passed carefully through the nostril to reach the back of the nasopharynx.

Collection Procedure for Cerebrospinal Fluid Specimens

CSF collection is done only by a physician. The phlebotomist may be asked to process and deliver samples after collection. Three to four tubes are collected in sterile plastic containers and numbered in the order of collection. Which laboratory department gets which tube is determined by your institution's policy unless the physician requests differently.

For some laboratories, the delivery of tubes is as follows: Tube 1 is delivered to the hematology laboratory for a cell count. Tube 2 is delivered to microbiology for a Gram stain and culture. Tube 3 is delivered to the chemistry laboratory for glucose and protein analysis. Tube 4 is used for repeat analysis or miscellaneous other tests.

For other laboratories the delivery is as follows: Tube 1 is reserved for nonroutine studies such as cytology. Tube 2 is used for immunology and chemistry testing such as glucose or protein. Tube 3 is delivered to microbiology for a Gram stain and culture and, if there is no fourth tube, also to hematology for a cell count. Tube 4 is delivered to hematology for a cell count. Hematology testing is important to account for any peripheral blood contamination of the sample during the lumbar puncture, which would otherwise give misleading results.

CSF specimens are always delivered to the laboratory immediately, and are analyzed as short turnaround time (stat) collections. When extra tubes are collected from a lumbar puncture, the tubes are refrigerated for any additional tests.

Amniotic Fluid Specimens

Why Collect an Amniotic Fluid Specimen?

Amniotic fluid is the fluid within the amniotic sac, developed within the uterus, that bathes and cushions the developing fetus. It is formed by the metabolism of fetal cells, by the transfer of water across the placental membrane, and in the third trimester by fetal urine. Amniotic fluid contains fetal cells, which may be analyzed for the presence of certain genetic disorders, such as Down syndrome. In the third trimester of pregnancy, the amniotic fluid can be analyzed for lipids that indicate the degree of development of the fetus's lungs. Bilirubin can also be determined at this stage to test for hemolytic disease of the newborn. Fluid may be tested for proteins associated with other abnormalities, such as spina bifida.

Collection Procedure for Amniotic Fluid Specimens

Amniotic fluid is collected by a physician in a procedure known as **amniocentesis**. The amniotic fluid is removed by a needle inserted through the mother's abdominal wall into the amniotic sac. The fluid is transferred into a sterile container protected from the light and is immediately transported to the laboratory for analysis. The phlebotomist may be responsible for transport.

REVIEW FOR CERTIFICATION

Nonblood specimens can provide valuable information about a patient's health or disease state. The most common procedure for urine specimen collection is the midstream clean catch, which can be done by the patient or assisted by the phlebotomist. Urine samples should be delivered to the laboratory within 1 hour of collection, except for timed specimens, which typically involve 24-hour collection,

TABLE 15-1	Common Body Fluid Collections	
Site	Fluid	Typical Reason for Collection
Joint space	Synovial fluid	Diagnosis of joint disorders and pain reduction
Peritoneal (abdominal) cavity	Peritoneal fluid	Diagnosis of ascites (abnormal increase of peritoneal fluid)
Pleural cavity (surrounding the lungs)	Pleural fluid	Diagnosis of pleural pneumonia
Pericardium (surrounding the heart)	Pericardial fluid	Diagnosis of pericarditis

or stat specimens. Fecal specimens are most commonly analyzed for the presence of O&P or occult blood. These specimens may be collected by the patient, who may also deliver the sample card to the laboratory for processing. Semen specimens are typically collected for fertility testing or rape determination. For fertility testing, prompt delivery is necessary for the determination of sperm viability. Throat culture swabs are carefully introduced through the mouth to the back of the throat; the specimens are used to culture infectious organisms. An NP sample is taken through the nostril to assess upper respiratory tract infections. Cystic fibrosis is diagnosed with the aid of a sweat electrolyte/chloride test, which a phlebotomist with special training may assist in performing. Internal body fluids, including CSF, joint fluids, peritoneal fluid, and amniotic fluid, are collected only by doctors. Phlebotomists may be involved in handling and transporting these samples.

BIBLIOGRAPHY

CLSI: *Sweat testing: Sample collection and quantitative chloride analysis; Approved guideline—Third edition.* CSLI document C34-A3. Wayne, Pa., 2009, Clinical and Laboratory Standards Institute.

CLSI: *Urinalysis; Approved guideline—Third edition.* CSLI document GP16-A3. Wayne, Pa., 2009, Clinical and Laboratory Standards Institute.

Family Practice Notebook: *Lumbar puncture,* 2014. Retrieved from www.fpnotebook.com/neuro/Procedure/LmbrPnctr.htm.

McPherson RA, Pincus MR: *Henry's clinical diagnosis and management by laboratory methods,* ed. 22, Philadelphia, 2012, Saunders.

Strasinger SK, Di Lorenzo MS: *Urinalysis and body fluids,* ed. 6, Philadelphia, 2015, FA Davis.

Turgeon ML: *Linné & Ringsrud's clinical laboratory science: The basics and routine techniques,* ed. 6, St. Louis, 2012, Mosby.

WHAT WOULD YOU DO?

In this case it would probably be best to ask your supervisor where you may store the urine sample while you finish your collection route. If it is nearby and convenient, you can use it. If not, and you would not be saving any time, it might be better to quickly deliver the urine sample to the laboratory after obtaining it and make up the lost time as the morning goes on. Here is a situation in which planning ahead can really help you do your job right. It is best to learn the location of resources, such as the sample refrigerator, *before* you need them. That way, when a situation comes up, you can smoothly work it into your routine.

STUDY QUESTIONS

See answers in Appendix F.

1. Define a random urine specimen and what it is used to screen for.

2. Explain the differences between a first morning specimen and a timed specimen.

3. Describe the procedure for collecting a midstream clean-catch specimen.

4. Explain why fecal specimens may be collected.

5. Explain why semen specimens may be collected.

6. Explain why NP specimens may be collected.

7. Explain the purpose of the SE test.

8. In CSF collections, how many tubes are collected, and which departments receive which tubes?

10. Explain why amniotic fluid may be collected.

11. Explain the difference between a throat culture and an NP culture.

12. Define the body areas where the following body fluids are found, and indicate whether the phlebotomist, the nurse, or the physician would be responsible for obtaining the specimen:
    a. Pleural fluid
    b. Synovial fluid
    c. CSF

13. Give some of the findings that a 24-hour urine specimen will yield and at least one method of yielding the results.

14. Explain two methods used to induce sweating in the SE test, and give the equipment used to collect, preserve, and process the specimen in the laboratory.

CERTIFICATION EXAMINATION PREPARATION

See answers in Appendix F.

1. An 8-hour urine specimen is typically collected
   a. in the morning.
   b. before going to bed.
   c. after a meal.
   d. any time during the day.

2. Which urine specimen is most commonly used to determine pregnancy?
   a. Random
   b. Fasting
   c. First morning
   d. Timed

3. The sweat electrolyte/chloride test is typically used to screen for
   a. multiple sclerosis.
   b. myasthenia gravis.
   c. cystic fibrosis.
   d. spina bifida.

4. A urine specimen is labeled
   a. before collection.
   b. after collection.
   c. by the patient.
   d. on the lid of the specimen.

5. A catheterized urine sample may be collected
   a. when a midstream clean-catch specimen is not obtainable.
   b. when the patient is unable to produce a specimen independently.
   c. by the physician, nurse, or medical assistant.
   d. all of the above.

6. A 72-hour stool specimen is collected to determine
   a. fat quantities.
   b. occult blood.
   c. protein concentrations.
   d. creatine levels.

7. A semen analysis must be
   a. delivered to the laboratory within 30 minutes of collection.
   b. kept refrigerated.
   c. collected in a condom.
   d. obtained after a 5-day period of abstinence.

8. The following body fluids are always treated as stat specimens, except for
   a. urine.
   b. peritoneal fluid.
   c. CSF.
   d. synovial fluid.

9. The test used to diagnose whooping cough, croup, and pneumonia is the
   a. SE test.
   b. NP culture.
   c. throat swab.
   d. urinalysis.

10. The following specimens are always collected by a physician, except for
    a. amniotic fluid.
    b. urine specimen.
    c. synovial fluid.
    d. CSF.

UNIT 4
Specimen Handling

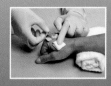

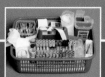

CHAPTER 16   Specimen Handling, Transport, and Processing

Proper handling of specimens after collection is critical to ensure the accuracy of the test results obtained from them. Analytes may change in composition and concentration over time and with temperature changes or exposure to light. The best drawing technique in the world is meaningless if the sample is not transported or processed according to established guidelines. Transport systems may be as simple as direct delivery to the laboratory or as complex as motorized carrier systems routed through a central distribution site. In the laboratory, the central processing department accessions the sample, centrifuges it, and prepares aliquots for distribution to other departments. Rejection of specimens can be avoided with proper attention to collection technique, handling, and transport.

OUTLINE

OBJECTIVES

After completing this chapter, you should be able to:

1. Discuss what might happen to a sample that is not properly handled and processed.
2. Describe four ways in which samples can be safely transported to the laboratory.
3. Explain why tubes should be transported in an upright position.
4. State the acceptable time between specimen collection and separation of cells from plasma or serum, and explain why this is necessary.
5. List two exceptions to time constraints, and state the maximum time that each may be held.
6. List two tests for which samples must be kept warm, and explain how to do this.
7. Describe how to handle samples that must be chilled.

8. List at least three analytes that are light sensitive, and explain how to protect them.
9. Describe the safety equipment that must be used when processing samples.
10. Explain why samples must be allowed to clot fully before processing, and state the average time for complete clotting to occur in a red-topped tube and when clot activators are used.
11. Explain the principle and proper operation of a centrifuge.
12. Describe the proper procedure for removing a stopper.
13. List at least five reasons for specimen rejection.

233

KEY TERMS

accession number

aerosol

aliquots

analytes

centrifuge

pneumatic tube system

ABBREVIATIONS

CBC complete blood count

CLSI Clinical and Laboratory Standards Institute

EDTA ethylenediaminetetraacetic acid

PPE personal protective equipment

OSHA Occupational Safety and Health Administration

QNS quantity not sufficient

stat short turnaround time

GENERAL GUIDELINES FOR SPECIMEN TRANSPORT

Tubes with additives should be inverted gently and completely 5 to 10 times immediately after being drawn. Thorough mixing allows the additives to be evenly distributed throughout the sample. Gentle inversion minimizes hemolysis. Do not mix together blood from different containers.

Specimens must be correctly labeled. Bar code labels are becoming the standard in most hospitals (Figure 16-1). An efficient and safe way to transport samples is in a leak-resistant bag with zip closure (Figure 16-2). Specimen bags are marked with a biohazard symbol and have a separate front pouch for requisitions to prevent contamination of the requisition should the specimen leak. Specimens transported from outside a hospital laboratory are carried in crush-resistant containers with absorbent material inside and biohazard labels outside the container. Government regulations require training for couriers who transport specimens in vehicles.

Tubes should remain upright during transport. This accomplishes several purposes: It promotes complete clot formation when there is no additive present; it prevents sample contamination due to prolonged contact with the stopper; and it reduces the likelihood of aerosol formation during uncapping, as there is no residual blood clinging to the stopper.

> **FLASH FORWARD**
>
> See section "Removing a Stopper" later in this chapter for a discussion of aerosols.

Time Constraints

The quality of test results depends heavily on the time between when the sample is drawn and when it is analyzed—the longer the interval, the more likely the results will be inaccurate. Ongoing glycolysis (metabolic sugar breakdown within cells) within the specimen is a primary cause of inaccurate test results. Many different tests can be affected by glycolysis, including those for glucose, potassium, calcitonin, phosphorus, aldosterone, and a number of enzymes.

As a general rule, an uncentrifuged blood sample should be delivered to the laboratory within 45 minutes of being drawn. Short turnaround time (stat) requisitions should be delivered to the laboratory immediately after being drawn.

According to the Clinical and Laboratory Standards Institute (CLSI), no more than 2 hours should pass between collection and separation by centrifugation of cells from plasma or serum. Separating the cells from the plasma prevents alteration of the levels of analytes in the serum or plasma as the cells continue to metabolize. Analytes (the substances being tested) may be elevated or decreased if cells are not separated; glucose is falsely decreased, potassium is falsely increased, and lactate dehydrogenase is falsely elevated. Once separated, the specimen can be held for longer periods. The appropriate storage temperature depends on the sample type and tests ordered.

A few sample types can wait longer before processing without loss of viability. Because fluoride inhibits glycolysis, glucose samples collected in gray-topped tubes can be held for 24 hours at room temperature and for 48 hours at 2° to 8° C. In this example, centrifugation can be delayed. Whole blood specimens collected in ethylenediaminetetraacetic acid (EDTA) for complete blood counts (CBCs) are stable for 24 hours. In this example, the sample is not centrifuged before testing because a well-mixed sample is tested. However,

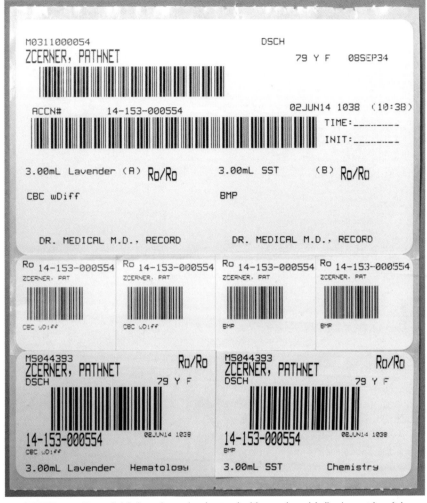

FIGURE 16-1 Bar code labels are becoming the standard for specimen labeling in most hospitals.

blood smears made from such samples must be done within 1 hour of collection because EDTA will eventually distort cell morphology.

Temperature Considerations

Temperature extremes can cause hemolysis. Samples that do not require cooling or warming should be kept at room temperature during transport.

Keeping Specimens Warm

Specimens that must be maintained at 37° C during transport and handling include cold agglutinins, cryoglobulins, and cryofibrinogen. The tubes for these specimens should be warmed using a heel-warmer packet before collection, and the sample should be transported wrapped in a heel-warmer packet as well. Heel warmers are effective up to

30 minutes. Some tests require warming of the sample in a 37° C heat block before testing. The phlebotomist should alert the laboratory staff of the arrival of a warm sample to make sure that it is held at the correct temperature until testing. Patients with certain types of blood disorders may have acquired cold agglutinins, which can cause problems with testing by automated instruments. To prevent this, the EDTA tube for a CBC must be prewarmed and kept warm. Specimens for cold agglutinin testing and cryofibrinogen must also be kept warm.

Keeping Specimens Cool

Chilling a specimen slows metabolic processes and keeps **analytes** stable during transport and handling. Samples that need to be chilled include

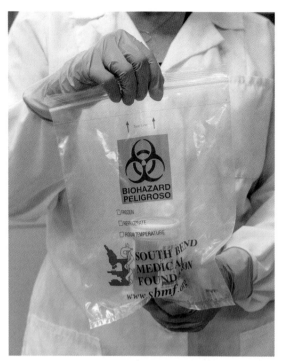

FIGURE 16-2 A leak-proof bag is an efficient and safe way to transport samples.

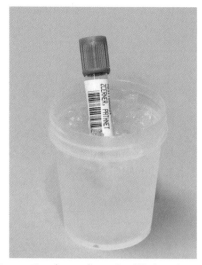

FIGURE 16-3 Samples needing to be chilled can be transported in shaved ice.

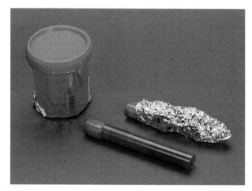

FIGURE 16-4 Samples needing to be protected from light exposure are collected in amber-colored microtubes or wrapped in aluminum foil.

pyruvate and lactic acid. A blood gas sample needs to be chilled if its delivery to the lab will be delayed. To chill a sample, place it in a slurry of chipped or shaved ice and water (Figure 16-3). This promotes complete contact between the sample and the ice bath. Avoid large ice cubes, as these may cause part of the sample to freeze. There are also commercially available systems that keep samples cold.

Keeping Specimens at Room Temperature

Some specimens must be kept at room temperature. If the specimen is being delivered outside the facility by courier, it may be placed in an insulated container to protect it from extreme heat or cold. Follow facility protocols for placing specimens in a transport device for delivery.

Protecting Specimens From Light

Exposure to light can break down light-sensitive analytes. Bilirubin is the most common light-sensitive analyte; others include vitamin B_{12}, carotene, folate, and urine porphyrin. To prevent light exposure, samples are collected in amber-colored microtubes, wrapped in aluminum foil, (Figure 16-4), or an amber/brown biohazard bag, and placed inside a brown

envelope or heavy paper bag. There are commercially available amber-colored sealable plastic bags that keep samples protected from light.

TRANSPORTING SAMPLES TO THE LABORATORY

How a sample is transported to the laboratory depends on the size of the institution and the degree of specialization within it. In many institutions, samples are hand-carried by the phlebotomist or another member of the laboratory team. Samples may be dropped off at designated areas within the hospital for transportation and delivery by the laboratory staff. This system works best when there are clear standards for documentation. A typical system uses a logbook at the drop-off and pickup area in which information about the specimen is documented. Minimum information should include the patient's name, hospital number and room number, specimen type, date and time of delivery to the drop-off area, and name of the person depositing it.

Larger hospitals may have a transportation department that is responsible for patient escort, as well as sample transport. In addition to the standard information concerning patient identification and sample type, specimens should be labeled with the laboratory as the destination.

Some institutions use a **pneumatic tube system**, in which samples are carried in sealed plastic carriers that travel within a network of tubes (Figure 16-5). Shock-absorbing foam inserts are placed in carriers to reduce the shaking and agitation of the sample during transport. Samples are first routed to a central station and then sent on to the lab. Pneumatic systems are often used for the delivery of paperwork and other items but are not always appropriate for blood samples, and the lab must assess how well this system meets its needs. Factors may include the reliability of the system, the speed of delivery, the likelihood of specimen damage during transport, and the cost of the alternative. Samples should always be bagged in sealable plastic bags, and the bag completely sealed, before being placed in the plastic carrier. When a spill occurs within the tube system, it must be closed down for decontamination.

Some larger laboratories may have self-contained motorized carriers that run on a track between departments within the laboratory for transporting specimens. There may also be tracks between different departments in the hospital to the laboratory, allowing for transport of specimens from outside of the laboratory.

Samples may arrive at the laboratory from sites outside of the hospital, such as a community clinic or private physician's office. These samples usually arrive by courier. Because of the short time allowed between collection and serum or plasma separation, the sample should be centrifuged at the collection site before transport. Samples also may arrive by overnight mail. Special containers are used to protect the sample and prevent contamination of other material during transport (Figure 16-6). Samples transported from outside the laboratory must adhere to both state and federal regulations that govern transportation of biological specimens.

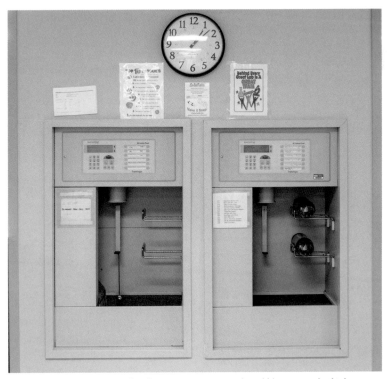

FIGURE 16-5 Pneumatic tube systems carry samples within a network of tubes.

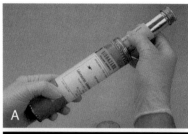

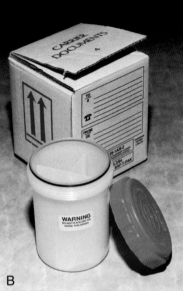

FIGURE 16-6 Courier and overnight mail services use a variety of specialized containers to protect samples and to prevent the contamination of other materials during transport. (**A,** From Zakus SM: *Clinical procedures for medical assistants,* ed. 4, St. Louis, 2001, Mosby; **B,** From Kinn ME, Woods MA: *The medical assistant: Administrative and clinical,* ed. 8, Philadelphia, 1999, Saunders.)

PROCESSING

Safety

The Occupational Safety and Health Administration (OSHA) requires personal protective equipment (PPE) to be worn during sample processing. Required equipment consists of gloves; a full-length lab coat, buttoned or snapped, with closed cuffs; and protective face gear, including either goggles and mask or a chin-length face shield.

> **«« FLASHBACK**
>
> You learned about OSHA's role in regulating workplace safety in Chapter 3.

Central Processing

Specimens entering the lab are usually first handled by central processing, an area devoted to accessioning and sorting samples as they arrive. The date and time of arrival are recorded, often with a time- and date-stamping machine. Alternatively, samples can be scanned in with a barcode reader, with the date and time recorded automatically in the laboratory's information system. Each sample is marked with an accession number, a unique identifying number used for cataloging the sample in the lab. In addition, samples are labeled with bar codes that are read by an electronic reader, which also records the time the sample is received and stores it in the computer system. Samples are then sorted by sample type and destination within the lab. Central processing is also usually responsible for centrifuging samples, to separate plasma or serum from cellular elements, and for preparing aliquots, which are small portions of the specimen transferred into separate containers for distribution to a variety of lab departments.

Before centrifuging, the stopper should remain on the sample to prevent its contamination or alteration. Cap removal releases carbon dioxide, which raises the pH and allows sample evaporation, causing increased concentration of analytes. An open tube is likely to pick up dust, sweat, powder from gloves, or other contaminants. It also creates the possibility of infectious aerosols during centrifugation.

Clotting

Serum specimens must be completely clotted before centrifugation. Incompletely clotted samples continue to clot after serum separation, interfering with testing. Plasma specimens, in contrast, can be centrifuged immediately because they have anticoagulants to prevent clotting.

Complete clotting may take 30 to 45 minutes at room temperature. Samples from patients on anticoagulants such as heparin or Coumadin (dicumarol) have longer clotting times, as do chilled specimens and those from patients with high white blood cell counts. Samples with clot activators (including serum separator tubes) clot within 30 minutes. If thrombin is used, complete clotting may occur within 5 minutes. Activators are also available that can be added to the tube after collection.

Centrifuging

A centrifuge spins the sample at a very high speed, separating components based on density. Cellular elements, which are denser, move to the bottom; the less dense plasma or serum is pushed to the top. Centrifuges come in a variety of sizes, from small tabletop models designed to hold six to eight specimens to large floor models that can hold 20 or more (Figure 16-7).

The most important principle of centrifuge operation is that every sample must be balanced by another of equal weight (Figure 16-8). Failure to balance the load causes the rotor of the centrifuge to spin out of center. This can damage the centrifuge and may allow it to move during operation, possibly causing it to fall off the table or move across the floor. In addition to the direct danger this poses to laboratory personnel, the resulting breakage of samples presents a biohazard. When necessary, an extra tube containing water should be added to balance an odd number of tubes. Repeated centrifugation of a specimen is not recommended because it may increase hemolysis of the sample and deterioration of analytes.

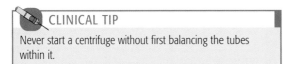

CLINICAL TIP

Never start a centrifuge without first balancing the tubes within it.

The lid of the centrifuge must be closed and secured during operation, and it must stay closed until the rotor comes to a stop. Never try to bring the centrifuge to a premature halt by touching the rotor; this is dangerous, and it can disrupt the sample. Repeated centrifugation of a specimen is not recommended because it may increase hemolysis of the sample and deterioration of analytes.

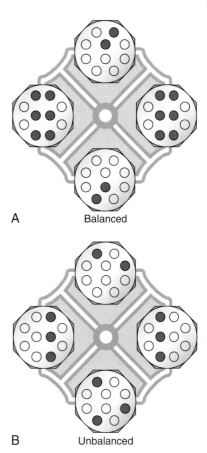

A   Balanced

B   Unbalanced

FIGURE 16-8 Tubes must be balanced in the centrifuge to avoid creating a hazard and damaging the machine. **A,** A balanced centrifuge arrangement. **B,** An unbalanced arrangement.

Removing a Stopper

The major risk of stopper removal is formation of an **aerosol**, a microscopic mist of blood that forms from droplets inside the tube. Aerosols are especially likely if the tube or rim has been contaminated by blood during collection or transport. Many automated instruments allow for testing without stopper removal. In these cases, the instrument removes the sample by piercing the stopper of the tube.

Careful stopper removal reduces the risk of aerosol formation. To remove a stopper, place a 4- × 4-inch piece of gauze over the top and pull the stopper straight up, twisting it if necessary. Do not rock it from side to side or "pop" it off. The Hemogard top is a plastic top that fits over the stopper to reduce aerosol formation and spattering. Commercial stopper removers are available as well.

When removing a top from a tube, always use a safety shield to prevent blood from accidentally spattering on you and to reduce the risk from aerosols. There are two types of safety shields.

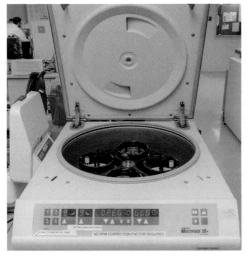

FIGURE 16-7 A tabletop centrifuge.

A personal shield has a headband that sits on your head like a hat. It has a clear plastic visor that you pull down over your face. A workstation shield attaches to the work counter from either above or below. Its height can be adjusted to offer the best protection to the person using it.

Preparing Aliquots

All tubes into which aliquots are placed should be labeled before filling and then capped before delivery to the appropriate department. Aliquots are not poured off because this may cause splashing and aerosol formation. Instead, an aliquot is removed with any one of several types of disposable pipetting systems (Figure 16-9). Aliquots may also be prepared automatically by an instrument in the laboratory. The system may include automated centrifuging and delivery of samples to testing instruments. A common task for the phlebotomist is to transfer serum or plasma to plastic transport tubes for testing at a commercial "send-out" laboratory. To prevent an identification error, you must label the transport tube before aliquoting the sample and then carefully match the patient information on the original tube with the transport tube label to be certain the aliquot is labeled correctly.

TRANSPORT AND PROCESSING OF NONBLOOD SPECIMENS

Microbiology samples must be transported to the laboratory immediately to increase the likelihood of recovering pathogenic organisms. Most specimens are collected in transport media and do not require

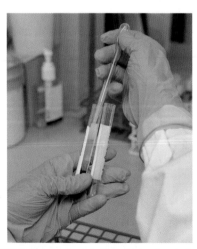

FIGURE 16-9 The specimen is divided into aliquots for distribution to laboratory departments. Several types of disposable pipetting systems are available for the removal of aliquots.

additional processing after collection. Most samples are plated immediately on culture media; often, the phlebotomist is trained to perform this task.

Twenty-four-hour urine samples must have their volume measured and recorded before aliquoting. It is important to write the total volume on the aliquot container, not the lid, and verify that the sample identifier on the main container and aliquot container are a match. Depending on the test being ordered, stool samples are kept at room temperature or refrigerated during transport and after delivery.

SPECIMEN REJECTION

All specimens received by the laboratory must be evaluated for acceptability before further processing. Criteria for rejection include the following:
1. Improper or inadequate identification
2. Hemolysis
3. Incorrect tube for the test ordered (e.g., EDTA for a chemistry test)
4. Tubes used past their expiration date
5. Inadequate ratio of blood to additive (e.g., a short draw for sodium citrate)
6. Insufficient volume for testing (known quantity not sufficient, or QNS)
7. Drawing a specimen at the wrong time (e.g., a therapeutic drug–level sample)
8. Contaminated specimen (e.g., urine for culture and sensitivity testing collected in a nonsterile container)
9. Improper handling (e.g., cold agglutinins not kept warm)
10. Bringing a sample to the laboratory outside the appropriate time frame

REVIEW FOR CERTIFICATION

Proper specimen handling is essential for obtaining accurate test results. Tubes with additives should be inverted gently and completely 5 to 10 times immediately after being drawn. All specimens must be properly labeled, and tubes should remain upright during transport. As a rule, a sample should be delivered to the laboratory within 45 minutes of being drawn, with no more than 2 hours between collection and centrifuging. Stat requisitions should be delivered to the laboratory immediately after being drawn. The phlebotomist should alert the laboratory staff regarding samples that must be kept warm to make sure that they are held at the elevated temperature until testing. Samples that require chilling should be placed in a slurry of chipped or shaved ice and water. To prevent light exposure, samples are collected in amber-colored microtubes or wrapped in aluminum foil. Transport systems vary in complexity, but all rely on scrupulous documentation at every stage. Samples may arrive at the laboratory via direct transport by the phlebotomist, pneumatic tube, collection department staff, courier, or overnight mail. Processing begins with assigning an accession number, centrifuging, and preparing aliquots. Safety precautions include the use of PPE and careful stopper removal to minimize the formation of and exposure to aerosols. Rejection of specimens can be avoided through careful attention to labeling, proper collection and handling techniques, and prompt delivery to the laboratory.

BIBLIOGRAPHY

CLSI: *Procedures for the handling and processing of blood specimens for common laboratory tests; Approved guideline—fourth edition.* CSLI document GP44-A4 (formerly H18-A4). Wayne, Pa., 2010, Clinical and Laboratory Standards Institute.

King D: Is your lab's specimen delivery system up to speed? *Advance Med Lab Prof* December:12-13, 2000.

McPherson RA, Pincus MR: *Henry's clinical diagnosis and management by laboratory methods,* ed. 22, Philadelphia, 2012, Saunders.

Turgeon ML: *Linné & Ringsrud's Clinical laboratory science: The basics and routine techniques,* ed. 6, St. Louis, 2012, Mosby.

STUDY QUESTIONS

See answers in Appendix F.

1. Describe how tubes with anticoagulant should be inverted.

2. What tests can be affected by glycolysis?

3. How soon after collection should cells be separated from plasma or serum?

4. How can specimens be maintained at 37° C during transport and handling?

5. What is the purpose of chilling a specimen?

6. What minimal documentation should be included with each specimen delivered to the laboratory?

7. What are some disadvantages to the pneumatic tube system?

8. What is the purpose of an accession number?

9. Explain why it is important that a centrifuge carry a balanced load.

10. Describe what aliquots are and how they are prepared.

11. Describe the procedure for removing a stopper.

12. How should stat specimens be transported to the laboratory, as opposed to routine specimens?

13. Explain the purpose of maintaining tubes in an upright position during transportation.

14. List the reasons specimens should be delivered under a time constraint to the laboratory.

15. Name the light-sensitive analytes, and describe how to handle these specimens.

CERTIFICATION EXAMINATION PREPARATION

See answers in Appendix F.

1. Which of these practices is NOT recommended during specimen transport?
   a. Placing the sample in a leak-proof bag
   b. Carrying the specimen upright
   c. Carrying the specimen at a 45-degree angle
   d. Labeling samples from outside the hospital with a biohazard symbol

2. Cold agglutinins and cryofibrinogen samples should be
   a. chilled before collection.
   b. transported on ice to the laboratory.
   c. warmed before collection and transported warmed.
   d. transported at room temperature.

3. Infant bilirubins are transported
   a. on ice.
   b. in amber-colored microtubes.
   c. in a heel-warmer packet.
   d. without special transport measures.

4. Once a cap is removed from a blood tube, the pH
   a. may decrease.
   b. may increase.
   c. will not change.
   d. becomes alkaline.

5. Which of the following can be centrifuged immediately after collection?
   a. Serum separator tubes
   b. Clot tubes
   c. Thrombin tubes
   d. Sodium citrate tubes

6. Which of the following specimens would not be rejected?
   a. A CBC collected in a lithium heparin tube
   b. An EDTA tube used for a chemistry test
   c. A sodium level collected in a sodium heparin tube
   d. A cold agglutinin sample transported in a heel-warmer packet

7. Complete blood clotting may take _____ at room temperature.
   a. 10 to 15 minutes
   b. 20 to 30 minutes
   c. 30 to 45 minutes
   d. 1 hour

8. The major risk of stopper removal is
   a. glycolysis.
   b. hemolysis.
   c. aerosol.
   d. clotting.

9. Which of the following is used to identify a patient specimen in the laboratory?
   a. Name of the collector of the specimen
   b. Accession number
   c. Specimen type
   d. Name of the person depositing specimen in the laboratory

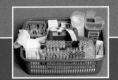

Point-of-care testing is the performance of analytic tests at the "point of care," which may be at the bedside, in the clinic, or even in the patient's home. Tests are done with small portable instruments that offer significant time and cost savings in many situations. Blood tests typically performed at the point of care include many tests in hematology, coagulation, and chemistry. In addition, the multiskilled phlebotomist may perform electrocardiography, occult blood analysis, urinalysis, pregnancy testing, and multiple tests for infectious diseases, including **rapid group A** *Streptococcus* ("strep") and HIV.

OUTLINE

OBJECTIVES

After completing this chapter, you should be able to:

1. Define point-of-care testing (POCT), and explain its advantages and disadvantages.
2. Discuss the importance of quality-assurance activities in POCT.
3. Describe the testing principle and clinical usefulness of the following:
   a. Activated coagulation time
   b. Blood gases and electrolytes
   c. Cardiac troponin T
   d. Cholesterol
   e. Dipstick urinalysis
   f. Glucose
   g. Hemoglobin
   h. Occult blood
   i. Pregnancy testing
   j. Prothrombin time
4. Perform the ancillary blood glucose test.
5. Describe the major features of an electrocardiogram and outline important points of patient preparation.

KEY TERMS

alternate site testing (AST)
ancillary blood glucose test
cardiac cycle
cardiac troponin T (cardiac TnT)
conduction system

depolarization
electrocardiogram (ECG or EKG)
electrocardiography
point-of-care testing (POCT)

P wave
Q-T interval
rapid group A *Streptococcus*
repolarization
sinoatrial node

ST segment
stylus
T wave

ABBREVIATIONS

ABGs arterial blood gases
ACT activated coagulation time
APTT activated partial thromboplastin time
AST alternate site testing
BNP B-type natriuretic peptide
CHD congestive heart disease
CLIA '88 Clinical Laboratory Improvement Act of 1988
COPD chronic obstructive pulmonary disease
EBV Epstein-Barr virus
ECG, EKG electrocardiogram
EDTA ethylenediaminetetraacetic acid
FDA Food and Drug Administration
g/dL grams per deciliter

Hb hemoglobin
hCG human chorionic gonadotropin
Hct hematocrit
HIV human immunodeficiency virus
NP nasopharyngeal
POC point of care
POCT point-of-care testing
PT prothrombin time
RBCs red blood cells
RSV Respiratory syncytial virus
TnT troponin T
WBCs white blood cells

ADVANTAGES OF POINT-OF-CARE TESTING

Point-of-care testing (POCT) refers to the performance of analytic tests immediately after obtaining a sample, often in the same room that the patient is seen in (the "point of care"). POCT is also known as alternate site testing (AST). POCT may be performed at the bedside, in the intensive care unit or emergency room, or in outpatient settings such as a clinic, physician's office, nursing home, assisted living center, or the patient's own home. Box 17-1 lists special considerations to keep in mind when drawing blood at a patient's home.

The advantages of POCT are considerable. By "bringing the laboratory to the patient," the turnaround time for obtaining test results is shortened, allowing more prompt medical attention, faster diagnosis and treatment, and potentially decreased recovery time.

BOX 17-1	Reminders for Performing Phlebotomy in a Patient's Home

1. When obtaining the specimen, always have the patient sitting or reclining in a safe, comfortable chair or bed.
2. Be aware of the nearest bathroom or sink. Carry antiseptic towelettes for handwashing.
3. Carry a cell phone for emergencies.
4. Always bring biohazard containers for specimen transport and removal of sharps.
5. Make sure that the patient has completely stopped bleeding before leaving.
6. Recheck the phlebotomy area to ensure that all materials used during the procedure have been removed and disposed of properly.
7. Preserve the specimen for transport at the proper temperature.

Most tests performed as POCT are tests waived by the Clinical Laboratory Improvement Act of 1988 (CLIA '88). Such tests are called "CLIA waived." The Food and Drug Administration (FDA) decides which tests are CLIA waived based on the ease of performing and interpreting the test. A CLIA-waived test is not subject to regulatory oversight by government authorities. The FDA website maintains a complete list of waived tests.

An essential feature of a CLIA-waived test is that the testing equipment and procedure are so simple and accurate that erroneous results are unlikely. Results are read directly from digital displays or monitors on the instrument. Although the direct cost per test is often more with these instruments, the total cost to the laboratory is often less when the time and cost for sample delivery or after-hours staffing of the laboratory are considered.

As the health care delivery landscape changes, and as more versatile and sophisticated devices are developed, POC testing is likely to become even more widespread and is likely to be used for more tests and in more settings. Becoming familiar with the newest POCT products will help you maintain an advantage in a changing health care system.

> **◄◄↰ FLASHBACK**
> You learned about CLIA '88 in Chapter 2.

Tests such as bleeding times have always been done at the bedside. The significant expansion of POCT in recent years has been possible because of the development of miniaturized analytic equipment and microcomputers. Instruments used in POCT are small, portable, and often handheld, with some tests requiring no instruments, only a card or reagent strip or "dipstick."

In general, POCT instruments are easy to use, the required training is simple, and they can be used by a variety of medical professionals, including phlebotomists, nurses, nurse assistants, and physicians.

Although these instruments are easy to use, the importance of carefully following the manufacturer's instructions cannot be overemphasized. For example, some manufacturers follow the traditional method of wiping away the first drop of blood from a dermal puncture and using subsequent drops for testing. However, a few instrument makers use the first drop of blood for their procedures. Using the second drop with such instruments would give false readings.

Quality assurance and controls are still essential for the use of POCT instruments, just as they are with laboratory based instrumentation. The laboratory is usually responsible for documentation and maintenance of POCT instruments. Finally, proper and adequate training for all personnel performing these procedures is critical to implement POCT successfully. Strict adherence to guidelines regarding calibrating equipment, running controls, performing maintenance, and keeping records is a must for a POCT program. Failure in any one of these areas can lead to erroneous test results and negative consequences for patients.

COMMON TESTS PERFORMED AT THE POINT OF CARE

Here we discuss some of the most common point-of-care tests likely to be performed by the phlebotomist. A more complete list is given in Box 17-2.

Hematology

Hemoglobin (Hgb) is the most common hematology test performed as a POC test. Hemoglobin testing is used to diagnose and monitor anemia. A simple, fast method of anemia testing uses a handheld hemoglobin analyzer (Figure 17-1). Such instruments can use arterial, venous, or dermal

blood specimens and typically give readouts in less than a minute. A whole blood sample is placed into a microcuvette or on a test strip, which is then inserted into the machine for a reading. The instrument determines the hemoglobin value in grams per deciliter (g/dL), which can be tracked over the disease course or be used to determine the response to therapy. Instruments are also available that provide readings of red blood cells (RBCs), white blood cells (WBCs), and platelets.

A hematocrit (Hct) reading is sometimes made at the bedside or, more commonly, in the clinic office. Blood is collected into a microhematocrit tube and spun down quickly using a tabletop centrifuge. Results are available within 2 minutes.

Coagulation

Coagulation monitoring is used to monitor patients with clotting disorders who are receiving therapy. Several handheld instruments are used for bedside measurement. Some use only a single drop of whole blood obtained from a dermal puncture; others use citrated blood obtained by venipuncture. Most give results in 5 minutes or less.

Heparin therapy may be monitored by determining the activated coagulation time (ACT). A small volume of blood is collected in a prewarmed tube that contains a coagulation activator. The tube is incubated at 37° C for 1 minute and then inspected by tilting the tube to determine whether a clot is present. If not, the tube is inspected every 5 seconds thereafter, with incubation continuing between observations. An automated ACT tester is available

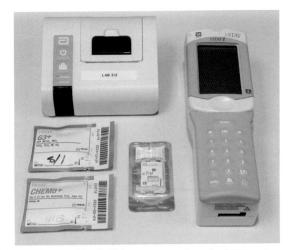

FIGURE 17-1 Handheld instruments such as the i-STAT system can perform chemistry analysis quickly and accurately. The test cards shown are for a chem 8 panel (basic metabolic panel), cTnI (troponin) and G3+ (blood gasses-pH, PCO$_2$, and PO$_2$).

BOX 17-2	Point-of-Care Tests

- B-type natriuretic peptide (BNP)
- Cardiac troponin T (TnT)
- Cholesterol
- Coagulation testing (ACT, PT, and APTT)
- Electrocardiography
- Glucose
- Hemoglobin
- Multiple chemistry panels (arterial blood gases, electrolytes, and blood urea nitrogen)

as well. The activated partial thromboplastin time (APTT) can also be used to monitor heparin therapy. With recent advances in POCT instrumentation, physicians now have a choice of tests for monitoring heparin therapy (Figure 17-2). Oral anticoagulant therapy using warfarin (Coumadin) is monitored by the prothrombin time (PT) test. CLIA-waived PT testing instruments are frequently used in physicians' offices and clinics (Figure 17-3). Antiplatelet medications, which are used to prevent stroke, and include aspirin and clopidogrel, may also require monitoring for their effect on coagulation.

Chemistry

Glucose

Bedside glucose monitoring is the most common chemistry test done by POCT. Glucose is determined with dermal puncture and reagent strips. The specimen tested is whole blood.

Ancillary Blood Glucose Test

The **ancillary blood glucose test** is performed at the bedside, most often for patients with diabetes mellitus. Steps for this test are shown in Procedure 17-1. Blood collected by dermal puncture is applied to a paper reagent strip or a microcuvette, depending on the instrument. Because different manufacturers have somewhat different procedures for their machines and test strips, be sure to read and understand the directions for the one you are using. Before any

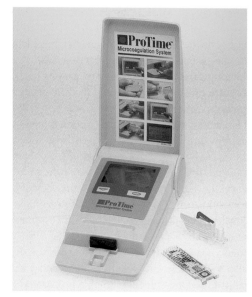

FIGURE 17-3 The ProTime Microcoagulation System for prothrombin time testing is designed to safely manage warfarin (Coumadin) therapy. (Courtesy ITC, Edison, N.J.)

patient sample can be tested, the instrument must be calibrated with materials provided by the manufacturer. This is usually performed by laboratory personnel at scheduled times. Control solutions must also be run using the same procedure as for the patient's test. These results are recorded as well. If any values fall outside the ranges provided by the manufacturer, troubleshooting must be performed until the values are correct. Proper calibration and control are critical for accurate results. Be sure to follow your institution's instructions exactly regarding performance and frequency.

Hemoglobin A1C

Hemoglobin A_{1c} can be analyzed as a CLIA-waived test, using a handheld portable testing monitor. It can be used at the bedside or other POC, providing immediate results. An example of a CLIA-waived device is the CHEK Diagnostics A1C now MultiTest A1c System. These devices are designed for clinics and physicians' offices to manage patients with diabetes. The test monitors the long-term effectiveness of diabetes therapy by providing a reading of A1c, a protein related to the average blood glucose level over a period of 4 to 6 weeks.

Cardiac Troponin T

Cardiac troponin T (cardiac TnT) is part of a protein complex in cardiac muscle that aids the interaction of actin and myosin. Damaged cardiac muscle releases

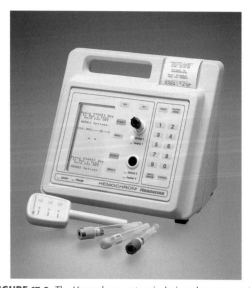

FIGURE 17-2 The Hemochron system is designed to manage the effects of anticoagulation drugs such as heparin. (Courtesy ITC, Edison, N.J.)

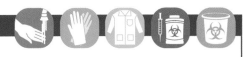

PROCEDURE 17-1

Ancillary Blood Glucose Test

1. **Perform a routine capillary collection**
   (presented in Procedure 10-1).
   Some manufacturers do not recommend wiping
   away the first drop of blood. Check the insert
   for the product you are using.

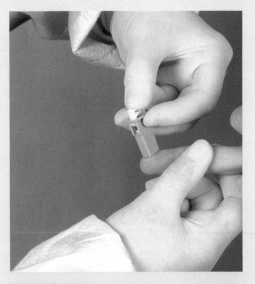

2. **Collect the sample.**
   Collect the blood drop directly onto the strip.
   Cover the appropriate area on the stick with a
   free-falling drop of blood. Be careful not to
   touch the strip yourself or allow the patient's
   skin to touch it because this can contaminate
   the strip.

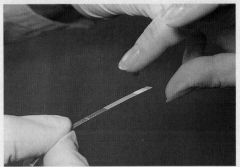

3. **Read and record the result.**
   Values that are well outside the range of normal
   (called "panic" values) should be reported
   immediately to the nursing staff or the
   physician in charge. Your laboratory should
   have a policy regarding the exact values that
   trigger such notification.

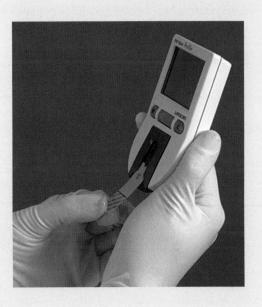

cardiac TnT, and the plasma level of cardiac TnT rises within 4 hours after an acute myocardial infarction (heart attack). It may stay elevated for up to 2 weeks, and its level may help determine the extent of damage and the patient's prognosis. Therefore monitoring cardiac TnT can provide valuable information for a patient with a possible myocardial infarction. Bedside determination is performed using anticoagulated whole blood, and results are available within 15 minutes (Figure 17-4).

Lipids

Cholesterol levels may be determined as part of a routine examination or to monitor therapy with cholesterol-lowering drugs. Some POCT determinations use a one-step, disposable color card test rather than a machine. These use whole blood from either a dermal puncture or a heparinized venous sample. Blood is applied to a card, and a color determination is made after the reaction takes place. Other cholesterol POCT methods use instrumentation (see Figure 17-1).

Blood Gases and Electrolytes

Several instruments are available that can analyze arterial blood gases (the concentrations of oxygen and carbon dioxide and the pH) and common electrolytes (sodium, potassium, calcium, chloride, and bicarbonate). Some systems are small enough to be handheld; others require a cart. They are particularly useful when frequent or rapid chemistry determinations must be made, such as in the emergency room or intensive care unit. Because of their complexity, all these instruments require careful calibration and

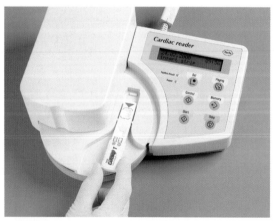

FIGURE 17-4 The Cardiac Reader system allows rapid determination of the cardiac markers troponin T and myoglobin from a single whole blood sample. (Courtesy Roche Diagnostics, Indianapolis, Ind.)

more training than do simpler instruments such as hemoglobin analyzers. The specimen tested is whole blood.

B-Type Natriuretic Peptide

B-type natriuretic peptide (BNP), also known as brain natriuretic peptide, is a hormone made by the heart in response to expansion of ventricular volume and pressure overload. Its production increases in patients with congestive heart disease (CHD). The measurement of BNP at the bedside allows the practitioner to quickly differentiate between chronic obstructive pulmonary disease (COPD) and CHD, which may have similar symptoms. BNP can also be monitored to determine the effectiveness of CHD therapy. The BNP test requires a whole blood sample collected in ethylenediaminetetraacetic acid (EDTA).

ELECTROCARDIOGRAPHY

Electrocardiography is a method for recording the electrical activity of the heart. The output of the electrocardiograph is a tracing, called an **electrocardiogram (ECG or EKG)**. The ECG is used to diagnose heart disease such as ischemia, myocardial infarction, or fibrillation.

With the increasing demand for multiskilled personnel, developing the ability to perform electrocardiography is a natural progression for phlebotomists. It is beyond the scope of this chapter to give a complete introduction to this topic. Instead, we give the broad outlines needed to understand electrocardiography and present the basics of patient preparation and ECG recording.

The Cardiac Cycle

As you learned in Chapter 7, each heartbeat cycle includes a contraction and relaxation of each of the four chambers of the heart. This contraction is triggered and coordinated by electrical impulses from the heart's pacemaker, called the **sinoatrial node**, located in the upper wall of the right atrium. Electrical impulses spread out from there through the heart's **conduction system**, triggering the coordinated contraction of the heart muscle. The **cardiac cycle** refers to one complete heartbeat, consisting of **depolarization** (contraction) and **repolarization** (recovery and relaxation) of both the atria and the ventricles. The electrical activity occurring during this cycle is recorded on the ECG.

The normal ECG consists of a tracing with five prominent points where the graph changes direction.

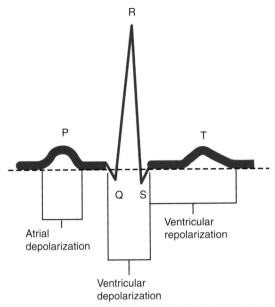

FIGURE 17-5 ECG tracing depicting P, Q, R, S, and T cycles. (Modified from Flynn JC, Jr: *Procedures in phlebotomy*, ed. 3, Philadelphia, 2005, Saunders.)

These are arbitrarily known as P, Q, R, S, and T (Figure 17-5). The regions immediately surrounding each point are known as the **P wave**, **T wave**, and so on. As shown in the figure, the sections joining these points are known variously as segments, complexes, or intervals. Each part of the graph corresponds to a particular portion of the cardiac cycle and can be analyzed to determine how the heart is functioning (Table 17-1).

Important parameters that can be determined from the ECG include the time intervals between different phases of the cardiac cycle, which indicate conduction efficiency, and the size of the electrical signals, which may be correlated with an increase or decrease of heart muscle mass. For instance,

ischemia may be associated with elongation of the **Q-T interval**, and myocardial injury may cause elevation of the **ST segment** above its normal position. The duration of the cardiac cycle can be read directly from the ECG because each small square represents a known unit of time (Figure 17-6).

Electrocardiogram Equipment

The electrical activity of the heart is recorded with 10 numbered electrodes that are placed in defined locations on the patient's chest, arms, and legs (Figure 17-7). The electrodes may be applied with an electrolyte solution to increase conductivity. A wire, is attached to each electrode. The wires pass to the ECG machine through a cable. The tracing is made on heat- and pressure-sensitive paper by a **stylus**.

Performing an Electrocardiogram

The machine and the patient should be positioned away from electrical equipment, including televisions, air conditioners, and other functioning appliances. The patient should be wearing a gown that opens in the front, and the lower legs must be exposed. The patient should be lying down and must remain still during the ECG (Figure 17-8). Electrode locations are cleaned with alcohol and shaved of hair, if necessary. Disposable adhesive electrodes are available, or electrolyte cream or gel is applied if reusable electrodes are being used. Electrodes are applied to the proper locations (as outlined in Box 17-3) and secured in place. The machine is turned on, and the recording is made. Many ECG machines automatically cycle through the 10 electrodes; alternatively, the technician switches the machine by hand to record from each electrode for a short time. After successfully recording from each electrode, the electrodes are removed, the skin is cleaned, and the patient can get dressed.

TABLE 17-1	Electrocardiogram Measurements
ECG Section	**Heart Activity**
P wave	Atrial depolarization
P-R interval	Time between atrial contraction and ventricular contraction
QRS complex	Ventricular depolarization
ST segment	Time between ventricular depolarization and beginning of repolarization
T wave	Ventricular repolarization
Q-T interval	Time between ventricular depolarization and completion of repolarization

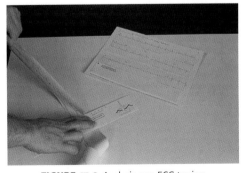

FIGURE 17-6 Analyzing an ECG tracing.

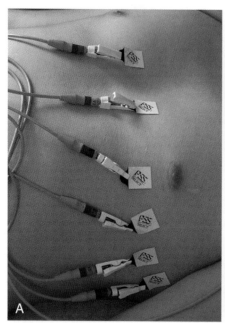
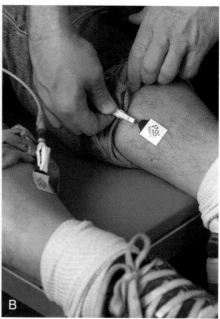

FIGURE 17-7 ECG electrodes are attached to the chest **(A)** and to the right and left legs **(B)**, as well as to the arms.

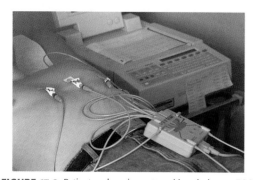

FIGURE 17-8 Patient and equipment position during an ECG.

BOX 17-3	Placement of Chest Electrodes

V_1, fourth intercostal space to the right of the sternum
V_2, fourth intercostal space to the left of the sternum
V_3, midway between position 2 and position 4
V_4, fifth intercostal space at the left midclavicular line
V_5, fifth intercostal space at the left anterior axillary line
V_6, fifth intercostal space at the left midaxillary line

OTHER CLIA-WAIVED TESTS

The number of CLIA-waived tests is growing because of both advances in bioanalytic chemistry and recognition that such tests allow more flexible delivery of care by a wider range of staff. The following tests are commonly performed as CLIA-waived tests, though not necessarily at the bedside or with handheld instruments.

Occult Blood

The occult blood test uses a card kit or slide and is a guaiac-based test. The stool specimen is placed on the card (two windows) or slide, and the reagent or developer solution (stabilized peroxide reagent) is added to the test area (Figure 17-9). Detection of occult blood in feces is used in the diagnosis of digestive tract diseases such as gastric ulcers or colon cancer. The patient must be informed of dietary restrictions that need to be followed before the test.

Urinalysis

Many commonly requested urine tests can be performed using a dipstick, a plastic strip with reagents embedded in it. Tests may include pH, protein, glucose, ketones, bilirubin, urobilinogen, blood, leukocyte esterase, nitrite, and specific gravity. Before testing begins, the urine specimen must be at room temperature and thoroughly mixed. The urine strip is briefly and completely immersed in a well-mixed fresh urine specimen (Figure 17-10). After removal, excess urine is blotted from the side of the strip (Figure 17-11). The color change on the strip is compared with the reference color chart on the bottle at the appropriate time (Figure 17-12). The change may be read by eye or with a tabletop

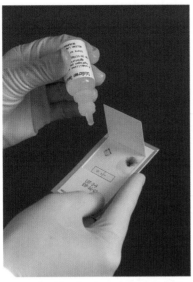

FIGURE 17-9 Applying developer to the occult blood card.

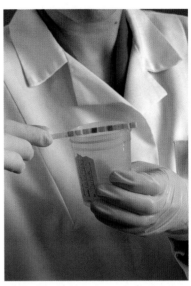

FIGURE 17-11 Remove excess urine by withdrawing the strip along the side of the container.

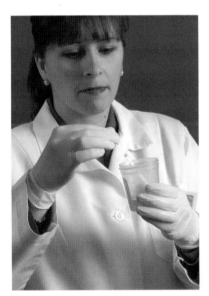

FIGURE 17-10 In a routine urinalysis procedure, the strip is completely immersed in the urine and then evaluated against the control, usually found in the bottle.

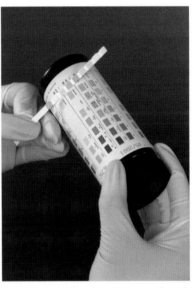

FIGURE 17-12 Compare the color change on the strip with the chart on the bottle.

instrument that reads the strip. The microscopic component of a urinalysis examination is NOT a waived test and must be performed by a qualified health care practitioner such as medical laboratory scientist (MLS) or medical laboratory technologist (MLT). MLS, MT, or MLT.

Pregnancy

A pregnancy test detects the presence of human chorionic gonadotropin (hCG), a hormone produced by the placenta after implantation of a fertilized egg. This hormone is present in both urine and serum, and test kits are available for each.

Infectious Disease

There are many POC tests used to detect infectious diseases. The tests are provided as kits that come with necessary reagents and test cassettes.

Rapid Group A *Streptococcus*

This test detects group A *Streptococcus (Streptococcus pyogenes)* from a throat swab. The procedure usually requires extracting the sample to isolate bacterial carbohydrates, followed by the addition of reagents and the development of a color change. Test results are generally available within 3 to 5 minutes (Figure 17-13).

Respiratory Syncytial Virus

Respiratory syncytial (sin-SISH-uhl) virus (RSV) infects the airways and may cause inflammation of the bronchioles, especially in young children. The POC test uses either a nasal wash or a nasopharyngeal (NP) swab.

Influenza A and B

Influenza (flu) is a viral disease of the respiratory system. There are two main types, A and B. The influenza A and B test detects both, and distinguishes between the two. The test is performed on a specimen collected by a nasal swab, nasopharyngeal swab, nasal wash or nasopharyngeal aspirate (in which fluid is withdrawn under suction from the rear of the nasal cavity). A single sample can be used to run both the test for A and B types.

Helicobacter pylori

Helicobacter pylori (H. pylori) is a bacterium found in the stomach that can cause ulcers. Antibodies to the bacterium can be detected with a POC test, with whole blood as the sample.

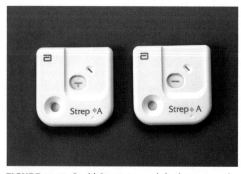

FIGURE 17-13 Rapid *Streptococcus* infection test results.

Infectious Mononucleosis

Infectious mononucleosis is caused by a virus, most commonly the **Epstein-Barr virus** (EBV). It causes sore throat, fever, and swollen glands. The POC test detects antibodies to EBV, with whole blood as the sample.

Human Immunodeficiency Virus

Human immunodeficiency virus (HIV) attacks T-helper cells in the immune system, which may cause acquired immunodeficiency syndrome (AIDS). The POC test detects antibodies to HIV, with whole blood as the sample.

REVIEW FOR CERTIFICATION

POCT refers to the performance of analytic tests immediately after obtaining a sample, often in the same room in which the patient is seen. Most tests performed as POCT are CLIA-waived tests, and the results are read directly from digital displays or monitors on the instrument. POCT instruments are easy to use, training is simple, and they can be used by a variety of medical professionals, including phlebotomists, nurses, nurse assistants, and physicians. Carefully following the manufacturer's instructions is important for obtaining accurate results. Hematology tests commonly performed as POCT include anemia and polycythemia evaluation by a handheld hemoglobin analyzer; coagulation monitoring; heparin therapy monitoring using the ACT or APTT; and oral anticoagulant therapy via the PT. Chemistry tests include glucose; cardiac TnT; cholesterol, using either a machine or a card test; arterial blood gases (ABGs); and electrolytes. Electrocardiography provides an ECG tracing that can be used to diagnose heart disease. The ECG includes waves and other features corresponding to particular portions of the cardiac cycle, which can be analyzed to determine how the heart is functioning. Numbered electrodes, called leads, are placed in defined locations on the patient's chest, arms, and legs. The machine and the patient should be positioned away from electrical equipment, and the patient should be lying down and must remain still during the ECG. Other tests performed as POCT include occult blood testing using a card kit, urinalysis with a dipstick or reagent stick, pregnancy testing for the presence of hCG, and multiple infectious disease tests, including rapid group A *Streptococcus*, Epstein-Barr virus, *H. pylori,* influenza, RSV and HIV.

BIBLIOGRAPHY

American Association for Clinical Chemistry: *The National Academy of Clinical Biochemistry Laboratory Medicine Practice Guidelines evidence-based practice for point-of-care testing published guidelines,* 2014. Retrieved from www.aacc.org/members/nacb/LMPG/OnlineGuide/PublishedGuidelines/poct/Pages/poctpdf.aspx#.

CliaWaived.com: *Diabetes A1c testing,* 2012. Retrieved from www.cliawaived.com/web/Diabetes_%28A1c_Testing%29.htm.

Kost GJ, editor: *Point-of-care testing: Principles, management, and clinical practice,* Philadelphia, 2002, Lippincott.

Santrach PJ: *Current and future application of point of care testing,* 2007. Retrieved from http://wwwn.cdc.gov/cliac/pdf/addenda/cliac0207/addendumf.pdf.

STUDY QUESTIONS

See answers in Appendix F.

1. Define POCT, and state four locales in which it may occur.

2. State an advantage and a disadvantage of POCT.

3. Describe the use of and the need for adherence to quality-assurance and quality-control procedures when performing POCT.

4. State two hematology tests that can be performed as POCT, and indicate how each test is done.

5. State four chemistry tests that can be performed as POCT, and indicate how each test is done.

6. Name the five waves that make up an ECG.

7. Name the heart activity that corresponds to the following:
   a. P wave
   b. QRS complex
   c. ST segment

8. Describe how to perform a dipstick urinalysis test.

9. Explain why it is important to follow the manufacturer's instructions when performing POCT.

10. Describe the POC test that can be used to evaluate the following:
    a. Anemia
    b. Warfarin therapy
    c. Cholesterol
    d. ABGs

11. List the common electrolytes that can be measured by POCT.

12. Describe the normal ECG pattern.

13. Relate ECG tracing to cardiac activity.

14. List the dipstick tests that are routinely performed on random urine specimens.

15. What types of specimens are used to determine pregnancy?

16. List the adherence guidelines for a POCT program. List the detrimental outcomes of failing to adhere to these guidelines.

17. The microcuvette tests and measures _____ and is essential in _____.

18. List the process used in ACT and the timed intervals if a clot does not form.

19. List the three analytes obtained in an ABG sample and the common electrolytes.

20. List the proper electrode placement for the precordial leads of an ECG.

CERTIFICATION EXAMINATION PREPARATION

See answers in Appendix F.

1. The percentage of packed red blood cells in a volume of blood is known as the
   a. hemoglobin.
   b. red blood cell count.
   c. packed cell volume.
   d. erythrocyte sedimentation rate.

2. A handheld hemoglobin analyzer gives a readout whose units are in
   a. grams per milliliter.
   b. grams per deciliter.
   c. kilograms per liter.
   d. kilograms per milliliter.

3. What POC test can be used to monitor heparin therapy?
   a. PT or APTT
   b. ACT or APTT
   c. ACT or PT
   d. PT or TT

4. What test can provide valuable information regarding whether a patient has experienced a myocardial infarction?
   a. Hemoglobin
   b. Cholesterol
   c. Cardiac TnT
   d. Glucose

5. What test can be used to screen for colon cancer?
   a. Hemoglobin
   b. Glucose
   c. Cholesterol
   d. Occult blood

6. Determination of hCG is used to evaluate
   a. liver disease.
   b. anemia.
   c. urinary tract infection.
   d. pregnancy.

7. What type of specimen is used for the occult blood test?
   a. Blood
   b. Urine
   c. Feces
   d. Saliva

8. What *Streptococcus* group is detected when performing a rapid strep test on a throat culture?
   a. Group A
   b. Group B
   c. Group C
   d. Group D

9. Before performing the dipstick test for a routine urinalysis, what two pretesting conditions must be met?
   a. Specimen must be at room temperature and well mixed.
   b. Specimen must be refrigerated and centrifuged.
   c. Specimen must be warmed to body temperature and well mixed.
   d. Specimen must be at room temperature and centrifuged.

10. For a POCT program to be successful, which of the following must be incorporated?
    a. Adherence to the manufacturer's instructions
    b. Use of quality-assurance and quality-control procedures
    c. Proper and adequate training of all personnel
    d. All of the above

Professional Issues

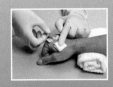
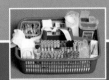

CHAPTER **18**   Quality Phlebotomy

Quality phlebotomy is a set of policies and procedures designed to ensure the highest-quality patient care and consistent specimen analysis. Continual, gradual improvement in the standard of care delivered is the goal of quality phlebotomy. The phlebotomist is best able to control preanalytic variables, which are those that influence patient care and sample integrity before analysis in the laboratory. Patient preparation, specimen collection, and transport and processing are critical areas for quality phlebotomy. Throughout this book, you have learned important precautions and techniques designed to maintain both the comfort and safety of the patient and the quality of the sample collected. We review those items here and discuss the laboratory procedures that have an impact on the quality of test results.

OUTLINE

Features of Quality Phlebotomy
Total Quality Management
Quality Assurance and Quality
   Control
Procedure Manual
Directory of Services
Monitoring of Variables
Preanalytic Variables
Requisition Handling

Equipment
Patient Identification
Patient Preparation and
Specimen Collection
Patient Preparation
Specimen Collection
Patient's Perception
Accidental Puncture
Transportation

Processing
Separation Times
Centrifuge Maintenance
Evaporation and Contamination
Refrigerators and Freezers
Aliquot Handling and Labeling
Analytical Variables
Postanalytical Variables
Review for Certification

OBJECTIVES

After completing this chapter, you should be able to:

1. Define quality assurance (QA), quality control (QC), total quality management, and continuous quality improvement, and discuss their differences and roles in quality phlebotomy.
2. Describe the contents of the procedure manual, and explain how the phlebotomist can use it.
3. Explain the role of the directory of services, and describe the information it contains.
4. List three types of analytic variables.
5. Describe at least five errors that may occur as a result of improper requisition handling, and explain QA procedures to monitor for them.
6. Describe procedures that should be followed for the QC of phlebotomy equipment.
7. Explain why expired tubes should not be used.
8. Define delta check, and explain its use in QA.

9. List nine patient activities that may affect laboratory test results, and give at least one example of a test affected by each.
10. List at least four blood collection sites that may lead to sample contamination, and list six sites that may result in pain or injury to the patient.
11. Discuss at least two errors that may result from improper tourniquet application.
12. Explain the risks of failing to cleanse the puncture site carefully, and discuss one method to monitor for such errors.
13. Describe precautions that must be taken when iodine is used as a cleansing agent, and list at least two laboratory tests that can be affected.
14. Discuss at least eight precautions that must be taken in collecting and labeling specimens.

15. Explain the phlebotomist's role in ensuring a positive patient perception of the level of care received.
16. Explain the steps to be followed in the case of an accidental needle stick, and describe QA procedures that may be used.
17. Discuss the monitoring of variables during sample transport.
18. Explain the effects of sample-processing variables on sample quality (e.g., separation times and centrifugation).
19. Describe how refrigerators and freezers are monitored.
20. Explain how multiple aliquots prepared from a single sample should be handled.

KEY TERMS

continuous quality improvement (CQI)
delta check

preanalytic variables
procedure manual
quality assurance (QA)

quality control (QC)
quality phlebotomy

total quality management (TQM)

ABBREVIATIONS

ABGs arterial blood gases
CLSI Clinical and Laboratory Standards Institute
CQI continuous quality improvement
IV intravenous
POCT Point-of-care testing
QA quality assurance

QC quality control
RBC red blood cells
stat short turnaround time
TQM total quality management
WBC white blood cells

FEATURES OF QUALITY PHLEBOTOMY

Quality phlebotomy refers to a set of policies and procedures designed to ensure the delivery of the highest-quality patient care and consistent specimen analysis. Quality phlebotomy ensures better patient care by reducing errors and increasing efficiency, making the delivery of care more cost efficient.

There are several aspects to quality phlebotomy. Quality control (QC) refers to the quantitative methods used to monitor the quality of procedures, such as regular inspection and calibration of equipment, to ensure accurate test results. QC is part of quality assurance (QA), the larger set of methods used to guarantee quality patient care, including the methods used for patient preparation and collection and transportation protocols. Both QC and QA are included in total quality management (TQM), the entire set of approaches used by the institution to provide patient satisfaction. Continuous quality improvement (CQI) is the major goal of TQM programs.

QA programs are mandated by the Joint Commission. Joint Commission standards require that a systematic process be in place to monitor and evaluate the quality of patient care. The direct involvement of workers is a requirement of TQM programs.

The team approach improves production by reducing errors and waste, thereby resulting in a reduction in health care cost.

Different health care organizations will have different programs in place to promote quality improvement. The Joint Commission stresses the collection and analysis of data to understand where the organization is weakest, and where to focus on improvements. Important aspects of any quality improvement program that you may be responsible for include:
- Patient wait time
- Accurate patient identification
- Duplicate test orders
- Technical proficiency
- Multiple attempts for a single collection
- Complication due to phlebotomy procedures
- Specimen re-collection due to collection errors
- Postcollection specimen handling

Total Quality Management

TQM focuses on gradual, continual improvements in the quality of services provided by the laboratory. Rather than merely setting a minimum standard to be met, the TQM philosophy sees the potential for improvement in every area, no matter how high the current performance level, to improve the services provided to "customers." For the clinical laboratory, the customers are the patients, the physicians and other health care providers who order tests, and the personnel who use test results to provide treatment. The phlebotomist is the member of the laboratory team with the most patient contact and is therefore most directly responsible for customer satisfaction in this area.

Quality Assurance and Quality Control

QA guarantees quality patient care through a specific program, including both technical and nontechnical procedures. QA programs use written documentation to set standards for the performance of procedures, monitor compliance with written procedures, and track patient outcomes with scheduled evaluations of all laboratory activities. Documentation provides written policies and procedures covering all services and provides evidence that standards have been met and that work is being performed efficiently. In the event of a problem, documentation provides a means of monitoring the actions taken to resolve the problem. Documentation includes a procedure manual for laboratory procedures, a floor book distributed to nursing departments detailing schedules and other information, the identification of variables that may affect patient care and test results, re-collection lists, hemolysis data, and continuing education for all members of the laboratory staff.

QC is part of QA. QC is the set of quantitative methods used to monitor the quality of procedures to ensure accuracy of test results. Its focus is on identifying the problems that may be preventing the delivery of quality phlebotomy. QC requires documenting equipment inspections, calibrating instruments, and monitoring the protocols used in each step of phlebotomy, from patient preparation and identification, through collection procedures and equipment, to transportation of specimens and distribution in the laboratory. Together, QC and QA help to ensure quality patient care.

Procedure Manual

The **procedure manual** is present in the department at all times. It contains protocols and other information about all the tests performed in the laboratory, including the principle behind the test, the purpose of performing it, the specimen type the test requires, the collection method, and the equipment and supplies required. QA procedures relevant to the procedure manual include updating the standards and protocols to comply with advances in the field, training for laboratory members in the proper

performance of procedures, scheduled testing of standard samples, and monitoring of results.

Directory of Services

The directory of services contains a variety of information pertinent to the smooth coordination of nursing staff and laboratory personnel. It may be available in hard copy or online at the laboratory website. It includes laboratory test schedules, early morning collection schedules, and written notification of any changes, plus information on patient preparation, specimen types and handling, and normal values. QA procedures relevant to the information in the directory of services include monitoring the numbers of incomplete or duplicate requisitions received, collecting statistics on the number of missed or delayed collections, and recording the time between a test request and a results report.

Monitoring of Variables

A variable is any factor that can be measured or counted that affects the outcome of test results and therefore patient care. Once identified, a variable is controlled through the institution of a set of written procedures. Monitoring of the variable is performed and documented to ensure that its impact on test results is minimized.

There are three types of variables: preanalytic, analytic, and postanalytic, each of which can affect test results. The phlebotomist is most responsible for controlling **preanalytic variables**, those that occur before analysis of the specimen (Figure 18-1). Venous blood specimen collection accounts for more than half of the errors in preanalytic variables. Analytic variables, those that occur during specimen analysis, can be affected by preanalytic variables, such as collection time or transport conditions. Postanalytic variables, such as delays in reporting results or improper entry of results in the data bank, also may be part of the phlebotomist's responsibilities.

PREANALYTIC VARIABLES

Requisition Handling

Preanalytic variables occur in each area of the phlebotomist's duties, beginning with test ordering and requisition handling. Requisitions must be accurately and completely filled out with the patient number, tests ordered, and priority (Figure 18-2). Variables to be controlled include duplicate or missing requisitions, tests left off the requisition, missing patient number, missing doctor name, or

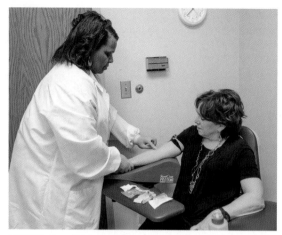

FIGURE 18-1 Phlebotomists are most responsible for controlling preanalytic variables, such as ensuring that the equipment they use is free of defects.

priority not indicated. When demographic, diagnostic, and insurance information is omitted or is inaccurate, there is a delay in reporting results, introducing a postanalytic variable. QA procedures for these variables include recording and counting the numbers of each type of requisition error.

Equipment

Phlebotomy equipment is designed and manufactured to be free of defects and minimize variability. Nonetheless, errors do occur, and it is up to the phlebotomist to identify and eliminate them before they interfere with patient care. QA procedures include the following:

- Tubes should be checked for lot number and expiration date. Never use an expired tube.
- Stoppers should be checked for cracks or improper seating. Reject any tube with a defective stopper.
- Tubes may lose vacuum without any visible sign of defect. When filling a tube, be aware of incomplete filling because of loss of vacuum. Clinical and Laboratory Standards Institute (CLSI) guidelines indicate that the volume should be ± 10% of the stated draw.
- Needles should always be inspected for defects, including blunted points or burrs (Figure 18-3). Never use a defective needle or one from a package with a broken seal.

- Syringe plungers must move freely in the barrel. Reject a syringe with a sticky plunger.

◀◀◀ FLASHBACK
You learned about venipuncture equipment in Chapter 8.

Patient Identification

It cannot be emphasized too strongly that proper patient identification is the most important procedure in phlebotomy. Improper identification can lead to injury or death. Proper identification is made when the patient number on the requisition matches the number on the patient's identification band *and* that band is attached to the patient (Figure 18-4). A further check on correct identification is to ask the patient to state his or her name and date of birth and to match that to the identification band and the requisition.

A **delta check** is a QA procedure that helps spot identification errors. This check compares previous patient results with current results. If the difference ("delta") between the two sets of results is outside the limit of expected variation, it alerts laboratory personnel to the possibility of an error.

PATIENT PREPARATION AND SPECIMEN COLLECTION

Many preanalytic variables arise during patient preparation and specimen collection. Although not all of them can be completely controlled in every procedure, developing skill as a phlebotomist largely means minimizing the effect of these variables to the greatest extent possible.

Patient Preparation

The patient's physical condition at the time of the collection has a significant effect on the sample quality. The phlebotomist has little or no control over most of these variables but may note their presence to aid in the interpretation of test results. Factors include the following:

- *Posture.* A sample collected from an erect patient has higher concentrations of large molecules such as enzymes and albumin, as well as white blood cells (WBCs) and red blood cells (RBCs), compared with a sample collected from a supine patient (Figure 18-5). This is due to a gravity-induced shift in fluids upon standing.

Lab Services

IMPORTANT
Patient instructions
and map on back

PHYSICIAN ORDERS

M ☐ Patient
F ☐ SS# __ __ __

Patient _____ _____ ____   D.O.B. _____
       Last Name   First   M.I.

Address _____ City _____ Zip _____ Phone # _____

Physician _____
         ATTACH COPY OF INSURANCE CARD

Date & Time of Collection: _____

Drawing
Facility: _____

Diagnosis/ICD-9 Code _____
                    (Additional codes on reverse)

☐ 789.00 Abdominal Pain   ☐ 414.9 Coronary Artery Disease (CAD)   ☐ 244.9 Hypothyroidism
☐ 285.9 Anemia (NOS)   ☐ 250.0 DM (diabetes mellitus)   ☐ 272.4 Hyperlipidemia
                             ☐ 780.7 Fatigue/Malaise   ☐ 401.9 Hypertension
                             ☐ 272.0 Hypercholesterolemia   ☐ 485.9 URI (upper respiratory infection)

☐ ROUTINE   ☐ PHONE RESULTS TO: # _____
☐ ASAP   ☐ FAX RESULTS TO: # _____
☐ STAT   ☐ COPY TO: _____

HEMATOLOGY	CHEMISTRY	CHEMISTRY	MICROBIOLOGY
☐ 1021 CBC, Automated Diff (incl. Platelet Ct.)	☐ 5550 Alpha Fetoprotein, Prenatal	☐ 5232 HBsAg	
☐ 1023 Hemoglobin/Hematocrit	☐ 3000 Amylase	☐ 3175 HIV (Consent required)	Source _____
☐ 1020 Hemogram	☐ 3153 B12/Folate	☐ 3581 Iron & Iron Binding Capacity	☐ 7240 Culture, AFB
☐ 1025 Platelet Count	☐ 3156 Beta HCG, Quantitative	☐ 3195 LH	☐ 7200 Culture, Blood x _____
☐ 1150 Pro Time Diagnostic	☐ 3321 Bilirubin, Total	☐ 3590 Magnesium	☐ Draw Interval _____
☐ 1151 Pro Time, Therapeutic	☐ 3324 Bilirubin, Total/Direct	☐ 3527 Phenobarbital	☐ 7280 Culture, Fungus
☐ 1155 PTT	☐ 3009 BUN	☐ 3095 Potassium	☐ Culture, Routine
☐ 1315 Reticulocyte Count	☐ 3159 CEA	☐ 3689 Pregnancy Test, Serum (HCG, qual)	☐ 7005 Culture, Stool
☐ 1310 Sed Rate/Westergren	☐ 3348 Cholesterol	☐ 3653 Pregnancy Test, Urine	☐ 7010 Culture, Throat
	☐ 3030 Creatinine, Serum	☐ 3197 Prolactin	☐ 7000 Culture, Urine
URINE	☐ 3509 Digoxin (recommend 12 hrs., after dose)	☐ 3199 PSA	☐ 7300 Gram Stain
☐ 1059 Urinalysis	☐ 3515 Dilantin	☐ 3339 SGOT/AST	☐ 7355 Occult Blood x _____
☐ 1082 Urinalysis w/Culture if indicated	☐ 3168 Ferritin	☐ 3342 SGPT/ALT	☐ 7365 Ova & Parasites x _____
Urine-24 Hr ____ Spot ____	☐ 3193 FSH	☐ 3093 Sodium/Potassium, Serum	☐ 7400 Smear & Suspension
Ht. ____ Wt. ____	☐ 3066 ▼ Glucose, Fasting	☐ 3510 Tegretol	(includes Gram Stain/Wet Mount)
☐ 3033 Creatinine	☐ 3061 Glucose, 1° Post 50 g Glucola	☐ 3551 Theophylline	☐ 7060 Rapid Strep A Screen (Negs confir by cult)
☐ 3036 Creatinine Clearance (also requires blood)	☐ 3075 ▼ Glucose, 2° Post Glucola	☐ 3333 Uric Acid	☐ 7065 Rapid Strep A Screen only
☐ 3398 Protein	☐ 3060 Glucose, 2° Post Prandial (meal)		☐ 7030 Beta Strep Culture
☐ 3096 Sodium/Potassium	☐ 3049 ▼ Glucose Tolerance Oral GTT		☐ 5207 GC by DNA Probe
☐ Microalbumin 24 Hr ____ Spot ____	☐ 3047 ▼ Glucose Tolerance Gestational GTT		☐ 5130 Chlamydia by DNA Probe
SEROLOGY	☐ 3650 Hemoglobin, A1C		☐ 5555 Chlamydia/GC by DNA Probe
☐ 8020 ANA (Antinuclear Antibody)			☐ 7375 Wright Stain, Stool
☐ 8040 Mono Spot			
☐ 3494 Rheumatoid Factor			
☐ 8010 RPR			
☐ 5365 Rubella	Additional Tests _____		

PANELS & PROFILES

☐ X 3309 CHEM 12
Albumin, Alkaline Phosphatase,
BUN, Calcium, Cholesterol, Glucose,
LDH, Phosphorus, AST, Total
Bilirubin, Total Protein, Uric Acid

☐ ▼ 3315 CHEM 20
Chem 12, Electrolyte Panel,
Creatinine, Iron, Gamma GT, ALT,
Triglycerides

☐ ▼ 3357 CARDIAC RISK PANEL
Cholesterol, HDL, LDL, Risk Factors,
VLDL Triglycerides

☐ X 3042 CRITICAL CARE PANEL
BUN, Chloride, CO2, Glucose,
Potassium, Sodium

☐ 3046 ELECTROLYTE PANEL
Chloride, CO2, Potassium, Sodium

☐ ▼ 3399 EXECUTIVE PANEL
Chem 20, Iron, Cardiac Risk Panel,
CBC, RPR, Thyroid Cascade

☐ 5242 HEPATITIS PANEL, ACUTE
HAVIgMAb, HBsAg, HBsAb, HBcAb, HCVAb

☐ ▼ 3355 LIPID MONITORING PANEL
Cholesterol, Triglycerides, HDL, LDL, VLDL,
ALT, AST

☐ 3312 LIVER PANEL
Alkaline Phosphatase, AST, Total Bilirubin,
Gamma GT, Total Protein, Albumin, ALT

☐ X 3083 METABOLIC STATUS PANEL
BUN, Osmolality (calculated), Chloride, CO2
Creatinine, Glucose, Potassium, Sodium,
BUN/Creatinine, Ratio, Anion Gap

☐ X 3376 PANEL B
Chem 12, CBC, Electrolyte Panel

☐ ▼ 3382 PANEL D
Chem 20, CBC, Thyroid Cascade

☐ X 3388 PANEL F
Chem 12, CBC, Electrolyte Panel,
Thyroid Cascade

☐ ▼ 3391 PANEL G
Chem 20, Cardiac Risk Panel, CBC,
Thyroid Cascade

☐ ▼ 3393 PANEL H
Chem 20, CBC, Cardiac Risk Panel
Rheumatoid Factor, Thyroid Cascade

☐ ▼ 3397 PANEL J
Chem 20, Cardiac Risk Panel

☐ 5351 PRENATAL PANEL
Antibody Screen ABO/Rh, CBC
Rubella, HBsAg, RPR
  ☐ 1059 with Urinalysis, Routine
  ☐ 1082 with Urinalysis w/Culture
       if indicated

☐ X 3102 RENAL PANEL
Metabolic Status Panel, Calcium,
Phosphorus

☐ 3188 THYROID CASCADE
TSH, Reflex Testing

▼ - patient **required** to fast
   for 12-14 hours

X - patient recommended to
   fast 12-14 hours

LAB USE ONLY	INIT
☐ SST	☐ PLASMA
☐ PURPLE	☐ SERUM
☐ YELLOW	☐ SWAB
☐ BLUE	☐ SLIDES
☐ GREEN	☐ DNA PROBE
☐ GREY	☐ B. CULT BTLS
☐ URINE	
☐ BLACK	
☐ OTHER:	

REC'V. SPECIMEN: ☐ FROZEN
                  ☐ AMBIENT   ☐ ON ICE

Special Instructions/Pertinent Clinical Information _____

Physician's Signature _____   Date _____
These orders may be FAXed to: 449-5288

LAB   7060-500 (7/96)

FIGURE 18-2 Laboratory requisition form. (From Proctor DB, Adams AP: *Kinn's the medical assistant: An applied learning approach,* ed. 12, St. Louis, 2014, Saunders.)

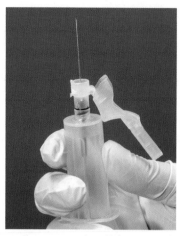

FIGURE 18-3 Always ensure that phlebotomy equipment is not defective.

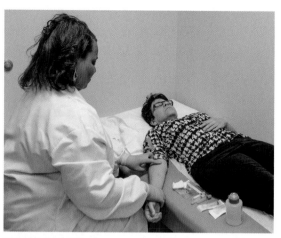

FIGURE 18-5 Collecting a specimen from an erect patient, as opposed to a supine patient, produces different test results.

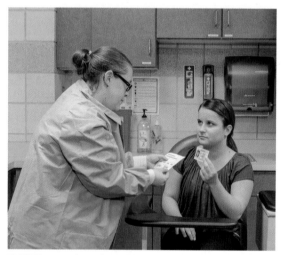

FIGURE 18-4 The patient's birth date should be documented by the phlebotomist on the requisition because the patient's age can affect laboratory values.

the administration of radiographic dyes, blood transfusions, or intravenous (IV) fluids, as these can affect test results. Anticoagulants (warfarin and heparin) cause prolonged bleeding after the puncture. It is important to know this, since it requires extra time after the puncture to apply pressure at the site and thus avoid compartment syndrome.

«↰   FLASHBACK

You learned about the risk of compartment syndrome in Chapter 11.

- *Short-term exercise.* Exercise increases levels of muscle enzymes such as creatine kinase, as well as WBCs, creatinine, and fatty acids.
- *Long-term exercise.* A prolonged exercise regimen increases sex hormones, as well as many of the values increased by short-term exercise.
- *Medications and medical treatments.* Certain medications affect test results directly. Aspirin is the most common one, prolonging bleeding times. Other treatments to be aware of include

- *Alcohol consumption.* Although moderate amounts of alcohol do not affect test results (except, of course, for the alcohol test), glucose is slightly elevated, and chronic consumption can lead to increased values on liver function tests, as well as interfering with platelet aggregation studies.
- *Smoking.* Smoking increases catecholamines, cortisol, WBCs, mean corpuscular volume, and hemoglobin, and it decreases eosinophils. Smoking also affects arterial blood gases (ABGs).
- *Stress.* Anxiety, crying, or hyperventilating may affect test results, including the stress hormones produced by the adrenal cortex. Prolonged crying or hyperventilating alters ABGs, and crying can increase WBCs.

- *Diurnal variation.* Certain specimens must be collected at specific times of day because of significant changes throughout the day. Such specimens include cortisol and iron.
- *Fasting.* Prolonged fasting increases bilirubin and fatty acids. Overnight fasting concentrates most analytes. A fasting specimen should be taken 8 to 12 hours after the last intake of food. It is the phlebotomist's responsibility to ascertain that the patient has had no food during that time. Caffeinated beverages, such as coffee, tea, and soda, must be avoided as well. Caffeine causes a transient rise in blood sugar levels. A patient not in the fasting state may produce a *lipemic sample,* in which the serum or plasma appears turbid. This turbidity, which is caused by an increase in blood triglycerides, interferes with many tests that rely on photometry, or the passage of light through the sample. A lipemic sample may cause clinically significant variances in results for phosphorus, creatinine, total protein and calcium. High-speed centrifugation may be used to pretreat lipemic specimens to overcome interference, but in cases of gross lipemia, the sample may have to be recollected.

> **◀◀◁ FLASHBACK**
> You learned about fasting specimens in Chapter 14.

- *Age.* Many laboratory values vary with age. For instance, because organ function declines with advancing age, values affected by kidney or liver function are different for the elderly than for younger patients. Cholesterol and triglyceride values increase with age, whereas the sex hormones may rise and then fall. Both RBC and WBC values are higher in infants than in adults. For all these reasons, it is important that the patient's date of birth be documented on the requisition form
- *Altitude.* Patients living at higher altitudes have less oxygen available to breathe, so the body compensates by producing a higher RBC mass. Therefore patients living in mountainous regions have higher counts of RBCs, hemoglobins, and hematocrits.
- *Dehydration.* Prolonged diarrhea or vomiting causes loss of fluid from the intravascular circulation. This results in hemoconcentration because of loss of water from plasma. Hemoconcentration produces a false increase in many analytes, including RBCs, enzymes, calcium, and sodium.

- *Sex.* The normal ranges of some analytes differ for males and females. Males, for example, have higher hemoglobin, hematocrit, and RBC counts than do females.
- *Pregnancy.* The changes that occur in pregnancy affect laboratory values. The presence of the fetus and increased water retention cause a dilution effect that is reflected in falsely lower hemoglobin and RBC counts, as well as other analytes.

> **◀◀◁ FLASHBACK**
> You learned about site selection, tourniquet application, and other aspects of collection in Chapter 9.

Specimen Collection

The phlebotomist has almost complete control over the variables that arise during specimen collection. These include the following:

- *Site selection.* Sites that can cause specimen contamination include hematomas or areas with edema and the side of the body that has undergone mastectomy or is currently receiving IV fluids. Sites that can cause pain or injury to the patient include burns or scars, previous puncture sites, the arm near a mastectomy, sites near fistulas or shunts, and the back of the heel or other regions close to the bone. In addition, accidental puncture of an artery during a venous procedure, or use of an artery for routine collection, carries a significant risk of infection.
- *Tourniquet application.* Tourniquets should be left on no longer than 1 minute to reduce hemoconcentration. Hemoconcentration causes the false increase of large molecules such as proteins and cholesterol and the false decrease of electrolytes like chloride and potassium (Figure 18-6). Once blood flow is established, the tourniquet must be released. Tourniquets applied too tightly can cause petechiae.
- *Site cleansing.* Proper cleansing reduces the risk of infection. Blood culture collections require special care to prevent contamination of the sample with skin flora. As part of its QA program, the microbiology department keeps records of blood cultures contaminated with normal skin flora. Iodine must be removed from the site after collection, because it can irritate the skin. Iodine should not be used for dermal puncture, because it is virtually impossible to keep it out of the sample. Iodine interferes with bilirubin, uric acid, and phosphorus tests.
- *Specimen collection.* Specimens must be collected in the right tube for the test ordered and in

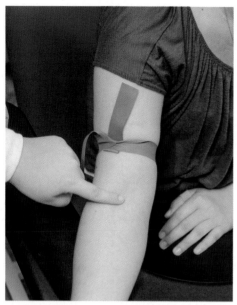

FIGURE 18-6 Application of the tourniquet is one preanalytic variable over which the phlebotomist has complete control.

the right order. The sample volume must be matched to the quantity of additives in the tube, and the tube size should be chosen to provide adequate volume for the test required. The specimen must be mixed gently and thoroughly by inversion immediately after being drawn.

«←¬ FLASHBACK
You learned the order of draw in Chapter 8.

- *Labeling.* Incorrect or incomplete labeling makes a specimen useless and requires redrawing the specimen at a later date. Label tubes immediately after they are drawn, before leaving the patient's room (Figure 18-7). Be sure that the labeling is complete, and note any special patient conditions on the requisition.

FIGURE 18-7 Make sure that all specimens are properly labeled.

«←¬ FLASHBACK
You learned about the elements of a complete label in Chapter 9.

Patient's Perception

The patient's perception of the level of care he or she receives is directly affected by the skill, professionalism, and care you show as a phlebotomist. This perception reflects not only on you but on the entire laboratory as well. You should strive to avoid painful probing, unsuccessful punctures, and repeated draws and be scrupulously careful regarding site selection, accidental arterial puncture, and nerve injury. In addition, infection control procedures must always be followed. Break the chain of infection by performing hand hygiene upon entering and leaving the room, and by wearing gloves during the procedure (Figure 18-8).

Accidental Puncture

Accidental puncture with a used needle must be reported immediately to a supervisor. Immediate and follow-up testing for bloodborne pathogens, plus counseling, is standard protocol for accidental needle sticks. QA procedures include monitoring the number of accidental punctures and instituting additional training or equipment modifications in the event of frequent accidents.

TRANSPORTATION

Specimen transportation variables include the method of delivery, the treatment of the sample during transportation, and the timing of delivery.

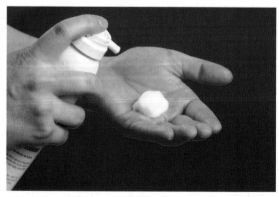

FIGURE 18-8 Infection control procedures are a vital part of quality phlebotomy. Hand hygiene and gloving should be performed for every procedure. (From Bonewit-West K: *Clinical procedures for medical assistants,* ed. 9, Philadelphia, 2015, Saunders.)

《《⤺ FLASHBACK

You learned about specimen transport and handling in Chapter 16.

Samples requiring either cold or warm temperatures during transport must be placed in the appropriate container and must be handled so that the appropriate temperature is maintained throughout the transport process (Figure 18-9). Aheel-warmer packet gradually loses its heat, for instance, and if the sample is not delivered before heat loss, the sample will be compromised. Short turnaround time (stat) specimens require prompt delivery and analysis, and the on-time record of the phlebotomist and the laboratory is analyzed in QA programs to determine whether changes must be made in transportation procedures.

Pneumatic tube systems require special monitoring to ensure that the sample is not overly agitated during transport, causing hemolysis. Some samples cannot travel by pneumatic tube, and it is the phlebotomist's responsibility to ensure their proper handling. The directory of services contains precisely this type of information.

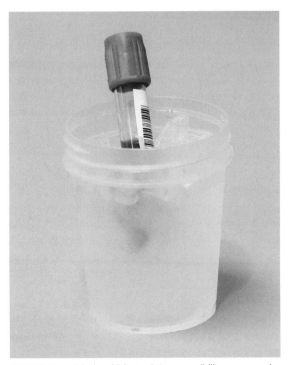

FIGURE 18-9 It is the phlebotomist's responsibility to ensure the proper handling of specimens.

PROCESSING

Specimen processing is another area in which the phlebotomist and other laboratory staff have almost complete control over the variables that arise. These include the time between collection and processing, the centrifugation process, the possibility of contamination and evaporation, the proper storage conditions, and the processing of aliquots.

Separation Times

No more than 2 hours should elapse between the time a specimen is collected and the time serum or plasma is separated from formed elements. After this time, the sample will begin to show falsely lowered glucose and falsely elevated potassium and lactate dehydrogenase. Even less time should be allowed for determinations of potassium, adrenocorticotropic hormone, or cortisol. Ammonia samples must be separated within 15 minutes of collection. The exception is for samples collected in serum separator tubes, which are stable once they are spun and a good gel seal is in place.

Centrifuge Maintenance

Centrifuges must be calibrated every 3 months with a tachometer to ensure that they are running at the reported speed. Variation may indicate the need to replace worn parts. Spinning samples below the required speed may result in incomplete separation of liquid from formed elements, affecting test results (Figure 18-10).

Evaporation and Contamination

Specimens should not be left uncovered any longer than necessary during processing. Evaporation of liquid, especially from small samples, can affect ABGs, alcohol, and ammonia, among other tests. Contamination may occur while the sample is uncovered, arising from airborne dust or talc from gloves. Contamination may also occur from incomplete separation, such as when RBCs are left in the sample after incomplete centrifugation.

Refrigerators and Freezers

Fluctuations in cold storage units can degrade sample quality. Temperatures of refrigerators and freezers must be monitored daily, with temperatures recorded either automatically or manually at specified times of day. Temperature readings that are too high or low indicate that the unit needs maintenance or replacement.

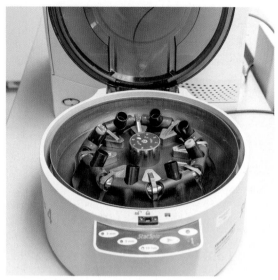

FIGURE 18-10 Correct use and maintenance of the centrifuge are important in quality specimen processing.

Aliquot Handling and Labeling

Multiple aliquots prepared from a single specimen allow different departments to share a single sample for multiple tests. Each aliquot must be properly labeled as to the source and additives present. Specimens with different additives should never be combined in a single aliquot.

ANALYTICAL VARIABLES

An analytical variable is any variable that affects the testing process. Although most samples are tested by MLS, MT, and MLT laboratory personnel, the phlebotomist may be trained to perform CLIA-waived testing. It is important to understand the analytical variables that can have a negative impact on test results. Point-of-care testing instruments require calibration and controls to be performed before testing patient samples. If the instrument is malfunctioning or the reagents are bad, calibration and control values will fall outside the predetermined range of acceptance. If pipetting of reagents is required for a test, improper pipetting technique may yield results that fall outside the expected range or falsely fall inside the expected range. No tests should be run until the instrument is working properly. Always follow the manufacturer's guidelines and any facility guidelines for ensuring that a POCT instrument is functioning properly before testing a patient sample.

POSTANALYTICAL VARIABLES

A postanalytical variable is any variable in the reporting and follow-up of test results. The phlebotomist may be responsible for reporting POCT results that he or she performed. Before a result is reported, it must be interpreted as being valid. A delta check, discussed earlier in this chapter, helps ensure that results generated are correct. If the result is outside the expected range, it may be necessary to perform the test again. If the phlebotomist is unsure, a MLS, MT, or MLT should be consulted. Once the result has been verified, the result is delivered to the physician ordering the test. The method of delivery is determined by the facility, and may include telephone, fax, computer, or hand delivery.

REVIEW FOR CERTIFICATION

Quality phlebotomy refers to a set of policies and procedures designed to ensure the delivery of consistent, high-quality patient care and specimen analysis. Quality phlebotomy includes quality control (QC), the group of quantitative methods used to monitor the quality of procedures. Quality control is part of quality assurance (QA), the larger set of methods used to guarantee quality patient care. Total quality management (TQM) is the entire set of approaches used by the institution to provide customer satisfaction. Continuing quality improvement (CQI) is the major goal of TQM programs. QA programs use written documentation to set standards for the performance of procedures and to monitor compliance. Two important documents are the procedure manual, which contains protocols and other information about all the tests performed in the laboratory, and the floor book, which contains a variety of information pertinent to the smooth coordination of nursing staff and laboratory personnel. Within the scope of TQM, the phlebotomist is most responsible for controlling preanalytic variables, those that occur before the specimen is analyzed. These variables include test ordering and requisition handling, equipment integrity, patient identification and preparation, specimen collection, and transportation. The patient's physical condition at the time of the collection has a significant effect on sample quality and may be influenced by fasting, dehydration, and other states. Specimen collection variables include site selection, tourniquet application, and site cleansing. Postcollection variables include labeling, method of delivery, treatment of the sample during transportation, and timing of delivery. Specimen processing variables include time between collection and processing, centrifugation process, possibility of contamination and evaporation, proper storage conditions, and processing of aliquots. In some situations, the phlebotomist may also be responsible for analytical variables and postanalytical variables.

BIBLIOGRAPHY

Bologna LJ, Mutter M: Life after phlebotomy deployment: Reducing major patient and specimen identification errors, *J Healthc Inf Manag* 16:65-70. Retrieved from http://www.himss.org/content/files/jhim/15-4/original02.pdf.

Calmarza P, Cordero J: Lipemia interferences in routine clinical biochemical tests, *Biochem Med (Zagreb)* 21(2):160-166, 2011.

CLSI: *Procedures for the collection of diagnostic blood specimens by venipuncture; Approved standard—sixth edition.* CSLI document GP41-A6 (formerly H03-A6). Wayne, Pa., 2007, Clinical and Laboratory Standards Institute.

CLSI: *Tubes and additives for venous and capillary blood specimen collection; Approved standard—Sixth edition.* CSLI document GP39-A6. Wayne, Pa., 2010, Clinical and Laboratory Standards Institute.

Drew N: Monitoring specimen collection errors, *Adv Med Lab Prof*, 2000.

Ernst DJ, Balance LO: Phlebotomy puncture juncture: Preventing phlebotomy errors—Potential for harming your patients, *Med Lab Obs*, September 2006.

Howanitz PJ, Renner SW, Walsh MK: Continuous wristband monitoring over 2 years decreases identification errors: A College of American Pathologists Q-tracks study, *Arch Pathol Lab Med* 126:809-815, 2002.

Kalra J: Medical errors: Impact on clinical laboratories and other critical areas, *Clin Biochem* 37:1052-1062, 2004.

Lippi G, Salvagno GL, Montagnana M, et al: Influence of short-term venous stasis on clinical chemistry testing, *Clin Chem Lab Med* 43:869-875, 2005.

Ogden-Grable H, Gill GW: CFIAC Authors and Disclosures, *Lab Med* 36(7):430-433, 2005.

STUDY QUESTIONS

See answers in Appendix F.

1. Explain the purpose of QA.

2. Describe how QA differs from QC.

3. What is the role of The Joint Commission in quality assurance?

4. List the four criteria that make up documentation processes.

5. What information does a procedure manual contain?

6. What is the purpose of a delta check?

7. If a patient presents with the smell of cigarettes on his or her breath, why should this be noted on the requisition?

8. What information should be labeled on aliquoted specimens?

9. Explain quality phlebotomy and its purpose.

10. Describe the philosophy, role, and purpose of TQM.

11. Explain the difference between the procedure manual and the floor logbook.

12. Explain preanalytic variables, and give examples of how to control or monitor such variables.

13. Describe a negative outcome of improper patient identification. Give two examples of how you would ensure that proper patient identification is achieved.

14. Give four variables of which a phlebotomist must be aware during a phlebotomy procedure and examples of how to control or prevent such variables.

CERTIFICATION EXAMINATION PREPARATION

See answers in Appendix F.

1. What organization mandates QA programs?
   a. Occupational Safety and Health Administration
   b. National Phlebotomy Association
   c. American Society for Clinical Pathology
   d. The Joint Commission

2. If there is a question concerning the principle behind a particular specimen collection, consult the
   a. QC logbook.
   b. floor book.
   c. policy manual.
   d. procedure manual.

3. If a phlebotomist wants to know the turnaround time for a specific procedure, it can be found in the
   a. policy manual.
   b. patient's chart.
   c. directory of services.
   d. *Physician's Desk Reference.*

4. Which of the following compares previous patient data with current data?
   a. Postanalytic variables
   b. Delta check
   c. Accession numbers
   d. Collection logbook

5. Fasting specimens should be collected
   a. 24 hours after the fast.
   b. 2 hours after waking up.
   c. 8 to 12 hours after eating.
   d. any time after midnight.

6. The phlebotomist usually does not have complete control over which of the following variables?
   a. Collection equipment
   b. Patient preparation
   c. Specimen collection
   d. Specimen labeling

7. No more than _____ should elapse between the time a specimen is collected and the time serum or plasma is separated from formed elements.
   a. 30 minutes
   b. 1 hour
   c. 2 hours
   d. 3 hours

8. _____ refers to a set of policies and procedures designed to ensure the delivery of consistent, high-quality patient care and specimen analysis.
   a. Quality phlebotomy
   b. QA
   c. QC
   d. TQM

9. The phlebotomist is most responsible for controlling
   a. analytic variables.
   b. postanalytic variables.
   c. TQM.
   d. preanalytic variables.

CHAPTER 19 Legal Issues in Phlebotomy

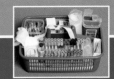

Legal and ethical considerations form an important underpinning to the practice of medicine, and phlebotomy is no exception. An increasingly complex and litigious health care environment has made familiarity with legal issues an important part of the phlebotomist's training. Medical malpractice is the most common legal claim in the health care field. Injuries that arise from failure to follow the standard of care may be grounds for a finding of malpractice. Careful observance of the standard of care, and documentation of that practice, is the best defense against malpractice. Comprehensive federal regulations governing the privacy of medical information have affected every sector of health care delivery. In addition to the legal requirement to protect patient confidentiality, there is an ethical duty to do so. Although full consideration of all the relevant legal issues is beyond the scope of this chapter, we introduce some important legal and ethical concepts that have an impact on the profession.

OUTLINE

Why Study Legal Issues?
The Legal System
 Laws
 Settlement and Judgment
Professional Liability
 Medical Malpractice

Other Examples of
 Potential Malpractice
 in Phlebotomy
Defense against
 Malpractice
Liability Insurance

Confidentiality
 Health Insurance Portability
 and Accountability Act
Review for Certification

OBJECTIVES

After completing this chapter, you should be able to:

1. Discuss why legal issues are important to the phlebotomist.
2. Differentiate the following types of laws: statutory, case, administrative, public, and private.
3. Define plaintiff, defendant, felony, misdemeanor, and tort.
4. Define liability, and give examples of situations in which a phlebotomist may be held accountable for the consequences of an action.
5. Explain how the accepted standard of care is determined, and give examples of these standards as they relate to phlebotomy.

6. Define malpractice, and explain what is necessary to prove it.
7. Differentiate between punitive and compensatory damages.
8. Describe steps the phlebotomist can take to avoid being accused of malpractice.
9. Explain the importance of confidentiality.
10. Define protected health information under Health Insurance Portability and Accountability Act (HIPAA) regulations.
11. Describe how the phlebotomist can safeguard a patient's privacy.

KEY TERMS

accepted standard of care
administrative law
assault
battery
case law
civil action
criminal action

damages
dereliction
event report
liability insurance
liable
malpractice
negligence

out-of-court settlement
plaintiff
private law
protected health
 information (PHI)
public law
scope of practice

statutory law
tort

ABBREVIATIONS

HIPAA Health Insurance Portability and Accountability Act

IRS Internal Revenue Service

OSHA Occupational Safety and Health Administration

PHI protected health information

WHY STUDY LEGAL ISSUES?

The health care system has become increasingly complex in the past two decades. This complexity stems from the interplay of technologic advances, associated increased costs of delivering care, and fear of litigation.

Several factors have led to the dramatic rise in health care costs in recent decades. First is the gradual inflation in the price of all goods and services. More important has been the growing sophistication of medical technology, with consequent higher costs for equipment purchase and maintenance, plus the need for highly trained operators at all levels of health care delivery. For instance, the cost of drawing a blood sample has risen significantly since the development of safety needles and other systems designed to protect the phlebotomist. The simple compound microscope that was used to do a differential blood count in the 1940s cost perhaps a few hundred dollars and required only occasional adjustment and cleaning. In contrast, today's automated cell counters cost thousands of dollars and require frequent calibration and regular maintenance, as well as a higher level of training to operate (Figure 19-1). Similarly, the fast pace of drug discovery and development has increased the cost of medical treatment for the typical patient. All these advances have enhanced the quality of patient care, but at a significant price. In addition to these sources of cost increase, more stringent regulations designed to safeguard health care providers have led to higher costs for service delivery.

Even more significantly, the availability of sophisticated technology has meant that more doctors order more tests on more patients, and that more patients expect them to order the tests. As the standard of care has risen, multiple sophisticated and expensive tests have been prescribed to supplement (and sometimes substitute for) a physician's clinical judgment. Increased fear of litigation has also fueled the rise in the use of multiple tests, often as much to protect against future lawsuits as to provide

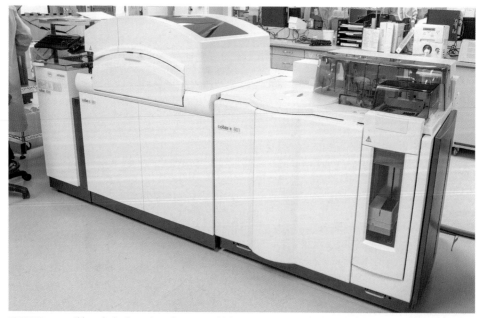

FIGURE 19-1 Although the invention of automated laboratory equipment has improved the quality of care, it has also contributed to the rising costs of health care.

crucial medical information. Such "defensive medicine" is understandable, given the very high cost of malpractice insurance and the potential for a ruinous liability judgment in the event of an oversight or mistake.

The rising cost of health care has led to efforts to keep costs under control, including reimbursement restrictions on diagnostic tests and limitations on prescription drugs. Meanwhile, the rights of patients have been increasingly recognized and expanded, and the level of care expected by patients has grown. The American Hospital Association has created the Patient Care Partnership, a statement of what patients should expect during a hospital stay with regard to rights and responsibilities (Box 19-1). It emphasizes the patient's right to quality care, a clean and safe environment, and protection of privacy, among other rights. Because of the conflicts arising from the interplay of these factors, along with the general rise in litigation in our society, the health care professions have been subjected to more and more lawsuits. Understanding your legal obligations and rights in this complex system is an important part of your professional training.

BOX 19-1	The Patient Care Partnership

Understanding Expectations, Rights, and Responsibilities

What to expect during your hospital stay:

- High-quality hospital care
- A clean and safe environment
- Involvement in your care
- Protection of your privacy
- Help when leaving the hospital
- Help with your billing claims

When you need hospital care, your doctor and the nurses and other professionals at our hospital are committed to working with you and your family to meet your health care needs. Our dedicated doctors and staff serve the community in all its ethnic, religious, and economic diversity. Our goal is for you and your family to have the same care and attention we would want for our families and ourselves.

The sections that follow explain some of the basics about how you can expect to be treated during your hospital stay. They also cover what we need from you to care for you better. If you have questions at any time, please ask them. Unasked or unanswered questions can add to the stress of being in the hospital. Your comfort and confidence in your care are important to us.

What to Expect During Your Hospital Stay

High-Quality Hospital Care

Our first priority is to provide you the care you need, when you need it, with skill, compassion, and respect. Tell your caregivers if you have concerns about your care or if you have pain. You have the right to know the identity of doctors, nurses, and others involved in your care, and you have the right to know when they are students, residents, or other trainees.

A Clean and Safe Environment

Our hospital works hard to keep you safe. We use special policies and procedures to avoid mistakes in your care and keep you free from abuse or neglect. If anything unexpected and significant happens during your hospital stay, you will be told what happened, and any resulting changes in your care will be discussed with you.

Involvement in Your Care

You and your doctor often make decisions about your care before you go to the hospital. Other times, especially in emergencies, those decisions are made during your hospital stay. When decision making takes place, it should include the following:

Discussing Your Medical Condition and Information About Medically Appropriate Treatment Choices

To make informed decisions with your doctor, you need to understand:

- The benefits and risks of each treatment.
- Whether your treatment is experimental or part of a research study.
- What you can reasonably expect from your treatment and any long-term effects it might have on your quality of life.
- What you and your family will need to do after you leave the hospital.
- The financial consequences of using uncovered services or out-of-network providers.

  Please tell your caregivers if you need more information about treatment choices.

Discussing Your Treatment Plan

When you enter the hospital, you sign a general consent to treatment. In some cases, such as surgery or experimental treatment, you may be asked to confirm in writing that you understand what is planned and agree to it. This process protects your right to consent to or refuse a treatment. Your doctor will explain the medical consequences of refusing recommended treatment. It also protects your right to decide if you want to participate in a research study.

Getting Information From You

Your caregivers need complete and correct information about your health and coverage so that they can make good decisions about your care. That includes the following:

- Past illnesses, surgeries, or hospital stays
- Past allergic reactions
- Any medicines or dietary supplements (such as vitamins and herbs) that you are taking
- Any network or admission requirements under your health plan

Continued

BOX 19-1	The Patient Care Partnership—cont'd

Understanding Your Health Care Goals and Values

You may have health care goals and values or spiritual beliefs that are important to your well-being. They will be taken into account as much as possible throughout your hospital stay. Make sure your doctor, your family, and your care team members know your wishes.

Understanding Who Should Make Decisions When You Cannot

If you have signed a health care power of attorney stating who should speak for you if you become unable to make health care decisions for yourself, or a living will or advance directive that states your wishes about end-of-life care, give copies to your doctor, your family, and your care team. If you or your family members need help making difficult decisions, counselors, chaplains, and others are available to help.

Protection of Your Privacy

We respect the confidentiality of your relationship with your doctor and other caregivers and the sensitive information about your health and health care that is part of that relationship. State and federal laws and hospital operating policies protect the privacy of your medical information. You will receive a Notice of Privacy Practices that describes the ways in which we use, disclose, and safeguard patient information and that explains how you can obtain a copy of information from our records about your care.

Preparing You and Your Family for When You Leave the Hospital

Your doctor works with hospital staff and professionals in your community. You and your family also play an important role in

your care. The success of your treatment often depends on your efforts to follow medication, diet, and therapy plans. Your family may need to help care for you at home.

You can expect us to help you identify sources of follow-up care and to let you know if our hospital has a financial interest in any referrals. As long as you agree that we can share information about your care with them, we will coordinate our activities with your caregivers outside the hospital. You can also expect to receive information and, where possible, training about the self-care you will need when you go home.

Help With Your Bill and Filing Insurance Claims

Our staff will file claims for you with health care insurers or other programs such as Medicare and Medicaid. They also will help your doctor with needed documentation. Hospital bills and insurance coverage are often confusing. If you have questions about your bill, contact our business office. If you need help understanding your insurance coverage or health plan, start with your insurance company or health benefits manager. If you do not have health coverage, we will try to help you and your family find financial help or make other arrangements. We need your help in collecting needed information and other requirements to obtain coverage or assistance.

While you are here, you will receive more detailed notices about some of the rights you have as a hospital patient and how to exercise them. We are always interested in improving. If you have questions, comments, or concerns, please contact: (relevant department here).

Reprinted with permission of the American Hospital Association, copyright 2003.

THE LEGAL SYSTEM

To understand your rights and obligations under the law, it is helpful to know a little bit about how the legal system operates.

Laws

Laws are created in a variety of ways. **Statutory law** is created by a legislative body. At the federal level, this is Congress, made up of the Senate and the House of Representatives. These laws are called statutes. State legislative bodies vary from state to state but usually follow the federal model.

Case law is law determined by court decisions, usually as an interpretation of existing statutory law. State courts rule on state laws, and federal courts rule on federal laws. The U.S. Supreme Court has ultimate jurisdiction over all laws, both federal and state.

Administrative law is created by administrative agencies, such as the Internal Revenue Service (IRS) or the Occupational Safety and Health Administration (OSHA). The regulations promulgated

by these agencies are given the force of law by the statutory laws that created the agencies.

Laws are also classified as either public or private. When a **public law** is violated, the offense leads to a **criminal action**, and the violator is prosecuted by the public in the person of the government's attorney (the district attorney). The offense may be either a felony or a misdemeanor, depending on the seriousness of the crime.

Phlebotomists can be charged with violations of public law. Failing to obtain informed consent from a patient before any procedure is example of this. Therefore blood must never be drawn without first obtaining the patient's consent. A patient can give consent either in writing or verbally. If a patient refuses to have his or her blood drawn, the phlebotomist must not attempt to force the patient to comply. To persist can lead to criminal charges of assault and battery. **Assault** is an unjustifiable attempt to touch another person, or the threat to do so. **Battery** is the intentional touching of another person without consent.

There are only a few situations in which the person whose blood is being drawn is not the person whose consent must be obtained. Parents have the right to give consent for a child to have his or her blood drawn, even though the child may refuse and may even be combative (Figure 19-2). Legally appointed guardians give consent for patients who are incapacitated. If there is any doubt about who is entitled to give consent, always ask the nurse or physician before proceeding with the draw.

In contrast to public law, when a **private law** is violated, the offense may lead to a **civil action**, in which the defendant is sued in civil court by the **plaintiff**, the person claiming to have been harmed by the defendant. Civil wrongs include torts. A **tort** is defined as any wrongful act that causes harm or injury to another person. Torts can be either intentional or unintentional. Unintentional torts are the basis for most medical malpractice suits. A malpractice suit may be brought against the individual causing the harm, or the institution employing the individual, or both. Supervisors may be held liable for the harms caused by an individual under their supervision.

A patient may choose to bring a civil action in a case for which a criminal action was also brought, whether or not the defendant was found guilty in the criminal action. For instance, a patient with a damaged nerve may sue for malpractice even if the case was not strong enough to sustain a criminal action. Other causes of action could include reusing needles, careless probing for a vein, accidental artery stick resulting in injury to patient, drawing

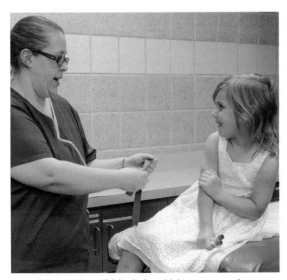

FIGURE 19-2 Child refusing phlebotomy procedure.

samples not requested by the physician, or releasing test results to someone not authorized to receive them. A patient must file a civil action within a specific time period after the damaged occurred, often within 2 years. This time period is called the statute of limitations.

Settlement and Judgment

Almost all civil and criminal actions are settled out of court. In an **out-of-court settlement**, the two parties reach an agreement without the intervention of a judge or jury. When a civil case is settled out of court, the settlement often includes a condition stating that neither party may discuss the amount of the settlement.

When the parties cannot reach agreement, the case goes to court for trial and judgment. A judgment against the defendant in a civil case usually results in a fine (known as damages), which may be only compensatory (to pay for costs incurred because of the injury, such as further medical care) or punitive. Headline-making damage awards are most often for punitive damages. Judgments in either civil or criminal actions can be appealed if the losing party feels that some part of the court proceeding was in error. Judgments may be upheld, reversed, or modified on appeal.

PROFESSIONAL LIABILITY

To be **liable** for an action means that you are legally responsible for it and can be held accountable for its consequences. As a medical professional, you are liable for both your actions (called an act of commission) and, in some cases, your failure to act (called an act of omission). For instance, if you damage a nerve while performing routine venipuncture, you may be held liable for an act of commission (i.e., something you did that you shouldn't have). If a physician orders a test that you fail to perform and, as a result, the patient suffers harm, you may be held liable for an act of omission (i.e., something you didn't do that you should have).

You are legally responsible for *any* action you perform as a medical professional, whether or not it is a duty assigned to you or you have received training for it (Figure 19-3). For instance, if you perform an arterial puncture, you are liable for any injuries that may result from it, whether or not you have been properly trained to perform it. Therefore *a professional should not attempt to perform duties for which he or she is not trained.* As a phlebotomist, you must perform only those procedures that

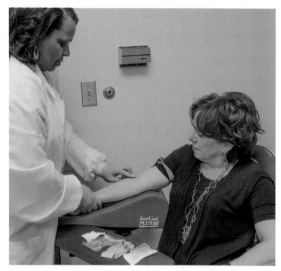

FIGURE 19-3 The phlebotomist is legally responsible for any injuries that result from venipuncture.

you have been properly trained to perform and that fall within your **scope of practice** as a phlebotomist. Your scope of practice is the set of procedures and responsibilities for which your training has prepared you and for which you have demonstrated competency. By performing a duty normally assigned to someone with a higher level of training and expertise, you are legally liable for that higher level of care. Your institution has policies and procedures regarding the duties you are expected to perform.

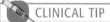

> **CLINICAL TIP**
>
> Never perform a procedure for which you have not received training.

Judgments regarding medical liability revolve around the concept of the **accepted standard of care**, which represents the consensus of medical opinion on patient care in a particular situation. The failure to perform an action consistent with the accepted standard of care is **negligence**. For example, phlebotomists violate the standard of care if a dirty needle is not properly disposed of and is used on another patient, or if the phlebotomist probes during the venipuncture to find the vein and damages nerves with improper drawing techniques. Cases have been prosecuted in which the phlebotomist did not correctly identify the patient and, as a result, the patient received incorrect test results and improper care. If the patient dies as a consequence, the

phlebotomist could be charged with murder or manslaughter.

When the standard of care is not followed, those professionals who were responsible for decision-making in that situation are liable for injuries incurred by the patient. For instance, most institutions allow a phlebotomist to make only two unsuccessful attempts at routine venipuncture before seeking the assistance of a more senior phlebotomist. If this is the accepted standard of care in your institution and you violate that policy, a patient who experiences harm or suffering as a result may have grounds to sue you and your hospital. The doctrine of respondeat superior means "Let the master answer." Under this doctrine, employers are held liable for the actions of their employees who are performing their responsibilities as delineated in the employee's scope of practice. As such, your actions as a phlebotomist can either protect the hospital against litigation or put it at risk. In a trial, the jury decides exactly what constitutes the accepted standard of care, whether that standard was followed, and whether the medical professionals were negligent. These decisions are usually made after listening to a variety of expert witnesses.

Medical Malpractice

Malpractice is the delivery of substandard care that results in harm to a patient. It is the most common liability in medicine and is sometimes called medical professional liability. A malpractice suit is brought by the plaintiff and usually names one or more professionals, as well as the institution, as the defendants. The suit alleges professional negligence as the cause of specific harms, which may include both physical and emotional distress, as well as lost income or potential income, as the result of specific actions.

In a civil suit, the plaintiff asks for **damages**, or monetary compensation. Damages may be awarded to cover only the actual costs of the injury, such as lost wages or further medical care. Damages can also be awarded to compensate for legal costs or pain and suffering. Punitive damages may be awarded to punish the defendant, usually for gross violations of accepted standards of care.

In a malpractice case, the burden of proof is on the plaintiff to show the four elements of negligence: duty, dereliction, injury, and direct cause.

Duty

The plaintiff must prove that the defendant owed the plaintiff a duty of care. For example, if a phlebotomist had a requisition for a patient and was expected by his or her supervisors to draw blood, the phlebotomist owed the patient a duty of care.

Dereliction

The plaintiff must prove that the defendant breached the duty of care to the plaintiff. This determination revolves around the accepted standard of care and the specific action or inaction of the plaintiff. For example, if a phlebotomist mislabeled the sample specified on the requisition, this may constitute dereliction or breach of duty.

Injury

The plaintiff must prove that a legally recognizable injury to the patient actually occurred. For instance, if mislabeling led to improper care that harmed the patient, injury occurred. If the time of draw for a therapeutic drug monitoring sample was written incorrectly, and the patient received too much medication as a result, the patient may be able to prove injury.

Direct Cause

The plaintiff must prove that the injury was sustained as a direct result of the defendant's actions or inactions. For example, if overmedication can be shown to be a direct result of mislabeling, direct cause is demonstrated.

Other Examples of Potential Malpractice in Phlebotomy

The standard of care when drawing blood from a patient is to perform no more than two unsuccessful punctures before calling for assistance. A phlebotomist who continues to attempt venipuncture without calling for assistance at this point is derelict in his or her duty. A patient who subsequently experiences pain and swelling in the arm may have a cause of action, if it can be shown that the injury resulted from the excess number of attempts.

The standard of care when drawing at a patient's bedside is not to place the phlebotomy tray on the bed. A phlebotomist who does so is derelict in his or her duty. If a patient's movements subsequently cause the tray to spill and filled tubes to break, the patient may be exposed to bloodborne pathogens (assuming the samples were from a different patient who was infected). In order to establish injury, the patient would then have to become infected. To establish direct cause, the patient would need to show that the infection was the result of the exposure (and not the result of exposure from some other source).

The standard of care when leaving a patient's bedside is to raise the bed rail if it was lowered for the draw. Therefore the phlebotomist has a duty to perform this action. If he or she fails to do so, this is a dereliction of duty. If the patient subsequently falls from bed and is injured, the question becomes whether the phlebotomist's failure to raise the bed rail was the direct cause of the injury. Mitigating factors might include whether the patient had been visited by a nurse in the meantime and whether the fall was the actual cause of the injury.

Other standards of care include proper patient identification, following the protocols for all blood collection processes in all procedures, and all non-blood collection procedures. Phlebotomists must also follow all institutional policies and procedures as they apply to their scope of practice. Phlebotomists must also comply with all HIPAA regulations and safeguard the privacy of their patients.

Defense Against Malpractice

As the preceding examples illustrate, deviation from the standard of care leaves the phlebotomist exposed to charges of malpractice. Conversely, the principal defense against a malpractice suit is to show that the standard of care was followed. This requires not only the actual practice of good care but the documentation of it as well. Clear, complete medical records are the cornerstone of the defense, because they show exactly what was done, when, by who, date, time, and witness if any. If good care is delivered and good medical records document this, a malpractice suit has little chance of succeeding.

Similarly, if a situation arises in which observation of the standard of care is called into question, all parties should carefully document exactly what happened—who did what when. For instance, if a patient complains of a shooting pain during a draw, you have a responsibility to follow institutional protocol to deal with the injury or the complaint; you should not try to avoid reporting it. Each institution has a set of protocols for reporting such incidents, which usually involve prompt and complete documentation of the circumstances of the incident in an event report.

CLINICAL TIP

Always maintain clear, complete medical records. Whenever an unusual incident occurs during a phlebotomy procedure, report it to your supervisor immediately and fill out an event report.

Patient communication is also an important aspect of preventing malpractice claims. For instance, clear communication with the patient is essential for obtaining informed consent for medical procedures (Figure 19-4). Procedures must be explained in a way that the patient can understand, and the patient must give positive consent ("Yes," or "I understand"), not merely a nod of the head or a look of agreement. If you and the patient do not speak the same language, an interpreter must be present to explain the procedure. As another example, you must remember to ask specifically whether the patient is taking blood-thinning medications such as heparin. Without this information, you may not apply pressure long enough after the draw, possibly leading to compartment syndrome, a potentially serious complication. The only time nonverbal consent is acceptable is in cases in which immediate action must be taken to save a patient's life. This is called implied consent. A medical emergency removes the need for informed consent. If a patient rolls up his or her sleeve and extends the arm after being told by the phlebotomist that he or she is there to draw the patient's blood, this too indicates implied consent.

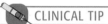

> **CLINICAL TIP**
>
> Always obtain positive informed consent before performing a procedure.

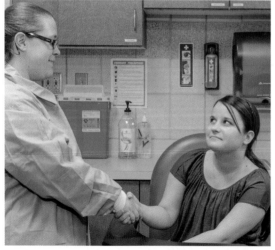

FIGURE 19-4 Clear communication with patients can help avoid malpractice claims.

> **FLASHBACK**
>
> You learned about asking about medications in Chapter 9.

Liability Insurance

Liability insurance covers monetary damages that must be paid if the defendant loses a liability suit. Most hospitals require a doctor to show proof of insurance before receiving admitting privileges. Phlebotomists are usually covered by their institution's liability insurance, although some phlebotomists also obtain their own.

CONFIDENTIALITY

In addition to your legal obligations, as a phlebotomist you are bound by both legal and ethical responsibilities, especially in the area of confidentiality. With the passage of the Health Insurance Portability and Accountability Act (HIPAA), the privacy of medical information has taken on legal ramifications as well.

Health Insurance Portability and Accountability Act

HIPAA defines a set of standards and procedures for protection of privacy of health information. **Protected health information (PHI)** is any part of a patient's health information that is linked to information that identifies the patient, such as date of birth, name, or address. PHI includes information in the patient's medical record, the results of tests, and other related information, in any form. Under HIPAA, patients have the right to control their protected health information, and disclosing PHI without the patient's consent is illegal. Upon intake, patients are informed of their rights under HIPAA. Your institution should have defined procedures for protecting private health information while allowing that information to be disclosed to those who need to know it and have a right to know it.

Safeguarding a patient's privacy requires several precautions:

- Never discuss a patient's condition, tests, or financial information in a public place, such as a hallway, elevator, or eating area. Be careful to keep phone conversations private. Avoid using the patient's name if possible.
- Never discuss information concerning a patient with someone not directly involved in that patient's care.

- Never release medical information concerning a patient to anyone not specifically authorized to acquire it. Disclosure of information to a third party (such as an employer, the news media, or a relative other than the parent of a minor) requires written authorization from the patient.
- Never leave patient records out where patients or visitors can glance at them.
- Always log off computers when tasks are completed.

In addition to protecting the patient's right to privacy, you have an obligation to maintain the integrity of the doctor-patient relationship. This means that you should not reveal test results to the patient but should leave this to the physician.

A patient is also entitled to privacy out of ethical considerations alone. As noted earlier, the Patient Care Partnership (Box 19-1) was developed by the American Hospital Association to encompass not only the right to confidentiality but also other important aspects of ethical patient care. While it does not carry the force of law, it represents an ideal that health care institutions may use to evaluate their own practices.

REVIEW FOR CERTIFICATION

The phlebotomist has a legal responsibility to follow standards of care in delivering health care services. Violation of public laws may lead to criminal prosecution, and violation of private laws may lead to civil suits. Injuries to patients that result from failure to follow the standard of care may result in a malpractice judgment or criminal prosecution. Medical malpractice is the most common civil action brought against health care professionals. Proof of malpractice requires findings of duty, dereliction, injury, and direct cause. The phlebotomist is usually covered by malpractice insurance carried by the institution. HIPAA establishes the legal right of the patient to have the privacy of his or her health information protected. Protection of patient confidentiality is not only a legal obligation under HIPAA but also an ethical duty to the patient. The phlebotomist should not discuss a patient's case with anyone who is not authorized to know and should never conduct discussions in public. Test results must not be released to anyone who is not authorized to receive them.

BIBLIOGRAPHY

American Hospital Association: *The patient care partnership*, 2014. Retrieved from http://www.aha.org/advocacy-issues/communicatingpts/pt-care-partnership.shtml.

Elsevier: *Legal and ethical issues in health professions*, ed. 6, St. Louis, 2015, Saunders.

Fremgen BF: *Medical law and ethics*, ed. 3, Upper Saddle River, N.J., 2008, Prentice Hall.

The Joint Commission: Patient safety: Facts about patient safety, 2014. Retrieved from http://www.jointcommission.org/facts_about_patient_safety/.

Judson K, Harrison C: *Law and ethics for the health professions*, ed. 6, New York, 2013, McGraw-Hill.

U.S. Department of Health & Human Services: Health information privacy, 2014. Retrieved from http://www.hhs.gov/ocr/privacy.

STUDY QUESTIONS

See answers in Appendix F.

1. List four reasons for why health care costs have increased.
2. Explain the type of laws OSHA creates.
3. Define plaintiff.
4. Give three scenarios in which a phlebotomist may be held liable.
5. Define negligence.
6. Define malpractice.
7. How can a phlebotomist fail to safeguard a patient's privacy?
8. What measures can phlebotomists take to protect themselves against malpractice suits?
9. Patient communication is an important aspect of malpractice claims. Give three examples of effective communication that may help to avoid a lawsuit.

10. Explain the difference between criminal actions and civil actions, and describe how each can pertain to phlebotomy.

11. Explain professional liability. Give at least three examples of duties that the phlebotomist can perform and three examples of patient care duties that the phlebotomist cannot perform.

12. Name three elements that a plaintiff must prove in a malpractice suit.

13. Describe the meaning of the following statement: "A phlebotomist who does so is derelict in his or her duty."

14. In defense against malpractice, what is the key in defending oneself?

15. What is liability insurance? Why would a phlebotomist have the need to carry liability insurance?

16. How does the phlebotomist maintain doctor-patient integrity?

17. Most judgments are settled in out-of-court settlements. Describe what happens when cases are not settled as easily.

18. Give at least one example of how a phlebotomist may commit a negligent act.

CERTIFICATION EXAMINATION PREPARATION

See answers in Appendix F.

1. Administrative agencies such as OSHA create which type of law?
   a. Statutory
   b. Case
   c. Administrative
   d. Federal

2. The failure to perform an action consistent with the accepted standard of care is
   a. negligence.
   b. assault.
   c. malpractice.
   d. dereliction.

3. The four elements of negligence are
   a. malpractice, tort, liability, and negligence.
   b. confidentiality, litigation, contract, and felony.
   c. duty, dereliction, injury, and direct cause.
   d. injury, direct cause, privacy, and tort.

4. The phlebotomist's duties and performance level should be outlined in the
   a. floor book.
   b. safety manual.
   c. OSHA guidelines.
   d. policies and procedure manual.

5. When a phlebotomist breaches the duty of care to a patient, this is known as
   a. direct cause.
   b. civil action.
   c. dereliction.
   d. assault.

6. A tort comes from a(n)
   a. out-of-court settlement.
   b. civil action.
   c. public law.
   d. criminal action.

7. _____ are the basis for most medical malpractice suits.
   a. Unintentional torts
   b. Criminal actions
   c. Felonies
   d. Misdemeanors

8. The principal defense against a malpractice suit is to
   a. show burden of proof.
   b. reach an out-of-court settlement.
   c. deny liability.
   d. show that the standard of care was followed.

9. The phlebotomist has a legal responsibility to do which of the following?
    a. Maintain the integrity of the doctor-patient relationship
    b. Maintain patient confidentiality
    c. Follow the standard of care
    d. All of the above

10. Medical information that is linked to a specific patient is called
    a. confidentially protected information.
    b. protected health information.
    c. private health information.
    d. protected confidential information.

11. Which of the following is not found in The Patient Care Partnership?
    a. The patient can expect protection of his or her privacy.
    b. The patient can expect high-quality hospital care.
    c. The patient can expect involvement in her or her care.
    d. The patient can expect the cheapest care possible.

Prefix	Meaning	Decimal	Exponent
deci-	tenth	0.1	10^{-1}
centi-	hundredth	0.01	10^{-2}
milli-	thousandth	0.001	10^{-3}
micro-	millionth	0.000001	10^{-6}
nano-	billionth	0.000000001	10^{-9}
deca-	ten	10	10^{1}
kilo-	thousand	1000	10^{3}
mega-	million	1,000,000	10^{6}

VOLUME UNITS

liter (L)
deciliter (dL)
milliliter (mL)
microliter (μL)
cubic centimeter (cc or cm^3)

VOLUME CONVERSIONS

1 L = 1000 mL
1 L = 10 dL
1 dL = 100 mL
1 mL = 1000 μL
1 mL = 1 cc

MASS UNITS

gram (g)
kilogram (kg)
milligram (mg)
microgram (μg)
nanogram (ng)

MASS CONVERSIONS

1 kg = 1000 g
1 g = 1000 mg
1 mg = 1000 μg

VOLUME-TO-MASS CONVERSIONS

Water has a density of 1 g/mL. Thus the volume of water in milliliters is equivalent to its weight in grams.

TEMPERATURE UNITS

	Degrees Fahrenheit	Degrees Centigrade
Freezing point of water	32	0
Room temperature	72	22
Normal body temperature	98.6	37
Boiling point of water	212	100

TEMPERATURE CONVERSIONS

To convert from centigrade to Fahrenheit:

$$(°C + 40) \times 9/5 - 40 = °F$$

Example:

$$(20° C + 40) \times 9/5 - 40 = 68° F$$

To convert from Fahrenheit to centigrade:

$$(°F + 40) \times 5/9 - 40 = °C$$

Example:

$$(110° F + 40) \times 5/9 - 40 = 43.3° C$$

Common English–Spanish Phrases for Phlebotomy

GENERAL RULES OF SPANISH PRONUNCIATION

Vowels: Pronunciation of vowels in Spanish is straightforward, since each vowel has one and only one sound:

a = ah
e = eh
i = ee
o = oh
u = oo

Emphasis: Emphasis goes on the last syllable unless the last letter is *n, s,* or a vowel. In those cases, it goes on the next-to-last syllable. Accent marks also indicate stressed syllables.

Each phrase is given in the following form:

English
    Spanish
    "Phonetic pronunciation"

Greeting the Patient
Please.
    Por favor.
    "Por fah-VOR"

Thank you.
    Gracias.
    "GRAH-see-as"

Good morning.
    Buenos días.
    "Bway-nos DEE-as"

Good afternoon.
    Buenas tardes.
    "Bway-nas TAR-des"

Good evening.
    Buenas noches.
    "Bway-nas NO-ches"

Checking Patient Identification
What is your name?
    ¿Cómo se llama usted?
    "CO-mo seh YA-ma oo-STED?"

May I see your identification bracelet?
    ¿Puedo ver su brazalete de identificación?
    "Poo-EH-do vair soo BRA-sa-LET-eh de ee-dent-ih-fi-cah-see-ON?"

Informing the Patient that you Need to Take a Blood Sample
Your doctor has ordered some laboratory tests.
    Su médico ha ordenado un análisis de laboratorio.
    "Soo MEH-dee-co ah OR-den-AH-doe oon ah-NAH-lee-sees de lah-BOR-ih-TOR-ee-o"

I have to take some blood for testing.
    Tengo que sacarle sangre para un análisis.
    "TENG-go keh sah-CAR-leh SANG-gray PAH-rah oon ah-NAH-lee-sees"

I am going to take a blood sample for testing.
    Voy a tomarle una muestra de sangre para análisis.
    "VOY ah to-MAR-lay OON-ah moo-ES-tra de SANG-gray PAH-rah ah-NAH-lee-sees"

Have you had anything to eat or drink in the last 12 hours?
    ¿Ha comido o bebido algo en las últimas doce horas?
    "Hah co-MEE-doh oh beh-BEE-doh AL-go en las UL-tee-mas DOH-seh OR-as?"

Collecting the Blood Sample
Please make a fist.
    Por favor haga un puño.
    "Por fah-VOR HAH-ga oon POON-yo"

Is the tourniquet too tight?
    ¿Está demasiado apretado el torniquete?
    "Eh-STAH deh-MAH-see-AH-doh AH-preh-TAH-doh el TOR-nih-KET-eh?"

You are going to feel a small prick.
    Usted va a sentir un pequeño piquete.
    "oo-STED vah ah sen-TEER oon peh-KEN-yo pih-KET-eh"

Please keep your arm straight.
    Por favor, mantenga su brazo firme.
    "Por fah-VOR, man-TENG-ah soo BRA-so FEER-meh"

You can now relax your arm and fist.
> *Usted puede relajar su brazo y puño.*
> "oo-STED PWED-eh REH-la-HAR soo BRA-zo ee POON-yo"

Asking the Patient to give you a Urine Sample

You need to give us a urine sample for testing.
> *Usted tiene que darnos una muestra de orina para análisis.*
> "oo-STED tee-EN-eh keh DARN-ohs OON-ah moo-ES-tra de oh-REEN-ah PAH-rah ah-NAH-lee-sees"

Useful Phlebotomy Terms

arm
> *brazo*
> "BRA-so"

blood
> *sangre*
> "SANG-gray"

finger
> *dedo*
> "DEH-doh"

finger stick
> *piquete del dedo*
> "pih-KET-eh del DEH-doh"

left arm
> *brazo izquierdo*
> "BRA-so IS-kee-AIR-doh"

needle
> *aguja*
> "ah-GOO-ha"

prick, stick
> *piquete*
> "pih-KET-eh"

right arm
> *brazo derecho*
> "BRA-so de-RESH-oh"

sample
> *muestra*
> "moo-ES-tra"

test, analysis
> *análisis*
> "ah-NAH-lee-sees"

tourniquet
> *torniquete*
> "TOR-nih-KET-eh"

urinalysis
> *análisis de la orina*
> "ah-NAH-lee-sees de la oh-REEN-ah"

urine
> *orina*
> "oh-REEN-ah"

Names of Laboratory Tests

blood test
> *análisis de la sangre*
> "ah-NAH-lee-sees de la SANG-gray"

glucose level
> *nivel de glucosa*
> "nee-VEL de glu-CO-sa"

blood count
> *recuento sanguíneo*
> "reh-KWEN-toh san-GEEN-ee-o"

electrolytes
> *electrólitos*
> "eh-lec-TRO-lee-toes"

cholesterol
> *colesterol*
> "co-LES-teh-ROL"

triglycerides
> *triglicéridos*
> "tree-glee-SEH-ree-dos"

pregnancy test
> *análisis de embarazo*
> "ah-NAH-lee-sees de EM-bar-AH-so"

liver enzymes
> *enzimas del hígado*
> "en-SEE-mas del EE-gah-do"

hepatitis C
> *hepatitis tipo C*
> "heh-pa-TEE-tis TEE-po say"

COMPETENCY CHECKLIST

Hand Washing

Name _____

Date _____

Instructions

1. Properly demonstrate aseptic hand-washing technique.
2. Demonstrate competency by performing the procedure of hand washing satisfactorily for the instructor. All steps must be completed as listed on the Competency Checklist.

Performance Standard

Properly wash hands using the aseptic technique. Maximum time to complete assignment: 5 minutes.

Materials and Equipment

- Sink with running water
- Soap dispenser
- Paper towels

Procedure

Record in the comments section any problems encountered while performing the procedure.

S = Satisfactory
U = Unsatisfactory

You Must:	S	U	Comments
1. Remove all hand and wrist jewelry, including rings.			
2. Wet your hands with warm water.			
3. Apply soap to your hands.			
4. Rub your hands together vigorously, working up a lather.			
5. Scrub palms, between fingers, under nails, and the back of hands for at least 15 seconds.			
6. Rinse in a downward position.			
7. Dry your hands thoroughly with paper towels.			
8. Turn off the faucet with paper towels.			
9. Discard paper towels.			

Performance Standard Met

_____ Yes
_____ No

Evaluator_____

Comments

Date _____

COMPETENCY CHECKLIST
Donning and Removing Personal Protective Equipment

Name _____

Date _____

Instructions

1. Properly demonstrate how to put on and take off personal protective equipment.
2. Demonstrate competency by demonstrating the correct order of putting personal protective equipment on and the appropriate order of removing and discarding it. All steps must be completed as listed on the Competency Checklist.

Performance Standard

Properly apply and remove personal protective equipment in the correct order. Maximum time to complete assignment: 8 minutes.

Materials and Equipment

- Hand-washing equipment
- Gown or lab coat
- Goggles, mask, or face shield
- Gloves
- Biohazard waste container

Procedure

Record in the comments section any problems encountered while performing the procedure.

S = Satisfactory
U = Unsatisfactory

You Must:	S	U	Comments

Apply Personal Protective Equipment

1. Wash your hands.
2. Put on a lab coat or gown and fasten buttons or ties appropriately.
3. Apply goggles, face mask, or face shield. If applying a mask, tie the mask at the top and then at the bottom.
4. Apply gloves over the cuffs of the lab coat or gown.

Remove Personal Protective Equipment

1. Untie and remove gown.
2. Remove gloves as you finish peeling off gown
3. Dispose of the gloves and gown in a biohazard waste container.
4. Remove the face mask, goggles, or face shield. If wearing a mask, untie the top ties and then the bottom ties, and discard the mask in a biohazard waste container.
5. Wash your hands.

Performance Standard Met   Comments

_____ Yes

_____ No

Evaluator _____   Date _____

COMPETENCY CHECKLIST

Venipuncture (Evacuated Tube Method)

Name _____

Date _____

Instructions

1. Perform a venipuncture using the evacuated tube method.
2. Demonstrate competency by demonstrating the procedure for performing a venipuncture satisfactorily for the instructor. All steps must be completed as listed on the Competency Checklist.

Performance Standard

Successfully and properly perform a venipuncture using the evacuated tube method. Maximum time to complete assignment: 10 minutes.

Materials and Equipment

- Hand-washing equipment
- Personal protective equipment
- Tourniquet
- Alcohol wipe
- Safety needle
- Disposable adapter
- Collection tubes
- Sharps container
- 2 × 2 gauze pad
- Bandage
- Biohazard waste container

Procedure

Record in the comments section any problems encountered while performing the procedure.

S = Satisfactory
U = Unsatisfactory

You Must:	S	U	Comments
1. Greet and identify the patient. Ask the patient to state his or her name. Use two identifiers to verify patient identity.			
2. Introduce yourself and explain the procedure to the patient.			
3. Verify the lab tests ordered against the requisition.			
4. Position and prepare the patient.			
5. Wash your hands and don personal protective equipment.			
6. Apply the tourniquet.			
7. Select vein by palpating the vein.			
8. Cleanse the site with an alcohol wipe and allow to air dry. Remove the tourniquet.			
9. Assemble the equipment.			
10. Reapply the tourniquet (if necessary).			
11. Examine the safety needle.			
12. Anchor the vein.			
13. Insert the needle into the vein at the appropriate angle.			
14. Advance and change tubes in the appropriate order of draw.			
15. Remove the tourniquet.			
16. Mix anticoagulated tubes as they are removed from the adapter.			
17. Remove the last tube from the adapter before removing the needle. Activate the safety device.			
18. Remove the needle and discard it in a sharps container.			
19. Apply pressure to the site with gauze.			
20. Label tubes with appropriate information.			
21. Check the site and apply a bandage.			
22. Thank the patient.			
23. Dispose of used supplies and materials.			
24. Remove personal protective equipment and wash your hands.			
25. Deliver specimens to appropriate departments.			

Performance Standard Met

Comments

_____Yes

_____No

Evaluator_____

Date _____

COMPETENCY CHECKLIST
Venipuncture (Syringe Method)

Name _____

Date _____

Instructions

1. Perform a venipuncture using the syringe method.
2. Demonstrate competency by demonstrating the procedure for performing a venipuncture satisfactorily for the instructor. All steps must be completed as listed on the Competency Checklist.

Performance Standard

Successfully and properly perform a venipuncture using the syringe method. Maximum time to complete assignment: 10 minutes.

Materials and Equipment

- Hand-washing equipment
- Personal protective equipment
- Tourniquet
- Alcohol wipe
- Syringe
- Safety needle
- 2 × 2 gauze pad
- Collection tubes
- Syringe transfer device
- Sharps container
- Bandage
- Biohazard waste container

Procedure

Record in the comments section any problems encountered while performing the procedure.

S = Satisfactory
U = Unsatisfactory

You Must:	S	U	Comments
1. Greet and identify the patient. Ask the patient to state his or her name. Use two identifiers to verify patient identity.			
2. Introduce yourself and explain the procedure to the patient.			
3. Verify the lab tests ordered against the requisition.			
4. Position and prepare the patient.			
5. Wash your hands and don personal protective equipment.			
6. Apply the tourniquet.			
7. Palpate the vein.			
8. Cleanse the site with an alcohol wipe and allow to air dry. Remove the tourniquet.			
9. Assemble the equipment.			
10. Reapply the tourniquet.			
11. Check the syringe plunger to verify free movement.			
12. Examine the safety needle.			
13. Anchor the vein.			
14. Insert the needle into the vein at the appropriate angle.			
15. Pull back the plunger evenly to withdraw blood.			
16. Remove the tourniquet.			

Continued

Procedure—cont'd

Record in the comments section any problems encountered while performing the procedure.	**S = Satisfactory** **U = Unsatisfactory**		
You Must:	S	U	Comments

17. Remove the needle and activate the safety device.
18. Apply pressure to the site with gauze.
19. Transfer blood to evacuated tubes in the correct order of draw using the syringe transfer device.
20. Mix any anticoagulated tubes as needed.
21. Discard the syringe and needle in a sharps container.
22. Label tubes with appropriate information.
23. Check the site and apply a bandage.
24. Thank the patient.
25. Dispose of used supplies and materials.
26. Remove personal protective equipment and wash your hands.
27. Deliver specimens to the appropriate departments.

Performance Standard Met	Comments

_____ Yes
_____ No

Evaluator _____   Date _____

COMPETENCY CHECKLIST
Capillary Puncture (Finger Stick)

Name _____

Date _____

Instructions

1. Perform a capillary puncture.
2. Demonstrate competency by demonstrating the procedure for performing a capillary puncture satisfactorily for the instructor. All steps must be completed as listed on the Competency Checklist.

Performance Standard

Successfully and properly perform a capillary puncture. Maximum time to complete assignment: 10 minutes.

Materials and Equipment

- Hand-washing equipment
- Personal protective equipment
- Alcohol wipe
- Skin puncture device
- Collection tubes (microtainers or capillary pipettes)
- Sealing caps or clay
- 2 × 2 gauze pad
- Bandage
- Sharps container
- Biohazard waste container

Procedure

Record in the comments section any problems encountered while performing the procedure.

S = Satisfactory
U = Unsatisfactory

You Must:	S	U	Comments
1. Greet and identify the patient. Ask the patient to state his or her name. Use two identifiers to verify patient identity.			
2. Introduce yourself and explain the procedure.			
3. Verify the lab tests ordered against the requisition.			
4. Wash your hands and don personal protective equipment.			
5. Assemble the equipment.			
6. Select the puncture site (and warm if necessary). Cleanse with alcohol and allow to air dry.			
7. Position and hold the finger and make the puncture in the appropriate area and position.			
8. Wipe away the first drop of blood.			
9. Collect the specimen in the appropriate containers, without air bubbles.			
10. Seal the specimen containers.			
11. Mix specimens with anticoagulant to prevent clot formation.			
12. Apply pressure to the puncture site with gauze.			
13. Bandage the puncture site appropriately based on the patient's age.			
14. Label the specimens.			
15. Thank the patient.			
16. Dispose of used supplies and materials appropriately.			
17. Remove personal protective equipment and wash your hands.			

Performance Standard Met

Comments

_____ Yes

_____ No

Evaluator _____

Date _____

COMPETENCY CHECKLIST
Bleeding Time

Name _____

Date _____

Instructions

1. Successfully perform the bleeding time test.
2. Demonstrate competency by demonstrating the procedure for bleeding time satisfactorily for the instructor. All steps must be completed as listed on the Competency Checklist.

Performance Standard

Determine platelet function, as well as the significance of the test result. Maximum time to complete assignment: 15 minutes.

Materials and Equipment

- Hand-washing equipment
- Personal protective equipment
- Alcohol wipe
- Blood pressure cuff
- Automated bleeding time puncture device
- Stopwatch or timer with second hand
- Filter paper
- Butterfly bandage
- Sharps container
- Biohazard waste container

Procedure

Record in the comments section any problems encountered while performing the procedure.

S = Satisfactory
U = Unsatisfactory

You Must:

	S	U	Comments
1. Greet and identify the patient. Ask the patient to state his or her name. Use two identifiers to verify patient identity.			
2. Identify yourself and explain the procedure.			
3. Verify the lab tests ordered against the requisition.			
4. Wash your hands and don personal protective equipment.			
5. Assemble the equipment.			
6. Position the patient's arm on a flat, steady surface.			
7. Select and cleanse the incision site with alcohol and allow to air dry.			
8. Apply the blood pressure cuff on the arm and inflate to 40 mm Hg.			
9. Position the incision device.			
10. Make the incision and start the timer.			
11. Wick blood onto the filter paper every 30 seconds after the timer starts.			
12. Stop the timer when blood is no longer absorbed by the filter paper and record the time.			
13. Deflate and remove the blood pressure cuff.			
14. Cleanse the puncture site and apply a butterfly bandage.			
15. Instruct the patient on puncture site and bandage care.			
16. Correctly dispose of used supplies and materials.			
17. Thank the patient.			
18. Remove personal protective equipment and wash your hands.			

Performance Standard Met

Comments

_____ Yes

_____ No

Evaluator _____   Date _____

COMPETENCY CHECKLIST
Venipuncture (Winged Infusion Method)

Name _____

Date _____

Instructions

1. Perform a venipuncture using the winged infusion method.
2. Demonstrate competency by demonstrating the procedure for performing a venipuncture satisfactorily for the instructor. All steps must be completed as listed on the Competency Checklist.

Performance Standard

Successfully and properly perform a venipuncture using the winged infusion method. Maximum time to complete assignment: 10 minutes.

Materials and Equipment

- Hand-washing equipment
- Personal protective equipment
- Tourniquet
- Alcohol wipe
- Winged infusion set
- Evacuated tubes or syringe
- 2×2 gauze pad
- Sharps container
- Bandage
- Biohazard waste container

Procedure

Record in the comments section any problems encountered while performing the procedure.

S = Satisfactory
U = Unsatisfactory

You Must:	S	U	Comments
1. Greet and identify the patient. Ask the patient to state his or her name. Use two identifiers to verify patient identity.			
2. Introduce yourself and explain the procedure to the patient.			
3. Verify the lab tests ordered against the requisition.			
4. Wash your hands and don personal protective equipment.			
5. Position the patient's hand and apply the tourniquet around the wrist.			
6. Choose the puncture site and palpate the vein.			
7. Cleanse the site with an alcohol wipe and allow it to air dry. Release the tourniquet.			
8. Assemble the equipment.			
9. Reapply the tourniquet (if necessary).			
10. Anchor the vein.			
11. Holding the butterfly wings, insert the needle into the vein at the appropriate angle.			
12. Advance the needle and hold it in place by one wing with the thumb of the opposite hand.			
13. Collect the sample in accordance with the method being used (evacuated tubes or syringe).			

Continued

Procedure—cont'd

Record in the comments section any problems encountered while performing the procedure.	**S = Satisfactory** **U = Unsatisfactory**		
You Must:	S	U	Comments
14. Release the tourniquet, remove the needle, and activate the safety device.			
15. Apply pressure to the site with gauze.			
16. Mix anticoagulated tubes if applicable.			
17. If using a syringe, transfer blood to evacuated tubes. Use a syringe transfer device.			
18. Discard the needle and tubing in a sharps container.			
19. Label tubes with appropriate information.			
20. Check the site and apply a bandage.			
21. Thank the patient.			
22. Dispose of used supplies and materials.			
23. Remove personal protective equipment and wash your hands.			
24. Deliver specimens to appropriate departments.			

Performance Standard Met   Comments

_____ Yes

_____ No

Evaluator _____   Date _____

COMPETENCY CHECKLIST
Modified Allen Test

Name _____

Date _____

Instructions
1. Properly perform the modified Allen test.
2. Demonstrate competency by demonstrating the procedure for determining collateral circulation satisfactorily for the instructor. All steps must be completed as listed on the Competency Checklist.

Performance Standard
Determine the presence of collateral circulation, as well as the significance of the test result. Maximum time to complete assignment: 5 minutes.

Materials and Equipment
- Towel

Procedure

Record in the comments section any problems encountered while performing the procedure.

S = Satisfactory
U = Unsatisfactory

You Must:	S	U	Comments
1. Extend the patient's wrist over a towel and position the hand palm up.			
2. Locate the radial and ulnar pulse sites by palpating with the appropriate fingers.			
3. Ask the patient to make a fist.			
4. Compress both arteries.			
5. Ask the patient to open and close the fist until the palm blanches.			
6. Release pressure on the ulnar artery and observe the color of the patient's palm.			
7. State and record a positive or negative result.			
8. Explain the significance and appropriate action to take for the test result.			

Performance Standard Met	Comments
_____ Yes	
_____ No	
Evaluator _____	Date _____

COMPETENCY CHECKLIST
Radial Artery Puncture

Name _____

Date _____

Instructions

1. Properly perform a radial artery puncture following the step-by-step procedure.
2. Demonstrate competency by demonstrating the procedure for performing a radial artery puncture for the instructor. All steps must be completed as listed on the Competency Checklist.

Performance Standard

Perform a radial artery puncture with accuracy and minimal discomfort. Maximum time to complete assignment: 12 minutes.

Materials and Equipment

- Hand-washing equipment
- Personal protective equipment
- Alcohol wipes
- Povidone-iodine tincture
- Local anesthetic
- Safety needle, needle block, and Luer cap
- Blood gas syringe (heparinized)
- 2 × 2 gauze pad
- Cup of ice chips
- Bandage
- Sharps container
- Biohazard waste container

Procedure

Record in the comments section any problems encountered while performing the procedure.

S = Satisfactory
U = Unsatisfactory

You Must:	S	U	Comments
1. Assemble the equipment.			
2. Greet the patient, introduce yourself, and explain the procedure. Ask the patient to state his or her name. Use two identifiers to verify patient identity. Introduce yourself and explain the procedure.			
3. Verify that the patient is in a respiratory steady state.			
4. Verify the lab tests ordered against the requisition.			
5. Wash your hands and don personal protective equipment.			
6. Perform the modified Allen test to assess collateral circulation in the hand.			
7. Locate the radial artery.			
8. Cleanse the puncture site with 70% isopropyl alcohol and allow to air dry.			
9. Cleanse the puncture site with povidone-iodine tincture and allow to air dry.			
10. Administer local anesthetic and wait 1 to 2 minutes.			
11. Cleanse your index finger with alcohol and place it above the area where the needle should enter the artery.			
12. Hold the syringe like a dart, bevel up, and insert the needle at a 45- to 60-degree angle distal to your finger until blood appears in the needle hub.			
13. Allow arterial pressure to fill the syringe.			
14. Remove the needle and apply direct pressure to the puncture site with folded gauze for at least 5 minutes.			
15. While applying pressure, expel air from the syringe, activate the safety device, and plant the needle into the rubber block.			

Procedure—cont'd

Record in the comments section any problems encountered while performing the procedure.   **S = Satisfactory**
U = Unsatisfactory

You Must:	S	U	Comments
16. Mix the specimen with heparin.			
17. Place the specimen in ice chips.			
18. Check the site and remove the povidone-iodine with an alcohol wipe.			
19. Apply a pressure bandage of gauze.			
20. Check for a pulse distal to the puncture site.			
21. Remove and discard the needle in a sharps container.			
22. Place the Luer cap on the syringe, label the specimen, and return it to the ice chips.			
23. Thank the patient.			
24. Dispose of used supplies and materials; remove personal protective equipment and wash your hands.			
25. Deliver the specimen immediately to the lab.			

Performance Standard Met   Comments

_____ Yes
_____ No
Evaluator _____   Date _____

COMPETENCY CHECKLIST
Blood Culture

Name _____

Date _____

Instructions

1. Properly perform a blood culture collection.
2. Demonstrate competency by demonstrating the procedure for collecting a blood culture satisfactorily for the instructor while adhering to aseptic technique. All steps must be completed as listed on the Competency Checklist.

Performance Standard

Collect a blood culture with accuracy. Maximum time to complete assignment: 10 minutes.

Materials and Equipment

- Hand-washing equipment
- Personal protective equipment
- Tourniquet
- Alcohol wipes
- Povidone-iodine tincture
- Aerobic blood culture bottle
- Anaerobic blood culture bottle
- Safety needle
- Disposable adapter
- 2 × 2 gauze pad
- Bandages
- Sharps container
- Biohazard waste container

Procedure

Record in the comments section any problems encountered while performing the procedure.

S = Satisfactory
U = Unsatisfactory

You Must:	S	U	Comments
1. Greet and identify the patient. Ask the patient to state his or her name. Use two identifiers to verify patient identity.			
2. Identify yourself and explain the procedure.			
3. Verify the lab tests ordered against the requisition.			
4. Wash your hands and don personal protective equipment.			
5. Apply the tourniquet, identify the puncture site, and remove the tourniquet.			
6. Vigorously scrub the site with alcohol and allow to air dry.			
7. Vigorously scrub the site with povidone-iodine and allow to air dry.			
8. Assemble the equipment.			
9. Cleanse the tops of the blood culture bottles.			
10. Reapply the tourniquet without contaminating the site.			
11. Perform the venipuncture.			
12. Inoculate each bottle in the correct order and mix the samples.			
13. Release the tourniquet, remove the needle, activate the safety device, and apply pressure to the site with gauze.			
14. Label the blood culture bottles correctly.			
15. Remove povidone-iodine from the patient's arm and apply a bandage.			
16. Discard used materials and supplies appropriately.			
17. Thank the patient.			
18. Remove personal protective equipment and wash your hands.			

Performance Standard Met   Comments

_____ Yes

_____ No

Evaluator _____   Date _____

COMPETENCY CHECKLIST
Blood Smear Preparation

Name _____

Date _____

Instructions

1. Successfully prepare a blood smear.
2. Demonstrate competency by demonstrating the procedure for preparing a blood smear satisfactorily for the instructor. All steps must be completed as listed on the Competency Checklist.

Performance Standard

Accurately prepare a peripheral blood smear. Maximum time to complete assignment: 5 minutes.

Materials and Equipment

- Hand-washing equipment
- Gloves
- Clean glass slides

Procedure

Record in the comments section any problems encountered while performing the procedure.

S = Satisfactory
U = Unsatisfactory

You Must:	S	U	Comments
1. Wash your hands and put on gloves.			
2. Apply a small drop of blood to the correct area of the slide.			
3. Place the spreader at the correct angle in front of the blood drop.			
4. Pull the spreader back to contact the blood drop.			
5. Move the spreader forward in a continuous motion.			
6. Repeat steps 2 through 5 to prepare a second slide.			
7. Allow the smears to dry.			
8. Properly label the smears.			
9. Examine the blood smears for quality and acceptability.			
10. Remove gloves and wash your hands.			

Performance Standard Met

Comments

_____ Yes

_____ No

Evaluator _____   Date _____

COMPETENCY CHECKLIST
Throat Swab

Name _____

Date _____

Instructions
1. Properly perform a throat swab.
2. Demonstrate competency by demonstrating the procedure for performing a throat swab satisfactorily for the instructor. All steps must be completed as listed on the Competency Checklist.

Performance Standard
Successfully and properly perform a throat swab. Maximum time to complete assignment: 5 minutes.

Materials and Equipment
- Hand-washing equipment
- Personal protective equipment
- Tongue depressor
- Flashlight
- Collection swab
- Transport tube with transport media
- Biohazard waste container

Procedure

Record in the comments section any problems encountered while performing the procedure.

S = Satisfactory
U = Unsatisfactory

You Must:	S	U	Comments
1. Greet and identify the patient. Ask the patient to state his or her name. Use two identifiers to verify patient identity.			
2. Introduce yourself.			
3. Verify the lab tests ordered against the requisition.			
4. Explain the procedure to the patient.			
5. Wash your hands and don personal protective equipment.			
6. Assemble the equipment.			
7. Position the patient.			
8. Depress the patient's tongue with a tongue depressor and inspect the back of the throat with the flashlight to locate inflamed areas.			
9. Quickly touch the tip of the swab to the tonsils and any other inflamed areas.			
10. Return the swab to the holder.			
11. Crush the ampule at the bottom of the holder containing the transport media.			
12. Thank the patient.			
13. Dispose of used supplies and materials.			
14. Remove personal protective equipment and wash your hands.			
15. Deliver the specimen to the appropriate department.			

Performance Standard Met

Comments

_____ Yes
_____ No

Evaluator _____

Date _____

2-hr PPBS	2-hour postprandial blood sugar
μL	microliter
ABG	arterial blood gas
ABN	Advance Beneficiary Notice of Noncoverage
ACA	American Certification Agency for Healthcare Professionals
ACE	angiotensin-converting enzyme
ACT	activated coagulation time
ACTH	adrenocorticotropic hormone
ADH	antidiuretic hormone
AIDS	acquired immunodeficiency syndrome
ALP	alkaline phosphatase
ALS	amyotrophic lateral sclerosis
ALT	alanine aminotransferase
AMT	American Medical Technologists
ANA	antinuclear antibody
aPTT	activated partial thromboplastin time
ASCLS	American Society for Clinical Laboratory Science
ASCP	American Society for Clinical Pathology
ASPT	American Society of Phlebotomy Technicians
AST	alternate site testing, aspartate aminotransferase
ATP	adenosine triphosphate
AV	arteriovenous, atrioventricular
BBP	bloodborne pathogen
BC	blood culture
BMP	basic metabolic panel
BNP	B-type natriuretic peptide
BT	bleeding time
BUN	blood urea nitrogen
BURPP	bilirubin, uric acid, phosphorus, and potassium
C&S	culture and sensitivity
CAP	College of American Pathologists
CBC	complete blood count
CBG	capillary blood gas
CCU	cardiac care unit
CDC	Centers for Disease Control and Prevention
CEUs	continuing education units
CHD	congestive heart disease
CHP	chemical hygiene plan
CK	creatine kinase
CK-BB	creatine kinase-BB
CK-MB	creatine kinase-MB
CK-MM	creatine kinase-MM
CLIA '88	Clinical Laboratory Improvement Act of 1988
CLS	clinical laboratory scientist
CLSI	Clinical and Laboratory Standards Institute
CLT	clinical laboratory technician

CMP	comprehensive metabolic panel
CNA	certified nursing assistant
CNS	central nervous system
COC	chain of custody
COPD	chronic obstructive pulmonary disease
CPR	cardiopulmonary resuscitation
CPT	certified phlebotomy technician
CQI	continuous quality improvement
CSF	cerebrospinal fluid
CT	computed tomography
CVC	central venous catheter
DIC	disseminated intravascular coagulation
diff	differential
DNA	deoxyribonucleic acid
DOB	date of birth
DOT	Department of Transportation
DVT	deep vein thrombosis
EBV	Epstein-Barr virus
ECG, EKG	electrocardiogram
EDTA	ethylenediaminetetraacetic acid
EMLA	Eutectic Mixture of Local Anesthetics
ENT	ear, nose, and throat
EP	expanded precaution
ER, ED	emergency room, emergency department
ESR	erythrocyte sedimentation rate
FBS	fasting blood sugar (glucose)
FDA	Food and Drug Administration
FDP	fibrin degradation product
FSH	follicle-stimulating hormone
FTA-ABS	fluorescent treponemal antibody absorption test
FUO	fever of unknown origin
g/dL	grams per deciliter
GGT	γ-glutamyltransferase
GH	growth hormone
GHS	Globally Harmonized System
GTT	glucose tolerance test
Hb A$_{Ic}$	glycated hemoglobin/glycosylated hemoglobin
HBsAG	hepatitis B surface antigen
HBV	hepatitis B virus
hCG	human chorionic gonadotropin
HCl	hydrochloric acid
Hct	hematocrit
HCV	hepatitis C virus
HDL	high-density lipoprotein
HEPA	high-efficiency particulate air
Hgb	hemoglobin
HIPAA	Health Insurance Portability and Accountability Act
HIV	human immunodeficiency virus
HLA	human leukocyte antigen

HMO	health maintenance organization
HTLV	human T-cell lymphotropic virus
ICD-9-CM	International Classification of Diseases, Ninth Revision, Clinical Modification
ICD-10-CM	International Classification of Diseases, Tenth Revision, Clinical Modification
ICU	intensive care unit
ID	identification
INR	international normalized ratio
IRDS	infant respiratory distress syndrome
IRS	Internal Revenue Service
IV	intravenous
KOH	potassium hydroxide
LDL	low-density lipoprotein
LH	luteinizing hormone
LIS	laboratory information services
LPN	licensed practical nurse
LTC	long-term care
LTT	lactose tolerance test
MCH	mean corpuscular hemoglobin
MCHC	mean corpuscular hemoglobin concentration
MCV	mean corpuscular volume
MHC	major histocompatibility complex
MI	myocardial infarction
MIS	manager of information services
MLS	medical laboratory scientist
MLT	medical laboratory technician
MPV	mean platelet volume
MRI	magnetic resonance imaging
MRSA	methicillin-resistant *Staphylococcus aureus*
MSH	melanocyte-stimulating hormone
MT	medical technologist
NAACLS	National Accrediting Agency for Clinical Laboratory Sciences
NFPA	National Fire Protection Association
NHA	National Healthcareer Association
NIDA	National Institute on Drug Abuse
NIOSH	National Institute for Occupational Safety and Health
NK	natural killer
NP	nasopharyngeal
NPA	National Phlebotomy Association
NSY	nursery
O&P	ova and parasites
OGTT	oral glucose tolerance test
OR	operating room
OSHA	Occupational Safety and Health Administration
PBT	phlebotomy technician by AMT
PCA	patient care assistant
P_{CO_2}	partial pressure of carbon dioxide
PCR	polymerase chain reaction
PCT	patient care technician
PE	protective equipment
PET	positron emission tomography
PFA	platelet function assay

PHI	protected health information
PICC	peripherally inserted central catheter
PID	pelvic inflammatory disease
PKU	phenylketonuria
PLT	platelets
PMN	polymorphonuclear
PMS	premenstrual syndrome
P_{O_2}	partial pressure of oxygen
POCT	point-of-care testing
POL	physician office laboratory
PPD	purified protein derivative
PPE	personal protective equipment
PPO	preferred provider organization
PSA	prostate-specific antigen
PST	plasma separator tube
PT	prothrombin time
PTH	parathyroid hormone
QA	quality assurance
QC	quality control
QNS	quantity not sufficient
RA	rheumatoid arthritis
RBC	red blood cell
RDW	red blood cell distribution width
RF	rheumatoid factor
RN	registered nurse
RPR	rapid plasma reagin
RPT	registered phlebotomy technician
RSV	respiratory syncytial virus
RT	respiratory therapist
SARS	severe acute respiratory syndrome
SCID	severe combined immune deficiency
SDS	safety data sheet
SE	sweat electrolytes
seg	segmented neutrophil
SLE	systemic lupus erythematosus
SPS	sodium polyanethole sulfonate
SST	serum separator tube
stat	short turnaround time
STI	sexually transmitted infection
T_3	triiodothyronine
T_4	thyroxine
TDM	therapeutic drug monitoring
TIBC	total iron-binding capacity
TLC	tender loving care
TnT	troponin T
t-PA	tissue plasminogen activator
TQM	total quality management
TSH	thyroid-stimulating hormone
TSS	toxic shock syndrome
URI	upper respiratory infection
UTI	urinary tract infection
VAD	vascular access device
VRE	vancomycin-resistant *Enterococcus*
WBC	white blood cell
WCS	winged collection set
WIS	winged infusion set

APPENDIX E   Mock Certification Exam

Pamela B. Primrose and Rachel Houston

1. What is phlebotomy?
   a. A trained professional in blood drawing
   b. The legal standards for a person who performs blood-drawing skills
   c. The process of drawing blood
   d. All of the above.

2. What is a phlebotomist?
   a. A trained professional in blood drawing
   b. The legal standards for a person who performs blood-drawing skills
   c. The process of drawing blood
   d. All of the above.

3. Which of the following is not part of a phlebotomist's point-of-care job-related duties?
   a. Taking blood pressure
   b. Instructing patients on urine specimen collection
   c. Performing a tracheostomy
   d. Performing POC testing

4. All of the following are considered hazards except:
   a. bending your knees when lifting heavy objects.
   b. airborne viruses and bacteria.
   c. handling broken glass when wearing gloves.
   d. All of the above are hazards.

5. All of the following are true about laboratory safety except:
   a. you may store food in the laboratory refrigerator.
   b. protect your feet from spills.
   c. always wear required personal protection equipment.
   d. All of the above are correct.

6. As written in the Patient Care Partnership from the American Hospital Association, the patient has the right to:
   a. high-quality care.
   b. protection of privacy.
   c. help with billing claims.
   d. All of the above.

7. Certification is evidence that:
   a. the phlebotomist is working in the field.
   b. the phlebotomist has demonstrated proficiency in the area of blood drawing.
   c. the phlebotomist is licensed in the field.
   d. the phlebotomist is accredited in the field.

8. Which of the following is not OSHA-required personal protection equipment?
   a. Steel-toe shoes
   b. Goggles
   c. Chin-length face shield
   d. Full-length lab coat

9. The Clinical Laboratory Improvement Act of 1988 follows guidelines and standards set by the:
   a. CLIA '88.
   b. CLSI.
   c. JCAHO.
   d. CDC.

10. Samples collected from a patient in a nursing home are sent to the:
    a. POL.
    b. CDC.
    c. reference laboratory.
    d. urgent care center.

11. Quality assurance for laboratory personnel includes all of the following except:
    a. specimen collection procedures.
    b. specimen transport processes.
    c. specimen-processing policies.
    d. the laboratory supervisor's home telephone number.

12. Personal protection equipment must be provided by the:
    a. CDC.
    b. OSHA.
    c. employee.
    d. employer.

13. Which of the following personal protection equipment must a phlebotomist use when performing a skin puncture or venipuncture?
    a. Goggles
    b. Gloves
    c. A mask
    d. Caps and booties

14. Under HIPAA, protected health information is defined as:
    a. information that the patient refuses to disclose to the physician.
    b. any test result.
    c. any part of a patient's health information that is linked to information that identifies the patient.
    d. information that summarizes the patient's insurance coverage.

15. Employers must provide vaccination against _____ free of charge.
   a. hepatitis A virus
   b. hepatitis B virus
   c. hepatitis C virus
   d. hepatitis delta virus

16. Which of the following would be a reason for rejection of a specimen by the laboratory?
   a. The patient's name, date of birth, and the date and time are written on the label and requisition slip.
   b. A specimen containing an additive has been inverted.
   c. An ESR has been collected in a red-topped tube.
   d. All of the above are reasons for rejections.

17. The quality of the test result depends on:
   a. the type of specimen.
   b. the source of the specimen.
   c. the time between collecting the specimen and analyzing the specimen.
   d. whether the sample is going to be analyzed for glucose or phosphate.

18. The purpose of Total Quality Management is to:
   a. check machinery with automated procedures.
   b. ensure that proper laboratory procedures are being followed.
   c. ensure that adequate patient care is being provided.
   d. All of the above.

19. A specimen may be rejected by the laboratory if:
   a. the tube was not initialed.
   b. the blood is hemolyzed.
   c. the tube was not transported properly.
   d. All of the above.

20. Transport bags have a separate compartment (pouch) for requisitions to:
   a. safeguard the requisition.
   b. keep the specimen from getting lost.
   c. prevent contamination if the specimen leaks.
   d. ensure the requisition goes to central receiving and the specimen to the processing laboratory.

21. _____ is the most important first step in phlebotomy and other testing procedures.
   a. Proper patient identification
   b. Proper hand washing
   c. Proper specimen handling
   d. Collecting sufficient blood

22. Acceptable method(s) of identifying a patient include:
   a. ask the patient to give his or her name and DOB.
   b. check the patient's ID band.
   c. ask the patient to present a photo ID.
   d. All of the above are acceptable.

23. When an admitted patient is not wearing an ID band, the phlebotomist must:
   a. ask the patient for a picture ID.
   b. not draw blood from this patient.
   c. question the patient and confirm the date of birth.
   d. not draw blood until nursing has placed an ID band on the patient.

24. What is the proper procedure for a phlebotomist to follow if a physician or member of the clergy is in the patient's room at the time of draw?
   a. Ask the physician or clergy member to step outside.
   b. Draw the blood with the physician or clergy member present.
   c. Return at another time if the specimen is not a stat request.
   d. Both a and c.

25. How should the phlebotomist proceed if there is a language barrier with the patient
   a. use hand gestures to communicate.
   b. leave the room and let the physician draw.
   c. draw the blood without consent.
   d. All of the above.

26. Most tubes containing additives should be inverted:
   a. once.
   b. three times.
   c. five to eight times.
   d. tubes containing additives should not be inverted.

27. The lavender-topped tube contains:
   a. no additive.
   b. heparin.
   c. SPS or ACD.
   d. EDTA.

28. The green-topped tube contains:
   a. no additive.
   b. heparin.
   c. SPS or ACD.
   d. EDTA.

29. The yellow-topped tube contains:
   a. no additive.
   b. heparin.
   c. SPS or ACD.
   d. EDTA.

30. The glass red-topped tube contains:
    a. no additive.
    b. heparin.
    c. SPS or ACD.
    d. EDTA.
31. Which of the following tubes contain(s) sodium fluoride and potassium oxalate?
    a. Red-topped tube
    b. Lavender-topped tube
    c. Gray-topped tube
    d. All tubes with splash guards
32. Which of the following tubes would hold a glucose specimen for 24 hours?
    a. Red-topped tube
    b. Lavender-topped tube
    c. Gray-topped tube
    d. All tubes with splash guards
33. In which tube(s) would a phlebotomist collect an erythrocyte sedimentation rate?
    a. Red-topped tube
    b. Lavender-topped tube
    c. Gray-topped tube
    d. All tubes with splash guards
34. Blood for serology testing should be drawn in a:
    a. red-topped tube.
    b. lavender-topped tube.
    c. gray-topped tube.
    d. all tubes with splash guards.
35. Which of the following tubes yield(s) a serum specimen?
    a. Red-topped tube
    b. Lavender-topped tube
    c. Gray-topped tube
    d. All of the above.
36. Coagulation studies should be drawn in a light blue tube containing which of the following additives?
    a. Clot activator
    b. Sodium citrate
    c. EDTA
    d. SPS
37. A blood donation given by a patient for use during his or her surgical procedure is called:
    a. an autologous donation.
    b. a cryoprecipitated donation.
    c. a Willebrand's collection.
    d. None of the above.
38. Why should a glass red-topped tube be drawn before a green-topped tube?
    a. Additives in the red-topped tube will not interfere with the tests performed on the green-topped tube.
    b. Red-topped tubes are always the first tube drawn.
    c. Since there are no additives in the red-topped tube, it cannot contaminate the green-topped tube.
    d. Green-topped tubes are always the last tube drawn.
39. Which of the following is false for blood culture collection?
    a. The culture must be collected in the red- and marbled-topped tube.
    b. The area must be prepped with iodine or another antibacterial agent before the draw.
    c. A tourniquet is not used for blood culture collection.
    d. Both a and c are false for blood culture collection.
40. Which of the following is correct for arterial blood gas collection?
    a. ABG must be collected in a red- and marbled-topped tube.
    b. The area must be prepped with iodine before the draw.
    c. A tourniquet is used in the collection.
    d. Both b and c are correct.
41. A heparinized needle and syringe are necessary in the collection of:
    a. blood culture.
    b. ESR.
    c. ABG.
    d. heparin levels.
42. A Hemogard top:
    a. is a plastic top that fits over the stopper.
    b. is only used on the lavender-topped tube.
    c. is used to reduce aerosol and splattering of blood.
    d. Both a and c.
43. Cold agglutinin test must be maintained at a temperature of:
    a. 37° F.
    b. 32° C.
    c. 32° F.
    d. 37° C.
44. Chilling a specimen will:
    a. speed up the metabolic process.
    b. maintain the stability of the specimen during transport.
    c. prevent problems in tubes containing EDTA.
    d. facilitate processing.

45. Specimens for which of the following tests must be kept chilled?
    a. Ammonia
    b. Pyruvate
    c. Lactic acid
    d. All of the above.

46. When labeling tubes, all of the following information must be placed on them except the:
    a. patient's name.
    b. date.
    c. time of draw.
    d. All of the above.

47. Which of the following is not needed for a routine phlebotomy procedure?
    a. Gloves
    b. Tourniquet
    c. Alcohol
    d. Iodine

48. What additional equipment may be needed when drawing blood from a patient in the premature nursery?
    a. Small butterfly needles
    b. Rewards, stickers, and toys
    c. Anesthesia
    d. Additional personal protection equipment

49. The depth of a heel puncture cannot exceed:
    a. 5.3 mm.
    b. 2.4 cm.
    c. 2.0 mm.
    d. 1.3 mm.

50. The tourniquet is placed _____ above the site of draw.
    a. 5-7 inches
    b. 3-4 inches
    c. 1-2 inches
    d. 4-6 inches

51. When a tourniquet is left on too tight, capillaries may rupture, causing:
    a. a rash.
    b. pain.
    c. urticaria.
    d. petechiae.

52. Which of the following is true when using a tourniquet during a phlebotomy procedure?
    a. Never tie a tourniquet on open sores.
    b. Tying a tourniquet too tightly can cause petechiae.
    c. Leaving a tourniquet on too long can cause hemoconcentration.
    d. All of the above are true.

53. A phlebotomist must inspect the needle for:
    a. burrs.
    b. expiration date.
    c. bevel facing up.
    d. All of the above.

54. Which of the following is the smallest needle?
    a. 18 gauge
    b. 19 gauge
    c. 20 gauge
    d. 21 gauge

55. A butterfly needle should be used:
    a. for patients with sclerosed veins and one tube being drawn.
    b. on adults' dorsal and metacarpal veins.
    c. on pediatric and geriatric patients.
    d. All of the above.

56. A tube holder is used to connect needle and evacuated tube to:
    a. prevent contact between the needle and tube.
    b. ensure a firm, stable connection between them.
    c. keep blood from entering the adapter.
    d. allow a syringe to be used.

57. The proper way to dispose of a needle is to:
    a. recap it and put it into a sharps container.
    b. throw it recapped into a biohazard bag.
    c. put it into a sharps container, after activating needle safety device, immediately after withdrawing it from a patient.
    d. collect it in a cup and dispose of it later.

58. In making a site selection, the phlebotomist should consider which of the following before a venipuncture?
    a. Scars or burns
    b. Edema
    c. Mastectomy
    d. All of the above.

59. Which of the following are correct for ending the phlebotomy procedure?
    a. Remove the needle, remove the tube, and remove the tourniquet.
    b. Remove the tourniquet, apply pressure, remove the needle, and discard the needle in the sharps container.
    c. Remove the tourniquet, remove the tube, place gauze, remove the needle, apply pressure, and discard the needle in the sharps container.
    d. Remove the needle, apply pressure, and discard the needle in a biohazard bag.

60. The area you are drawing blood from begins to swell and fill with blood. This is a common complication occurring in phlebotomy known as:
    a. convulsions.
    b. short draw.
    c. hypovolemia.
    d. hematoma.

61. A tourniquet that has been left on too long can cause:
    a. petechiae.
    b. hemolysis.
    c. hemoconcentration.
    d. All of the above.

62. What should a phlebotomist do first if a patient has syncope during a phlebotomy procedure?
    a. Go quickly for help
    b. Apply a cold compress
    c. Remove the needle and tourniquet, and apply pressure
    d. Attempt to wake the patient by speaking loudly

63. Which of the following is a sign or symptom of syncope?
    a. Small red dots at the site of draw
    b. Black and blue discoloration at the site
    c. Cold, damp, clammy skin
    d. All of the above.

64. Blood that has seeped from a vein into tissue is called:
    a. hemoconcentration.
    b. hematoma.
    c. petechiae.
    d. short draw.

65. Which of the following may cause vein occlusion?
    a. Dermal puncture
    b. CABG
    c. Sphygmomanometer
    d. Chemotherapy

66. Which of the following complications may occur if the phlebotomist punctures a bone?
    a. Hematoma
    b. Hemoconcentration
    c. Arteriosclerosis
    d. Osteomyelitis

67. Veins that are hard and cordlike are called:
    a. thrombosed.
    b. sclerosed.
    c. collapsed.
    d. tortuous.

68. The term that means the rupturing of red blood cells is:
    a. hemostasis.
    b. hemoglobin.
    c. hemolysis.
    d. hematoma.

69. High bilirubin levels can lead to:
    a. mismatched blood groups.
    b. breakdown of antibodies.
    c. jaundice, which can lead to brain damage.
    d. All of the above.

70. Thrombosis is:
    a. an autoimmune reaction.
    b. blood pooled in the legs.
    c. clot formation within a blood vessel.
    d. inflammation of the thyroid gland.

71. Which of the following will cause a shortened bleeding time in a bleeding time test?
    a. Aspirin
    b. Infection
    c. Hair at the incision site
    d. Scratching of a capillary

72. A hematoma can be prevented if:
    a. pressure is applied on the vein until bleeding stops completely.
    b. a bandage is immediately placed on the vein.
    c. the needle is removed before the tourniquet is released.
    d. All of the above.

73. Aspirin may affect a patient's:
    a. HCG.
    b. CBC.
    c. bleeding time.
    d. heparin time.

74. In a CSF collection, the phlebotomist will:
    a. obtain the specimen from the physician after it has been collected from the patient.
    b. transport the specimen to the laboratory.
    c. process the microbiology specimen under the microscope.
    d. All of the above.

75. Midstream clean catch urine collections are:
    a. obtained by a phlebotomist or other trained health care professional.
    b. always a stat specimen.
    c. collected in a sterile container.
    d. Both a and c.

76. The process for collecting amniotic fluid is known as:
    a. an amniocentesis.
    b. an amnioectomy.
    c. an amniotomy.
    d. an amniology.

77. The amniotic fluid must be:
    a. transferred into a sterile container.
    b. protected from light.
    c. transported immediately to the laboratory for analysis.
    d. All of the above.
78. Prompt delivery to the laboratory of semen samples is necessary to determine _____ in fertility testing.
    a. viability
    b. volume
    c. V_{max}
    d. All of the above.
79. Fecal specimens are collected for:
    a. ova and parasite testing.
    b. testing for digestive abnormalities.
    c. occult blood analysis.
    d. All of the above.
80. What is the best sample to determine blood pH and blood gases?
    a. Capillary blood
    b. Venous blood
    c. Arterial blood
    d. Cerebrospinal fluid
81. An un-iced ABG must be delivered to the laboratory within:
    a. 1 hour.
    b. 5-10 hours.
    c. 5-10 minutes.
    d. 2 hours.
82. Arterial blood gas must be processed immediately to minimize:
    a. blood loss into tissue.
    b. hematoma.
    c. petechiae.
    d. changes in the analyte.
83. All of the following are safety equipment for arterial blood gas collection except a:
    a. small rubber block.
    b. fluid-resistant gown.
    c. transport container.
    d. face shield.
84. If the result of the modified Allen test is negative,
    a. another artery must be selected for blood collection.
    b. the patient does not have hepatitis B.
    c. dermal puncture may proceed.
    d. sweat electrolytes are unlikely to be positive for cystic fibrosis.
85. The NP culture is used to diagnose:
    a. whooping cough.
    b. croup.
    c. upper respiratory infections.
    d. All of the above.

86. The SE test is used to diagnose:
    a. whooping cough.
    b. elevated levels of salt.
    c. cystic fibrosis.
    d. All of the above.
87. Which procedure is normally collected by a nurse or respiratory therapist?
    a. Glucose tolerance test
    b. Routine blood collection
    c. Arterial blood gas
    d. Capillary or dermal punctures
88. When drawing from an adult, dermal punctures can be used as an alternate for all of the following except a(n):
    a. CBC.
    b. glucose tolerance test.
    c. ESR.
    d. arterial blood gas determination.
89. For which of the following patients should a dermal puncture be performed?
    a. Patients who require frequent blood draws
    b. Patients with burns on the arms
    c. Patients who are at risk for venous thrombosis
    d. All of the above.
90. Which of the following is the reason for cleansing the first drop of blood in a dermal puncture?
    a. To rid the sample of arterial blood
    b. To rid the specimen of fluid from tissue
    c. To rid the specimen of potassium
    d. All of the above.
91. When collecting blood from a child, the phlebotomist should:
    a. consider the psychological aspect of the draw.
    b. log the amount of blood collected to avoid depletion.
    c. collect dermal punctures whenever possible.
    d. All of the above.
92. Which of the following should a phlebotomist *not* do when drawing blood from a child?
    a. Use the patient identification process
    b. Explain the procedure
    c. Tell the child that the procedure will not hurt
    d. During the draw, tell the child "just a few more seconds"
93. What does the phlebotomist look for when identifying a newborn?
    a. The first and last name on the ID band
    b. The hospital identification number and the last name
    c. The date of birth
    d. The mother's ID bracelet

94. Improper cleansing of a venipuncture site can cause:
    a. hematoma.
    b. infection.
    c. petechiae.
    d. All of the above.

95. A pathogen is:
    a. the invasion and growth of a microorganism.
    b. an infectious, disease-causing microorganism.
    c. always a bacterium.
    d. never a virus.

96. Which of the following components is needed to make what is known as the chain of infection?
    a. Reservoir
    b. Means of transmission
    c. Susceptible host
    d. All of the above

97. A health care–associated infection is:
    a. an infection contracted within a health care institution.
    b. an infection that requires hospitalization.
    c. an infection that is only significant when a patient is immunocompromised.
    d. All of the above.

98. When a patient has a highly contagious disease, he or she is placed:
    a. in standard isolation.
    b. in expanded precautions isolation.
    c. in tier 1 isolation .
    d. in protective environment.

99. A patient who is known to have tuberculosis is placed:
    a. in expanded precautions isolation.
    b. in a protective environment.
    c. in standard isolation.
    d. in Airborne Precautions.

100. A patient who has diarrhea and bacterial gastroenteritis is placed:
    a. in Contact Precautions.
    b. in a protective environment.
    c. in standard isolation.
    d. in tier 1 precautions.

101. Patients within a neonatal ICU/burn unit or the recovery room are:
    a. in enteric isolation.
    b. in a protective environment.
    c. in strict isolation and on blood and body fluid precautions.
    d. on wound and body fluid precautions.

102. The most infectious health care–associated disease is:
    a. HIV.
    b. HBV.
    c. HCV.
    d. HAV.

103. An infection is:
    a. a disease-causing microorganism.
    b. the invasion and growth of a pathogen.
    c. always caused by bacteria.
    d. never caused by a virus.

104. Microorganisms that cause disease are:
    a. pathogenic.
    b. normal flora.
    c. nonpathogenic.
    d. None of the above.

105. Which of the following are causative agents?
    a. Only bacteria
    b. Airborne vectors
    c. Bacteria, viruses, protozoa, and fungi
    d. Direct and indirect vectors

106. Elevation of _____ is an indication of an infection.
    a. erythrocytes
    b. leukocytes
    c. thrombocytes
    d. megakaryocytes

107. Red blood cells are:
    a. erythrocytes.
    b. leukocytes.
    c. thrombocytes.
    d. platelets.

108. The primary function of a red blood cell is to:
    a. fight infections.
    b. carry iron.
    c. carry iodine.
    d. carry hemoglobin.

109. The most abundant white blood cell is the:
    a. lymphocyte.
    b. basophil.
    c. neutrophil.
    d. megakaryocyte.

110. The fluid portion of blood is:
    a. serum.
    b. hemoglobin.
    c. the sediment.
    d. plasma.

111. The average adult has approximately how much blood?
    a. 0.05 L
    b. 5 L
    c. 0.5 L
    d. 15 L

112. The vein most commonly used for venipuncture is:
    a. the antecubital.
    b. the basilic.
    c. the median cubital.
    d. All of the above.
113. Veins carry:
    a. deoxygenated blood away from the heart.
    b. oxygenated blood away from the heart.
    c. blood back to the heart.
    d. All of the above.
114. Arteries carry:
    a. deoxygenated blood away from the heart.
    b. oxygenated blood away from the heart.
    c. deoxygenated blood back to the heart.
    d. oxygenated blood back to the heart.
115. The outermost layer of the heart is the:
    a. epicardium.
    b. myocardium.
    c. endocardium.
    d. mesocardium.
116. The contractile layer of the heart is the:
    a. epicardium.
    b. myocardium.
    c. endocardium.
    d. mesocardium.
117. The upper receiving chamber of the heart is the:
    a. atrium.
    b. ventricle.
    c. aorta.
    d. valves.
118. Which valve separates the right atrium and the right ventricle to prevent the backflow of blood?
    a. The right atrioventricular valve
    b. The tricuspid valve
    c. The bicuspid valve
    d. Both a and b are correct
119. Which of the following are the semilunar valves?
    a. The mitral valve and the bicuspid valve
    b. The aortic valve and the pulmonary valve
    c. The tricuspid valve
    d. Both a and c
120. Which of the following are atrioventricular valves?
    a. The mitral or bicuspid valve
    b. The aortic valve and the pulmonic valve
    c. The tricuspid valve
    d. Both a and c
121. The aorta is:
    a. the major vein.
    b. the major artery.
    c. a peripheral artery.
    d. a systemic vein.
122. The pulmonary vein will carry blood:
    a. to the heart from the lung.
    b. to the lung from the heart.
    c. to the heart from the brain.
    d. to the lung from the brain.
123. The exchange of oxygen and carbon dioxide occurs in:
    a. the capillaries.
    b. the loops of Henle.
    c. the bronchi.
    d. All of the above.
124. Anatomy is:
    a. the structure of the human body.
    b. the function of the human body.
    c. homeostasis.
    d. hemostasis.
125. Physiology is:
    a. the structure of the human body.
    b. the function of the human body.
    c. homeostasis.
    d. hemostasis.
126. Renal failure is:
    a. the inability of the kidneys to maintain blood homeostasis.
    b. treatable with dialysis or transplantation.
    c. life threatening.
    d. All of the above.
127. Blood in the urine is called:
    a. hemostasis.
    b. hemoconcentration.
    c. hematuria.
    d. hemoccult.
128. A loss of pituitary gland function:
    a. is likely to be very serious, since this gland regulates many others.
    b. is likely to be very serious, since this gland produces digestive enzymes.
    c. is unlikely to be very serious, since this gland only affects fertility.
    d. is unlikely to be very serious, since this gland only affects hair growth.
129. Homeostasis is:
    a. the dynamic steady state of the body in good health.
    b. the ability of the blood to clot whenever necessary.
    c. when a person has had adequate sleep and has not eaten in 12 hours.
    d. the ability of the body to recognize an invading organism.

130. Hemostasis is:
    a. the dynamic steady state of the body in good health.
    b. the process by which blood vessels are repaired after injury.
    c. when a person has had adequate sleep and has not eaten in 12 hours.
    d. the ability of the body to recognize an invading organism.

131. Formation of blood cells is known as:
    a. homeostasis.
    b. hemostasis.
    c. hematopoiesis.
    d. hemopoiesis.

132. The building blocks of all living things are:
    a. cells.
    b. systems.
    c. nuclei.
    d. organs.

133. The blood cells that carry oxygen are:
    a. white blood cells.
    b. platelets.
    c. red blood cells.
    d. tissue cells.

134. Groups of cells working together to perform the same job are called:
    a. organs.
    b. systems.
    c. ligaments.
    d. tissues.

135. The location where bones come together is called:
    a. pivot.
    b. joint.
    c. ligament.
    d. tendon.

136. There are three sectional planes that are used to depict internal organs. Which of the following is a horizontal plane dividing the body into top and bottom portions?
    a. Sagittal plane
    b. Transverse plane
    c. Frontal plane
    d. Midsagittal plane

137. All of the following structures are located in the abdominal cavity except:
    a. rectum.
    b. spleen.
    c. liver.
    d. stomach.

138. The three kinds of muscles in the body are:
    a. skeletal, striated, and voluntary.
    b. involuntary, smooth, and striated.
    c. cardiac, involuntary, and smooth.
    d. skeletal, smooth, and cardiac.

139. The muscle of the circulatory system can be classified as which type of muscle?
    a. Striated voluntary
    b. Nonstriated voluntary
    c. Striated involuntary
    d. Nonstriated involuntary

140. Which kind of muscle straightens a part of the body?
    a. Flexor
    b. Extensor
    c. Striated
    d. Involuntary

141. The stomach passes food into the:
    a. large intestines.
    b. gallbladder.
    c. esophagus.
    d. small intestines.

142. Compared to arteries, veins:
    a. have thinner walls.
    b. carry blood under lower pressure.
    c. may be closer to the surface of the skin.
    d. All of the above.

143. Substances that speed up digestion are called:
    a. chemicals.
    b. enzymes.
    c. compounds.
    d. elements.

144. Tissue fluid is returned to the circulation through the:
    a. lymphatic system.
    b. digestive system.
    c. nervous system.
    d. endocrine system.

145. Which is the correct ratio of plasma to formed elements in the blood?
    a. 45% plasma, 55% formed elements
    b. 50% plasma, 50% formed elements
    c. 55% plasma, 45% formed elements
    d. 60% plasma, 40% formed elements

146. Digestion begins in the:
    a. esophagus.
    b. stomach.
    c. small intestine.
    d. mouth.

147. When you exhale you rid the body of:
    a. oxygen.
    b. carbon dioxide.
    c. nitrogen.
    d. electrolytes.

148. The organs of the urinary system are the:
    a. kidneys, ureter, bladder, and urethra.
    b. kidneys, skin, lungs, and large intestines.
    c. skin, lungs, small intestines, and large intestines.
    d. liver, heart, kidneys, and large intestines.

149. Tiny microscopic hairs called _____ are found in all of the air passages of the body.
    a. alveoli
    b. mucus
    c. flagella
    d. cilia

150. The master gland(s) in the endocrine system is/are the:
    a. ovaries or testes.
    b. thyroid.
    c. pituitary.
    d. thymus.

151. The phlebotomist dropped a tube of blood on the floor and it broke on impact. The proper way to clean up the blood and broken glass includes all of the following except:
    a. don PPE as required by facility.
    b. pick up the glass using forceps.
    c. dispose of glass in waste container.
    d. saturate site with bleach.

152. Mary the phlebotomist brought in ice cream bars in celebration of passing her certification exam. She put them in the freezer thinking it was alright because only test reagents, no blood or body fluids, were stored inside. She was reprimanded for all of the following reasons except:
    a. test reagents can contain blood or body fluids.
    b. no food or drink is allowed in the laboratory without permission.
    c. laboratories are designated as biohazardous.
    d. OHSA regulations were violated.

153. The phlebotomist prepares to draw blood on a child that doesn't want to have her blood drawn. The phlebotomist can gain the child's trust by doing all of the following except:
    a. use a soothing tone of voice.
    b. explain the procedure in terms the child understands.
    c. tell the child it will not hurt.
    d. give the child choices when possible.

154. The phlebotomist donned gloves, gown, and goggles before performing an ABG procedure. She is still at risk for which type of exposure?
    a. Cutaneous
    b. Permucosal
    c. Percutaneous
    d. All of the above

155. A patient in open heart recovery has an order for an H&H (hemoglobin and hematocrit), electrolytes, glucose, and ABGs. The phlebotomist tells the nurse to collect all of the specimens through the arterial line because:
    a. arterial blood and venous blood values are equivalent.
    b. blood samples will be labeled as arterial samples.
    c. she will dispense blood into tubes and an ABG syringe.
    d. arterial blood will yield more accurate values.

156. While in the ER performing a venipuncture, you, the patient, and the patient's family clearly overhear two nurses outside the room discussing the patient next to you. You should:
    a. ignore the conversation and focus on drawing your patient.
    b. report the breach of confidentiality to your supervisor.
    c. talk loudly to distract attention away from the nurses.
    d. tell the family to close the door if it happens again.

157. You are working quickly to complete your early AM draws when you encounter a difficult draw on a newborn that will surely take longer. You should call down to the laboratory for assistance because you:
    a. do not have the appropriate materials to shield the specimen from light.
    b. need a slurry of ice to transport the temperature sensitive specimen.
    c. are nearing the acceptable time lapse between collection of the specimen and analysis.
    d. need another phlebotomist to take over so you can end your shift on time.

158. While performing QC on a point-of-care instrument for glucose testing prior to the 10-PM patient glucose testing, the phlebotomist records a QC value for the normal control that is in range and a value for the abnormal control that is two points out of range. The appropriate course of action is to:
    a. continue with patient testing because the normal control was in 6 2S.D.
    b. continue with patient testing because the abnormal control did not exceed 6 2S.D.
    c. initiate trouble-shooting protocol for out-of-range controls.
    d. perform venipuncture draws in lieu of POCT collection for the 10 PM glucoses.

159. While processing a specimen, the phlebotomist accidently spills a tube of blood on the table. The phlebotomist should:
    a. disinfect the contaminated area with 10% bleach.
    b. allow bleach to remain in contact with contaminated area for 20 minutes.
    c. clean up visible blood first.
    d. All of the above.

160. The phlebotomist has an order for a blood draw on his father who is in the hospital. The phlebotomist can identify his father by:
    a. greeting and acknowledging the patient as "Dad."
    b. greeting and acknowledging the patient by first and last name.
    c. asking the patient to state his first and last name.
    d. asking the patient to state his name and checking the requisition against the patient's armband.

161. As you are putting away the new order of Vacutainer tubes, you should:
    a. place them on the bottom shelves to prevent chemical spills.
    b. rotate the stock putting the later expiration dates in the front.
    c. position current stock so it will be used up first.
    d. leave the shipment unopened until needed so it remains fresh.

162. Why is it important that the patient see the phlebotomist wash his or her hands before and after the draw?
    a. So the patient is assured that infection-control policies are being followed
    b. To ensure that the laboratory achieves high marks on the patient satisfaction surveys
    c. So the phlebotomist does not get reported to the director of nursing and laboratory supervisor
    d. To prevent compromising glove fit and glove integrity during the venipuncture procedure

163. The ER nurse hands the phlebotomist an ID bracelet to put on a trauma patient so the phlebotomist can draw stat labs. The phlebotomist should:
    a. put the arm band on the patient and complete the stat draw in an emergency situation.
    b. inform the nurse that he or she is not allowed to do so and request that the patient put it on.
    c. attach the armband to the gurney rail and perform the stat draw.
    d. ask the patient to verify their information and to put the armband on themselves.

164. The phlebotomist receives an order for the following tests: glucose, PT/INR, and a CBC. Which of the following lists the correct tubes in the correct order?
    a. Red, green, lavender
    b. Light blue, lavender, gray
    c. Lavender, gray, light blue
    d. Red, light blue, lavender

165. You have received an order to draw a CBC and cholesterol level on Mr. Smith. He states he is in a rush. Which of the following actions is appropriate to take to speed the process along?
    a. Blow on the site to get the alcohol to dry faster
    b. Draw only a green-topped tube
    c. Leave the tourniquet tied the entire time
    d. None of the above are appropriate.

166. You are on your last patient for the AM draws only to find that you have almost depleted your supply of tubes. The order is for a CBC and electrolytes, and you only have lavender and red tops left on your tray. The proper course of action is to:
    a. draw two lavender top tubes and deliver one to Chemistry and one to Hematology
    b. call down to the laboratory to have SST tubes delivered to you in the patient's room
    c. draw the blood in a syringe and transfer to the appropriate tubes when you get to the laboratory
    d. draw one lavender tube for Hematology and one red top tube for Chemistry

167. You receive a specimen from a physician's office dated yesterday. The specimen is now 18 hours old, but you do not reject it because it was:
    a. a glucose test drawn in a gray top
    b. an ammonia level that remained uncapped
    c. a stool culture for *C. difficile* kept at room temperature
    d. B$_{12}$ at room temperature in a red top tube

168. When processing the specimens that the courier just dropped off, you find that there are four tests ordered but only two tubes received: one lavender and one SST tube. The requisition is marked for a CBC, RPR, BUN, and creatinine. The phlebotomist should:
    a. inform the physician's office the patient needs to have two more tubes drawn.
    b. make aliquots from the SST tube for the RPR and BUN/Creatinine tests.
    c. mark QNS on the requisition for the RPR test and process the others.
    d. process all tubes and inform Chemistry the tube needs to be routed to Immunology.

169. After putting a tourniquet on a patient, the phlebotomist noticed the development of petechiae. She verified correct application of the tourniquet and should now:
    a. stop the procedure and refer the patient back to her physician.
    b. get the supervisor's permission to continue the venipuncture.
    c. continue the procedure and expect a longer clotting time at the puncture site.
    d. remove the tourniquet and perform the procedure on the patient's other arm.

170. The phlebotomist removed the cap from the needle, proceeded to anchor the vein, and noticed he forgot to reapply the tourniquet. The appropriate course of action would be:
    a. to insert the needle anyway because the vein is visible without a tourniquet.
    b. discard the Vacutainer and needle unit and start the procedure over.
    c. set the Vacutainer and needle unit in an upright position and reapply tourniquet.
    d. have the patient hold the Vacutainer and needle unit while he applies the tourniquet.

171. The patient has one small, visible, palpable median cephalic vein in the left arm. The phlebotomist will select which needle combination as the best option for the venipuncture procedure?
    a. 18 g with a 10-mL syringe
    b. 20 g with a butterfly
    c. 22 g with a Vacutainer
    d. 25 g with a 5-mL syringe

172. The phlebotomist is trying to fill the second tube but the tube is not filling. There is no visible hematoma, the needle did not move during the tube switch, and the first tube filled just fine. The appropriate course of action is to:
    a. end the draw and restick the patient in a new site.
    b. remove the tube as it seems the vacuum is depleted and try another tube of the same type.
    c. end the draw and advise the physician you could not complete the requisition.
    d. move on to the next tube and document that the second tube could not be collected.

173. The patient has an order for a CBC and a PT, both of which only require a small amount of blood. She had a mastectomy on the left side and scars from a serious burn on the antecubital site of the right arm. The phlebotomist should:
    a. call the physician for permission to draw from the left arm.
    b. check the patient for possible alternate venipuncture sites.
    c. collect the blood by performing a fingerstick on the right hand.
    d. perform an arterial draw using a small gauge needle and Vacutainer.

174. The phlebotomist enters a patient's room and says, "Hi, John. I need to draw some blood again." The phlebotomist's identification of the patient is:
    a. okay because the phlebotomist has already drawn the same patient twice today.
    b. okay because the patient and the phlebotomist are long-time friends.
    c. okay because the patient has been in the hospital for a month and everyone knows him.
    d. not okay because proper identification of the patient must be adhered to at all times.

175. An extremely obese patient with tiny, virtually nonpalpable veins requires a CBC. The best option for obtaining the blood sample is:
    a. venipuncture using a 22 Vacutainer and a 2-mL tube.
    b. venipuncture using 21-gauge needle and syringe.
    c. dermal puncture using a microtainer tube.
    d. dermal puncture using a Natelson tube.

176. The phlebotomist is preparing to perform a venipuncture on a child who is extremely upset and crying, and the mother is becoming extremely frustrated and upset with the child. The best course of action is to:
    a. ask the mother to calm down so she can be more effective in soothing the child.
    b. ask the mother to step out of the room if possible and get another phlebotomist to assist.
    c. ask the mother to tell the child it won't hurt and will be over quickly if the child sits still.
    d. ask the mother to grab the child, sit in the chair, and hold his arm securely during the draw.

177. The phlebotomist blows her nose into a tissue prior to entering the patient's room. She moves the patient's telephone, water cup and pitcher over to the side of the bed table so she can put the tray on it. The phlebotomist then goes into the restroom to wash her hands before beginning the procedure. The phlebotomist's actions:
    a. were the correct procedure for performing a venipuncture in a patient's room.
    b. might have compromised the patient had she not washed her hands.
    c. left the patient at risk for a health care-associated infection.
    d. inappropriate because the phlebotomist should never touch the patient's belongings.

178. The phlebotomist tells the nurse who stopped by the laboratory that Mary Jones in room 630, who had a blood glucose of 1200 mg/dL, must continue to have venous draws instead of performing POCT due to the high glucose level. This conversation is *or* is not appropriate because:
    a. it violates patient confidentiality.
    b. both are medical professionals and the nurse need the information to treat Ms. Jones.
    c. the information is not protected personal information.
    d. the nurse does not need the information to treat the patient.

179. While performing a stack of afternoon draws, the sleeve of the phlebotomist's lab coat is contaminated with a splatter of blood. The appropriate course of action is to:
    a. wipe off the blood with an alcohol swab.
    b. get bleach from the nurse's station and spray the area.
    c. discard the coat and get a fresh one from the laboratory.
    d. roll up the sleeve so the blood is not visible.

180. The patient's requisition says Mary Smith. She verifies her date of birth but informs you that she just got married and her name is now Mary Jones and requests that you change the name on the form. The phlebotomist should:
    a. call the physician's office for verification and have a new requisition faxed.
    b. honor the patient's request since her insurance card says Mary Jones.
    c. check the patient's driver's license or picture ID to verify the name Mary Jones.
    d. cross out Smith and write in Smith-Jones, her initials, date, and time.

181. A patient comes to the laboratory stating that the physician called and told her to get a stat CBC drawn. You have no requisition so you should:
    a. call the physician and get a verbal order.
    b. transcribe the verbal order onto a requisition.
    c. have the physician fax over the request.
    d. All of the above.

182. You receive an order for a blood gas on a 10-day-old baby in the pediatric unit. You check your phlebotomy cart for the following equipment:
    a. heparinized syringe and 25-gauge needle.
    b. 2-mL green top tube for venous blood gases.
    c. Natelson tube and plastic end caps.
    d. heparinized capillary tubes and clay.

183. The phlebotomist is processing a chain of custody specimen and is called to a code blue when she has not yet completed the process. The appropriate course of action is to:
    a. seal the specimen and place it in the courier pick-up basket.
    b. sign the specimen over to another tech to finish up the process.
    c. go to the code and then call the client to come back for a recollection.
    d. put the specimen on the phlebotomy cart and take it to the code blue.

184. You are performing a therapeutic phlebotomy on a patient with polycythemia. After collection of the unit of blood you will:
    a. discard the unit according to laboratory policy.
    b. process the unit for delivery to the blood bank.
    c. separate the unit into pack cells, plasma, and platelets.
    d. prepare the RBCs for re-infusion into the patient.

185. The phlebotomist enters the room of an elderly patient who tells her she had difficulty manipulating the cup while collecting her midstream clean-catch specimen, so she just voided all of the urine into the collection cup. The phlebotomist should:
    a. take the specimen back to the laboratory for analysis.
    b. give the patient a new kit and tell her to recollect it correctly.
    c. inform the nurse so that he or she can assist the patient or collect a cath specimen.
    d. inform the physician so he or she can perform a suprapubic collection.

186. A child suspected of having whooping cough comes in for testing. The phlebotomist will perform a:
    a. blood draw.
    b. urine collection.
    c. throat swab.
    d. nasopharyngeal swab.

187. The phlebotomist is up on the obstetrics floor and is given an amniotic fluid to transport back to the laboratory. He should:
    a. wrap the specimen in foil or place in a brown bag.
    b. place the specimen on a slurry of ice.
    c. wrap the specimen in a heel warmer.
    d. separate the specimen into three tubes.

188. The phlebotomist receives a specimen for bilirubin testing from the courier about 1.5 hours after collection, and notices that the tube is clear and has not been packaged to be protected from light. This is or is not an appropriate example of transport because:
    a. the tube was delivered on time.
    b. the specimen needed to be protected from light.
    c. the specimen is too old.
    d. bilirubin specimens do not need to be protected from light.

189. The phlebotomist completes a difficult venipuncture on a very angry patient. After returning to the laboratory the phlebotomist should:
    a. document what occurred during the procedure and interaction with the patient.
    b. tell the other phlebotomists about how angry the patient was as she drew his blood.
    c. call her friend to vent and calm down before going out to collect the remaining draws.
    d. forget about it because she followed proper protocol and procedure.

190. The phlebotomist completes a draw in the ER. She is then asked to perform a stat ABG on another patient. She has never performed an ABG but has been observing other phlebotomists over the past week or so. She is the only phlebotomist available so she goes ahead and performs the arterial draw. The phlebotomist had a duty to the patient for all of the following except:
    a. performing the arterial procedure because it was a stat.
    b. getting someone who was qualified to perform an arterial draw.
    c. making sure all of the necessary equipment was available.
    d. relieving the other phlebotomist so he or she could perform the draw.

191. The phlebotomist was preparing to deliver pathology reports to the doctors' mailboxes when she noted her neighbor had been diagnosed with prostate cancer. She promptly called her neighbor who had been anxiously awaiting the news. All of the following apply to the phlebotomist's action except:
     a. violation of HIPAA.
     b. created a liability issue for the laboratory.
     c. okay because her neighbor asked for the information.
     d. violated physician-patient integrity.

192. While restocking the phlebotomy cart, the phlebotomist finds a labeled specimen in the rack. The phlebotomist should:
     a. check the time and date of collection and process accordingly.
     b. discard the specimen in the biohazardous waste.
     c. leave it on the tray until someone comes looking for it.
     d. reprint the label and go redraw the patient.

193. While processing specimens, the phlebotomist finds a tube labeled with the patient's name, medical record number, DOB, date, and time. The phlebotomist should:
     a. reject the specimen because it does not have the phlebotomist's ID on the label.
     b. process the specimen and deliver it to the appropriate department for analysis.
     c. relabel the tube because it contains protected personal information.
     d. call the floor and ask who the physician is and write it on the label.

194. The phlebotomist performed an I-STAT electrolyte test on a patient. The results were abnormal but within linearity of the instrument. The phlebotomist should:
     a. rerun the controls before reporting the result.
     b. enter the results into the computer and report out.
     c. draw a venous blood sample for testing in the laboratory.
     d. recalibrate the instrument and then retest the patient.

195. While performing a venipuncture procedure, the phlebotomist checks the expiration date of the tube being used. This action is considered part of:
     a. quality assurance.
     b. a delta check.
     c. a point of care check.
     d. quality control.

196. When performing POCT, the phlebotomist must make sure the cartridge is seated properly in the instrument. This is an example of:
     a. a preanalytic variable.
     b. an analytic variable.
     c. a postanalytic variable.
     d. a delta check variable.

197. When completing a butterfly draw on a pregnant woman, the phlebotomist accidentally scratches the top of her hand through the glove as she withdrew the needle. The phlebotomist should:
     a. not worry about it because the woman is pregnant and therefore not a risk.
     b. wash it off and not report it because it is a superficial wound and not a puncture wound.
     c. complete an accidental exposure report form after performing first aid.
     d. get a complete history on the woman to give to her supervisor.

198. While in the middle of performing a difficult venipuncture, the patient states that she feels like she is going to vomit. You observe her and note that she is pale and diaphoretic. You should:
     a. withdraw the needle and grab an emesis basin and cool cloth.
     b. continue drawing the blood quickly so you do not have to restick the patient.
     c. tell the patient to put her head down on her other arm and continue the draw.
     d. pull the needle out and go get someone from the laboratory to help you.

199. A 10-year-old child comes into the laboratory with an insurance card and a requisition for a blood draw, stating his mother is in the car. The phlebotomist or patient representative should:
    a. call the physician to verify the information on the requisition.
    b. draw the blood because the child is a mature minor.
    c. send the child home without performing the venipuncture.
    d. ask the child to go and get his mother from the parking lot.

200. A physician brings in her elderly mother who is in a wheelchair. She states that her mother is a difficult draw and that she will perform the procedure. She cleanses the arm and proceeds to insert the syringe needle multiple times in multiple sites along the elderly woman's arm until she finally gets blood. The phlebotomist should:
    a. do nothing because the physician knows what she is doing.
    b. keep quiet because the patient was a relative and gave consent.
    c. document the incident and inform her supervisor.
    d. take the syringe away from the physician and do the procedure herself.

CHAPTER 1

STUDY QUESTIONS

1. Phlebotomy is the practice of drawing blood samples for analysis.

2. Six steps in routine blood collection are:

    1. Correctly and positively identify the patient.

    2. Choose the appropriate equipment for obtaining the sample.

    3. Select and prepare the site for collection.

    4. Collect the sample, ensuring patient comfort and safety.

    5. Correctly label the sample.

    6. Transport the sample to the laboratory in a timely manner, using appropriate handling procedures.

3. A phlebotomist must adhere to safety regulations, interact with patients, keep accurate records, and operate computers.

4. Certification is evidence that an individual has demonstrated proficiency in a particular area of practice.

5. CEUs are required to remain certified and provide updates on new regulations and techniques to help refresh skills.

6. Organizations that provide accreditation for phlebotomy programs are the American Medical Technologists (AMT), the National Accrediting Agency for Clinical Laboratory Sciences (NAACLS), the National Phlebotomy Association (NPA), and the American Society of Phlebotomy Technicians (ASPT).

7. Organizations that provide certification for phlebotomists are the American Society for Clinical Pathology (ASCP), the NPA, the American Certification Agency for Healthcare Professionals (ACA), the AMT, and the ASPT.

8. Phlebotomists may wish to become members of a professional organization to follow changes in the field and learn new techniques.

9. A patient must be informed of intended treatments and their risks and must give consent before these treatments are performed; this is known as informed consent.

10. HIPAA violations would include providing protected health information with anyone not authorized to receive it, allowing PHI in your control to be viewed by nonauthorized people, and discussing PHI in a public place where it may be unintentionally overheard.

11. Ancient phlebotomy procedures included bloodletting and the use of leeches. These practices were used to bleed a person and thus rid that person of his or her ailment.

12. Both ancient and modern phlebotomy involve blood and the veins, but unlike ancient phlebotomy, modern phlebotomy has set protocols, procedures, and guidelines. Phlebotomy is used in the diagnosis and treatment of disease and as a therapeutic procedure.

13. Job-related duties in the phlebotomist's job description may include correctly and positively identifying the patient, choosing the appropriate equipment for obtaining the sample, selecting and

preparing the site for collection, collecting the sample, ensuring patient comfort and safety, and correctly labeling the sample.

14. Required personal characteristics for a phlebotomist include dependability, honesty, integrity, positive attitude, professional detachment, professional appearance, interpersonal skills, telephone skills, and communication skills.

15. (This answer is up to the student's discretion and class discussion.)

16. The two most important legal aspects to a phlebotomist are obtaining informed consent and maintaining patient confidentiality.

CERTIFICATION EXAM PREPARATION

1. b		**4.** c	
2. b		**5.** d	
3. a		**6.** d	

CHAPTER 2

STUDY QUESTIONS

1. The four branches of support personnel in the hospital organizational system are fiscal, support, nursing, and professional services.

2. The two main areas of the laboratory are the anatomic and clinical areas; the phlebotomist works in the clinical area.

3. A physician specializing in pathology oversees the laboratory.

4. Laboratory tests performed in the coagulation department:

Test	Therapy Monitored
PT	Coumadin
INR	Coumadin
APTT	Heparin

5. The immunology department performs tests to monitor the immune response through the detection of antibodies.

6. Molecular diagnostics characterize genetic and biochemical techniques used to diagnose genetic disorders, analyze forensic evidence, and track diseases.

7. The following are liver function tests: ALT, AST, GGT, ALP, enzymes, and bilirubin.

8. The microbiology department performs culture and sensitivity testing.

9. CLIA '88 mandates that facilities that perform patient testing meet performance standards to ensure the quality of procedures.

10. The Joint Commission and College of American Pathologists.

11. The Clinical Laboratory Standards Institute sets laboratory standards and guidelines.

12. A phlebotomist may also be employed in HMOs, PPOs, POLs, nursing homes, urgent care centers, or reference laboratories.

13. The blood bank or immunohematology department is the laboratory that has a special patient or specimen identification process. Mislabeling or mishandling these specimens may result in a patient's death.

14. The technologist looks for agglutination of specimens; if the specimen agglutinates, the blood type is not compatible and cannot be transfused to the patient. If the blood does not agglutinate, the blood type is compatible with that of the patient and can be transfused.

15. Professional services are services that are provided at the request of the physician to aid in the diagnosis and treatment of a patient. Examples of professional services are physical therapy, occupational therapy, and respiratory therapy.

CERTIFICATION EXAM PREPARATION

1. d
2. c
3. c
4. a
5. b
6. d
7. c

8. c
9. b
10. a
11. b
12. a
13. c

CHAPTER 3

STUDY QUESTIONS

1.

Safety Hazard	Example
Biological	Bacteria, viruses
Sharps	Needles, lancets, broken glass
Electrical	High-voltage equipment
Chemical	Lab reagents, preservatives
Latex sensitivity	Gloves
Physical	Wet floors, lifting heavy objects
Fire, explosive	Oxygen, chemicals
Radioactive, x-ray	Equipment, reagents

2. Safety precautions include wearing personal protective equipment; never storing food with biohazard substances; protecting feet from spills, slips, and falling; avoiding putting things in the mouth in the work area; avoiding eye-hand contact in the work area; and not wearing loose clothing, hair, or jewelry that can get caught in equipment or contaminated.

3. Never recap after collection; needle sticks can occur.

4. Hazardous material labels must display a warning to alert you to the hazard, the manufacturer or other responsible party, an explanation of the hazard, a list of precautions to reduce risk, and first aid measures to take in case of exposure.

5. A safety data sheet provides information on the chemical, its hazards, the procedure for its cleanup, and first aid in case of exposure.

6. A chemical hygiene plan describes all safety procedures, special precautions, and emergency procedures used when working with chemicals.

7. If a chemical spills on your arm, proceed to the safety shower, flush the area for 15 minutes, and go to emergency room for treatment.

8. In the event of electric shock to someone, turn off the equipment or break contact between the equipment and the victim using a nonconductive material, do not touch the victim until the risk of further shock is removed, call 911, start CPR if indicated, and keep the victim warm.

9.

Extinguisher Type	Contains
A	Pressurized water or soda and acid
BC	Carbon dioxide or foam
ABC	Dry chemical
Halon	Chlorofluorocarbons

10. The protocol for assistive breathing is as follows: determine consciousness; if there is no response, call 911 and begin rescue breathing; make sure the victim is flat on a firm surface; check the airway; position the victim's head; if the victim is not breathing, pinch the nose shut, place your mouth over the victim's mouth, and exhale; check to see whether the victim's chest rises, indicating a clear airway; give two full ventilations and check for breathing; and continue until breathing occurs or until assistance arrives.

11. Skin conditions associated with latex use include the following:
    • Irritant contact dermatitis: redness, swelling, itching
    • Allergic contact dermatitis: the body's immune system reacts to proteins absorbed through the skin
    • Anaphylaxis: rapid severe immune reaction; airway may swell shut, heart rate increases, and blood pressure decreases

12. The Occupational Safety and Health Administration (OSHA) regulates all work environments to prevent accidents. It provides guidelines for accident prevention.

13. To control a bleeding emergency, you *must* apply pressure to the area or wound, elevate the limb unless it is fractured, and maintain pressure until medical help arrives.

14. The early signs of shock include pale, cold, clammy skin; tachycardia (rapid pulse); shallow breathing; weakness; and nausea, vomiting, or both. In case of shock, keep the victim warm and lying down with the airway open, and call for professional assistance.

15. The plan to follow during a disaster emergency varies from institution to institution. It is important to learn and know your institution's disaster plan.

16. No answer provided.

CERTIFICATION EXAM PREPARATION

1. c

2. a

3. b

4. c

5. b

6. d

7. a

8. d

9. d

10. c

11. d

12. c

CHAPTER 4

STUDY QUESTIONS

1. Infection is the invasion and growth of disease-causing microorganisms in the human body.

2. Four classifications of pathogens are viruses, bacteria, fungi, and protists.

3.

Disease	Causative Infectious Organism
AIDS	Human immunodeficiency virus (HIV)
Gonorrhea	*Neisseria gonorrhoeae*
Hepatitis	Hepatitis virus (A-E and G)
Malaria	*Plasmodium*
Oral and genital herpes	Herpes simplex
Strep throat	*Streptococcus*
Syphilis	*Treponema pallidum*
Trichomoniasis	*Trichomonas vaginalis*
Tuberculosis	*Mycobacterium* tuberculosis

4. Health care-related infections are contracted by a patient during a hospital stay as the result of direct contact with other patients or by failure of hospital personnel to follow infection control protocols.

5. The chain of infection is made up of a source, a means of transmission, and a susceptible host.

6. The chain of infection is broken by preventing transmission, which can be achieved by hand washing, using personal protective equipment, isolating patients at risk of spreading or contracting infections, and using standard precautions.

7. Direct contact involves the transfer of microorganisms from an infected person to a susceptible host by body contact; indirect contact involves contact between a susceptible host and a contaminated object.

8. Fomites are objects, whereas vectors are organisms.

9. Hand washing is the most effective way to prevent the spread of infection.

10. Personal protective equipment includes fluid-resistant gowns, masks, respirators, face shields, gloves, and shoe covers.

11. Standard Precautions are an infection control method that uses barrier protection and work control practices to prevent direct skin contact with biohazardous materials.

12. Bloodborne pathogens include syphilis, HIV, hepatitis A through E, HTLV types I and II, malaria, babesiosis, and Colorado tick fever.

13. Hepatitis B may be stable in dried blood for at least 7 days.

14. Bleach should be in contact with a contaminated area for 20 minutes for complete disinfection.

15. In 1992 OSHA issued Standard Precautions, which dictated that employers must have a written bloodborne pathogen exposure control plan and provide personal protective equipment to all workers (health care and others) at no charge to the employee. The Standard Precautions also dictated that employers must provide hepatitis B vaccine, free follow-up care for accidental exposure, and yearly safety training and ensure that needles are not being recapped.

CERTIFICATION EXAM PREPARATION

1. d
2. b
3. c
4. d
5. c
6. c

7. c
8. c
9. b
10. c
11. b
12. a

CHAPTER 5

STUDY QUESTIONS

1. The parts of a word always include a root and may include a suffix or prefix.

2.

Prefix	Meaning
ante-	before
anti-	against
brady-	slow
cirrho-	yellow
cyan-	blue
epi-	on, over
erythro-	red
hemi-	half
hyper-	above
hypo-	below
inter-	between
intra-	within
leuko-	white
lute-	yellow
micro-	small
nano-	billionth
neo-	new
peri-	around
poly-	many
post-	after
rube-	red
tachy-	fast
tetra-	four

3.

Root	Meaning
agglut-	clump together
angio-	vessel
arthro-	joint
bili-	bile
cardio-	heart
derm-	skin
heme-	blood
hepato-	liver
nephr-	kidney
oste-	bone
phago-	eat
phlebo-	vein
-pnea	breath
pulmon-	lung
ren-	kidney
thromb-	clot
tox-	poison

4.

Suffix	Meaning
-ectomy	surgical removal
-emia	blood condition
-genous	originating from
-itis	inflammation
-oma	tumor, growth
-pathy	disease
-penia	deficiency
-plasty	shape
-plegia	paralysis
-stasis	stopping
-tomy	cut

5.

Abbreviation	Meaning
AIDS	acquired immunodeficiency syndrome
ASAP	as soon as possible
BP	blood pressure
CCU	cardiac care unit
COPD	chronic obstructive pulmonary disease
CPR	cardiopulmonary resuscitation
CV	cardiovascular
CVA	cerebrovascular accident
DM	diabetes mellitus
DOB	date of birth
DVT	deep vein thrombosis
Dx	diagnosis
ECG/EKG	electrocardiogram
FUO	fever of unknown origin
GI	gastrointestinal
hypo	hypodermically

Abbreviation	Meaning
ICU	intensive care unit
ID	identification
IM	intramuscular
IV	intravenously
LMP	last menstrual period
MI	myocardial infarction
NB	newborn
NPO	nothing by mouth
O_2	oxygen
OB	obstetrics
OR	operating room
pp	post-prandial
prep	prepare
pt	patient
q	every
qns	quantity not sufficient
Rx	prescription
SOB	shortness of breath
stat	immediately
STI	sexually transmitted infection
TB	tuberculosis
URI	upper respiratory infection
UTI	urinary tract infection

6.

Singular	Plural
appendix	appendices
larynx	larynges
papilla	papillae
scapula	scapulae
testis	testes
vertebra	vertebrae

CERTIFICATION EXAM PREPARATION

1. a		**12.** a	
2. d		**13.** c	
3. b		**14.** d	
4. b		**15.** d	
5. c		**16.** d	
6. d		**17.** b	
7. a		**18.** a	
8. b		**19.** d	
9. b		**20.** b	
10. c		**21.** a	
11. b		**22.** c	

CHAPTER 6

STUDY QUESTIONS

1. Homeostasis is the steady state of good health.

2.

Tissue	Example
Epithelial	Lining of gut, surface of the eye
Muscle	Heart
Nerve	Neurons, spinal cord
Connective	Bone, blood

3. c. The nucleus contains DNA.

4. a. The plasma membrane regulates the flow of materials in and out of the cell.

5. b. Mitochondria are "power plants" of the cell.

6. d. Cytoplasm contains cellular material.

7. The anatomic position is the body erect, facing forward, arms at the sides, and palms forward.

8. Body cavities are spaces within the body that contain major organs.

9. e. Ventral is the front surface of the body.

10. g. Posterior is the back surface of the body.

11. b. Lateral is toward the side.

12. c. Medial is toward the middle.

13. a. Prone is lying on the abdomen facing down.

14. h. Supine is lying on the back.

15. d. Extension is straightening the joint.

16. f. Inferior is below.

17. The three body planes are as follows:

Frontal: vertical division (front and back)

Sagittal: vertical division (left and right)

Transverse: horizontal division (top and bottom)

18. Hematopoiesis is the formation of blood cells.

19. The following laboratory tests are used to assess for bone and joint disorders:

Lab Test	Tests For
ALP	Bone metabolism marker
ANA	Systemic lupus erythematosus
Calcium	Mineral calcium imbalance
ESR	General inflammation test
Magnesium mineral	Magnesium imbalance
RF	Rheumatoid arthritis
Synovial fluid analysis	Arthritis
UA	Gout
Uric acid	Gout

20. Osteomyelitis is a bone infection that can be caused by improper phlebotomy technique.

21. The following laboratory tests are used to assess for muscle disorders: aldolase, AST, troponin, myoglobin, CK, CK-MM, CK-MB, and lactate dehydrogenase.

22. The divisions of the central nervous system are the brain and spinal cord.

23. Lab tests used to assess for digestive disorders include the following: CBC, amylase, lipase, ALP, ALT, AST, GGT, bilirubin, HBsAg, ammonia, hepatitis antibody, carotene, O&P, gastrin, occult blood, and stool culture.

24. External respiration is the exchange of gases in the lungs, whereas internal respiration is the exchange of gases at the cellular level.

25. The endocrine system maintains homeostasis in conjunction with the nervous system by producing hormones.

26.

Joint Type	Examples
Immovable	Facial bones, cranium (synarthrosis)
Partially movable	Vertebrae (amphiarthrosis)
Free moving	Elbow, shoulder, knee (diarthrosis)

CERTIFICATION EXAM PREPARATION

1. c
2. b
3. a
4. b
5. b
6. a
7. c
8. c
9. b
10. d

11. b
12. a
13. d
14. c
15. c
16. d
17. c
18. a
19. b
20. b

CHAPTER 7

STUDY QUESTIONS

1. The circulatory system transports blood containing oxygen and nutrients throughout the body and picks up metabolic waste products for disposal.

2. Pulmonary circulation carries blood between the heart and lungs for gas exchange, whereas systemic circulation carries blood between the heart and the rest of the body.

3. Veins carry blood toward the heart; arteries carry blood away from the heart.

4. The four valves of the heart are atrioventricular, pulmonary semilunar, bicuspid, and aortic semilunar.

5. Contraction of the heart is known as systole, and relaxation is known as diastole.

6. The three layers surrounding the lumen of veins and arteries are tunica adventitia, media, and intima.

7. The yellow liquid portion of whole blood, containing fibrinogen, is called plasma.

8. The formed elements constitute 45% of blood volume.

9. A phagocyte attacks and digests bacteria.

10. B cells produce antibodies.

11. The extrinsic pathway begins with the release of tissue factor by endothelial cells. The intrinsic pathway begins when the plasma coagulation factors contact materials exposed when blood vessels are damaged.

12. Autoimmunity is an attack by the immune system on the body's own tissues. Examples include rheumatoid arthritis, systemic lupus erythematosus, myasthenia gravis, and multiple sclerosis.

13. The lymph organs include lymphatic vessels, lymph nodes (the tonsils are the largest lymph nodes in the body), the spleen, the thymus, and the thoracic and right lymphatic ducts. Lymphedema is one lymphatic disorder; it constitutes an accumulation of fluid blocking a lymphatic vessel. Lymphoma is another disorder; it characterizes a tumor of a lymph gland. Hodgkin's disease is a type of lymphoma.

14. The types of immunity include nonspecific and specific immunity. Nonspecific immunity refers to the defense against infectious agents independent of the specific chemical markers on their surfaces. Nonspecific immunity encourages inflammation and phagocytosis. Specific immunity involves the molecular recognition of antigens on the surface of a foreign agent. Specific immunity involves the antigen or antibody response, also called humoral immunity.

15. In the coagulation process, enzymes enter the common pathway, reacting with factors X and V to convert circulating inactive prothrombin to active thrombin.

CERTIFICATION EXAM PREPARATION

1. a
2. a
3. c
4. b
5. c
6. b
7. a
8. c
9. b
10. b
11. b
12. c
13. d
14. a
15. b

CHAPTER 8

STUDY QUESTIONS

1. A tourniquet prevents venous flow out of the arm.
2. The gauge of a needle indicates the diameter of the needle's lumen.

3. If a large-gauge needle is used in venipuncture, collection is slower and blood cells may be hemolyzed (destroyed) as they pass through the narrower opening.

4. The rubber sleeve on the multisample needle keeps the needle from becoming contaminated or injuring you or the patient, and it keeps blood from leaking onto or into the adapter or tube holder, especially when changing tubes.

5. An advantage of the syringe method is that blood appears in the hub when the vein has been entered. A disadvantage of the syringe method is that there is the potential for needle stick when depositing blood into the collection tube.

6. When blood tubes are evacuated, a vacuum is created within the tube so that a measured amount of blood will flow in easily.

7. Unused blood tubes must be discarded when they expire because out-of-date tubes may have decreased vacuum, preventing a proper fill, or they may have additives that degrade over time.

8. SPS is sodium polyanetholesulfonate. It is an additive that prevents blood from clotting.

9. Blood collected in a tube with an anticoagulant must be mixed thoroughly after collection by gently and repeatedly inverting the tube.

10. Thixotropic gel forms a barrier between blood cells and serum or plasma, thus preventing contamination and allowing easy separation.

11. Glycolysis is a cellular reaction used to harvest energy from glucose.

12. Blood specimens used for analysis are whole blood, serum, and plasma.

13. b. Tan is used for lead analysis.

14. a. Red is for a blood bank.

15. i. Light blue is for coagulation.

16. g. Lavender is used for a CBC.

17. c. Gray is used for a glucose tolerance test.

18. e. Black is used for the sedimentation rate.

19. d. Gold BD Hemogard is used for chemistry testing.

20. f. Green is used for ABGs.

21. h. Dark (royal) blue is used for trace metals.

22.

2	light blue
6	lavender
5	green
3	red (plastic tube)
1	yellow (sterile)
7	gray
4	gold BD Hemogard

CERTIFICATION EXAM PREPARATION

1. a		11. a	
2. c		12. d	
3. a		13. b	
4. c		14. b	
5. b		15. a	
6. d		16. a	
7. b		17. d	
8. b		18. b	
9. b		19. a	
10. b		20. d	

CHAPTER 9

STUDY QUESTIONS

1. It is extremely important to correctly and positively identify the patient in any phlebotomy procedure.

2. To properly identify a patient, match the information on the requisition with the information on the patient's identification band (for inpatients) or with information provided by the patient (for outpatients).

3. Information typically found on a requisition form includes the patient's name, date of birth, the patient's hospital ID number (for inpatients), the patient's room number and bed (for inpatients), the patient's physician's name or code, the type of test requested, and the test status.

4. When requisitions are received, you should examine them for the necessary information, check for duplicates or errors, group them together for the same patient, prioritize them, and gather all the equipment you will need to perform the collections.

5. Hemoconcentration is an increase in the ratio of formed elements to plasma caused by leaving the tourniquet on too long.

6. The three veins in the antecubital area suitable for venipuncture are the median cubital, cephalic, and basilic.

7. The median cubital vein is the first choice for venipuncture because it is large and well anchored and does not move when the needle is inserted.

8. Veins feel spongy, bouncy, and firm on palpation; arteries pulsate; and tendons feel rigid.

9. To help locate a vein, tap the arm, have the patient make a fist, or warm the site with a warm towel or hot pack.

10. A hematoma is a reddened, swollen area in which blood collects under the skin. It can form when the extra pressure from the tourniquet forces blood out through the puncture.

11. The correct position for the arm after venipuncture is straight or slightly bent, but not bent back over the puncture site.

12. To correctly label blood tubes, label them at the bedside using a pen or permanent marker. The label must have the patient's name and identification number, the date and time of collection, and the collector's initials or identification number. If labels are computer generated, make sure all the information is present, and then add the collector's initials or identification number.

13. The requisition slip must contain the patient's identification or chart number, the patient's last and first names, the patient's date of birth, the physician's name, and the test(s) ordered.

14. Phlebotomists must prepare the patient and then wash their hands so that when it is time to perform the venipuncture, the gloves and everything they touch are as free from contamination as possible. If phlebotomists wash their hands, put on gloves, and then prepare the patient, they may inadvertently pick up contaminants from the patient, which can then be transferred to the puncture site.

15. An Advance Beneficiary Notice of Noncoverage is a Medicare form. The phlebotomist may be required to present it to the patient for his or her signature. It must be presented to the patient far enough in advance of the service that the patient has time to understand its implications and make an informed decision.

CERTIFICATION EXAM PREPARATION

1. d
2. b
3. c
4. c
5. b
6. d
7. c
8. c
9. b
10. a
11. c
12. b
13. b
14. b
15. c

CHAPTER 10

STUDY QUESTIONS

1. Sites commonly used for adult capillary collection are the palmar surface of the distal segments of the third and fourth fingers and the big toe.

2. Dermal puncture is preferred for children because the young child's smaller veins and lower blood volume make standard venipuncture difficult and potentially dangerous.

3. Dermal puncture may be advisable for patients undergoing frequent glucose monitoring or frequent blood tests, obese patients, patients with IVs in place, geriatric patients, patients with burns or scars, patients at risk for venous thrombosis, restrained patients, and patients at risk for anemia, hemorrhage, infection, organ or tissue damage, arteriospasm, or cardiac arrest.

4. The first drop of blood in a dermal puncture is wiped away with clean gauze to prevent contaminating the sample with tissue fluid.

5. Micropipets are typically used for the collection of samples for arterial blood gas determinations.

6. Warm washcloths or heel-warmer packets can be used to stimulate blood flow to the capillaries.

7. Specific areas of the skin to avoid when performing a capillary stick include areas with scars, cuts, bruises, rashes, or edema and callused, burned, bluish, and infected areas, as well as previous puncture sites.

8. Heel sticks are preferred to finger sticks in children under the age of 1 year.

9. Unless alcohol air-dries before a capillary stick, stinging, hemolysis, and contamination can occur. Alcohol also can interfere with the formation of rounded drops of blood on the skin surface.

10. Povidone-iodine may elevate test results for bilirubin, uric acid, phosphorus, and potassium and therefore is not recommended for use with capillary collection procedures.

11. The third and fourth fingers are acceptable to use for dermal puncture.

12. The order of collection for a dermal puncture is (1) blood smears; (2) platelet counts, CBCs, and other hematology tests; and (3) other tests.

13. The bleeding time test measures the length of time required for bleeding to stop after an incision is made. It helps assess the overall integrity of primary hemostasis, involving the vascular system and platelet function.

14. Small children may remove bandages and choke on them; therefore it is not recommended that bandages be used on children younger than 2 years.

CERTIFICATION EXAM PREPARATION

1. a		8. b	
2. d		9. b	
3. d		10. e	
4. b		11. d	
5. d		12. d	
6. b		13. c	
7. c			

CHAPTER 11

STUDY QUESTIONS

1. If a patient is not in the room when you come to collect a specimen, every effort must be made to locate that patient by checking with the nursing station.

2. If a patient is not wearing an ID bracelet, contact the nursing station so that one can be attached by the nurse on duty. Unless an ID band is on the patient, you must not draw blood. Specific policies regarding the resolution of patient identification problems may vary from institution to institution, so be sure to follow the policy of your institution.

3. Unconscious patients should be treated just as you would conscious ones: identify yourself and describe the procedure. They may be able to hear you, even if they cannot respond.

4. Potential barriers to communicating with a patient include sleeping or unconscious patients; the presence of physicians, members of the clergy, or visitors; apprehensive patients; language problems; and patient refusal.

5. Hemolysis is the destruction of red blood cells, resulting in the release of hemoglobin and cellular contents into the plasma.

6. Veins that are occluded are blocked. Occluded veins feel hard or cordlike and lack resiliency.

7. When performing a dorsal hand stick, the tourniquet is applied around the wrist below the antecubital fossa.

8. Povidone-iodine must be used when collecting for a blood alcohol test. Alcohol can adversely affect test results.

9. Hemoconcentration can be caused by a tourniquet that is on longer than 1 minute, pumping of the fist, sclerosed or occluded veins, long-term IV therapy, or dehydration.

10. Before syncope, a patient's skin often feels cool, damp, and clammy.

11. If a needle's bevel has stuck to the vein wall, slightly rotate the needle to correct its position.

12. Too much vacuum on a small vein can cause it to collapse during a blood draw. During the syringe method, it may occur when the plunger is pulled too quickly.

13. The policy at most institutions is that a second try is acceptable. After a second unsuccessful try, another phlebotomist should be found to draw blood from the patient.

14. Reflux of an additive during collection can be prevented by keeping the patient's arm angled downward so that the tube is always below the site, allowing it to fill from the bottom up. Also, remove the last tube from the needle before removing the tourniquet or needle.

15. Reasons specimens may be rejected include no requisition form; unlabeled or mislabeled specimens; incompletely filled tubes; defective tubes; collection in the wrong tube; hemolysis, or clotted blood in an anticoagulated specimen; contaminated specimens and containers; and improper special handling.

CERTIFICATION EXAM PREPARATION

1. c	9. c
2. d	10. b
3. d	11. d
4. a	12. b
5. a	13. c
6. c	14. b
7. a	15. b
8. d	

CHAPTER 12

STUDY QUESTIONS

1. To reduce a child's anxiety before a draw, prepare your material ahead of time; perform the procedure in a room that is not the child's hospital room; be friendly, cheerful, and empathetic; explain the procedure in child's terms; do not say that the procedure will not hurt, but say that it is okay to say "ouch"; and give children choices whenever possible, such as which arm or finger they want to use or the type of bandage they prefer.

2. When performing venipuncture on patients younger than 2 years, use shorter needles, if possible, and use the smallest gauge consistent with the requirements of the tests. Butterflies and smaller tube sizes should be used. If the patient is younger than 1 year, a heel stick should be performed, rather than venipuncture.

3. EMLA is a topical anesthetic cream used in pediatric patients to numb the venipuncture site.

4. Children can be immobilized during a draw by wrapping newborns or infants in receiving blankets. Older children need to be restrained. They may be seated in the lap of a parent or assistant who hugs the child's body and holds the arm not being used in the draw, or they may be lying down with the parent or assistant leaning over the child, holding the unused arm securely.

5. Bilirubin is light sensitive. Bili lights should be turned off during collection, and the specimen should be shielded from light.

6. A PKU sample is collected via capillary stick onto a special filter paper supplied in a kit provided by the state agency responsible for PKU tests.

7. Physical changes in older adults include skin that is less elastic and thinner; a tendency to bruise more easily; longer healing times; more fragile, less elastic, and narrower blood vessels; loss of supporting connective tissue, leading to "loose skin"; loss of muscle tissue, allowing veins to move from their usual locations; and arteries that are closer to the surface.

8. To perform a draw on an older adult patient, be especially careful with patient identification; be aware of the frequency of blood draws; be especially gentle; do not apply the tourniquet as tightly; place the arm on a pillow and have the patient grip a washcloth while the arm is supported by rolled towels; do not "slap" the arm to find a vein; anchor the vein firmly; and apply pressure longer to ensure bleeding has stopped.

9. VAD is the acronym for vascular access device. It is a tube that is inserted into either a vein or an artery and is used to administer fluids or medications, monitor blood pressure, or draw blood.

10. To draw blood from a patient who has an IV line, have the nurse turn off the IV drip before the draw (less than 2 minutes); apply the tourniquet distal to the IV insertion site; select a vein distal to the IV insertion site and in a different vein; discard the first 5 mL of blood drawn, since it will be contaminated with IV fluid; and on the requisition, note that the specimen was drawn from an arm with an IV and identify the IV solution.

11. Types of VADs include CVC (Broviac, Groshong, Hickman, or triple lumen), implanted port, PICC, arterial line, heparin or saline lock, and AV shunt (external or internal).

12. In a phlebotomy procedure, a child may experience a fear of the unknown and a fear of pain. As a phlebotomist, you must explain the procedure in detail to the child, using words the child understands. The phlebotomist should speak to the child during the entire procedure, letting the child know how much longer the procedure will last.

13. Since a newborn is under reverse isolation, additional protection equipment is needed. Blood should be drawn from the infant's heel. The amount collected, tests, and their frequency must be recorded to prevent blood depletion.

14. Besides the PKU test, neonates are screened for hypothyroidism, galactosemia, homocystinuria, maple syrup disease, biotinidase deficiency, and sickle cell anemia.

15. Common disorders affecting older adults include hearing loss, stroke, arthritis, and tremors, all of which can make blood collection difficult. Extra care should be taken appropriate to each condition.

16. The collection site should be rotated in HIV patients to avoid damaging veins and tissues by performing frequent draws.

CERTIFICATION EXAM PREPARATION

1. c		**9.** d	
2. c		**10.** a	
3. c		**11.** c	
4. a		**12.** c	
5. c		**13.** d	
6. b		**14.** c	
7. c		**15.** b	
8. b			

CHAPTER 13

STUDY QUESTIONS

1. Arterial collection is most often used for testing ABGs.

2. Abnormal ABG values can be produced by COPD, lung cancer, diabetic coma, shock, cardiac or respiratory failure, and neuromuscular disease.

3. Normal blood pH is 7.35.

4. Acidosis is indicated by a lower pH, whereas alkalosis is indicated by a higher pH.

5. A syringe used for venipuncture is not heparinized, whereas a syringe used for arterial puncture is pretreated with heparin (glass or gas-impermeable plastic) to prevent coagulation.

6. Povidone-iodine must be used, in addition to alcohol, for arterial puncture.

7. Lidocaine may be used to numb an arterial puncture site.

8. Safety precautions to take when collecting arterial blood include wear a fluid-resistant gown, face protection, and gloves; use a puncture-resistant container for sharps; use a small rubber or latex block for the needle.

9. For blood gas collection, 21- or 22-gauge needles are most often used.

10. Collateral circulation is the accessory supply of blood to a region by more than one artery. Collateral circulation is tested for using the modified Allen test.

11. The needle should be inserted at an angle 45 to 60 degrees above the plane of the skin for an arterial collection.

12. Pressure should be applied to the puncture site for 5 minutes after an arterial collection.

13. An arteriospasm is the spontaneous constriction of an artery in response to pain.

14. ABG sampling errors include using too much or too little heparin; insufficient mixing; allowing air bubbles to enter the syringe; using an improper plastic syringe; using an improper anticoagulant; puncturing a vein instead of an artery; and exposing the specimen to the atmosphere after collection.

15. ABG specimens may be rejected due to inadequate volume of specimen for the test, clotting, improper or absent labeling, using the wrong syringe, air bubbles in the specimen, failure to ice the specimen, and too long a delay in delivering the specimen to the laboratory.

16. Capillary blood gas testing is most commonly performed on pediatric patients because they generally should not be subjected to the deep punctures required for ABG testing. This procedure is usually performed on the heel.

17. Capillary blood is not as desirable as arterial blood for testing blood gases because capillary blood is a mixture of blood from the capillaries, venules, and arterioles, and it is mixed with tissue fluid. In addition, this method of collection is open to the air, and the specimen may exchange gases with room air before it is sealed.

CERTIFICATION EXAM PREPARATION

1. b
2. a
3. d
4. c
5. d
6. d

7. c
8. b
9. a
10. c
11. a

CHAPTER 14

STUDY QUESTIONS

1. Basal state is the body's state after 12 hours of fasting and abstinence from strenuous exercise.

2. Blood composition is influenced by age, altitude, dehydration, environment, gender, pregnancy, stress, diet, diurnal variation, drugs, exercise, body position, and smoking.

3. Timed specimens are most often used to monitor medication levels, changes in a patient's condition, and normal diurnal variation in blood levels at different times of the day.

4. GTT is the acronym for glucose tolerance test. It is a test used to screen for diabetes mellitus and other disorders of carbohydrate metabolism.

5. TDM means therapeutic drug monitoring. It is often used to adjust drug dosing in patients.

6. Blood cultures are ordered to test for the presence of microorganisms in the blood.

7. Aseptic collection technique and drawing the correct volume are critical for meaningful BC results.

8. A potential blood donor must (1) register by providing identifying information and written consent, (2) interview with a trained interviewer and provide a medical history, and (3) submit to a physical exam, which includes hemoglobin testing.

9. Cold agglutinins must be kept warm until the serum is separated from the cells. They can be wrapped in an activated heel-warmer packet or placed in the incubator.

10. Tests that require the sample be transported on ice include ABGs, ammonia, lactic acid, pyruvate, glucagon, gastrin, adrenocorticotropic hormone, and parathyroid hormone.

11. Chain of custody (COC) is a protocol that ensures that a sample is always in the custody of a person legally entrusted to be in control of it. The chain begins with patient identification and continues through every step of the collection and testing process. COC documentation includes special containers, seals, and forms, as well as the date, time, and identification of the handler.

12. For blood alcohol testing, the site must not be cleaned with alcohol, as this will falsely elevate the result (use soap, water, and gauze or another nonalcoholic antiseptic solution instead); tubes must be filled as full as the vacuum allows to minimize the escape of alcohol from the specimen into the space above; and the specimen should not be uncapped, because that also allows alcohol to escape and compromises the integrity of the sample before testing.

13. To prepare a blood smear, place a drop of blood on a clean slide ½ to 1 inch from the end, centered between the two slides; place the spreader onto the first slide at a 25- to 30-degree angle and draw it back to just contact the blood drop; and then move the spreader forward in one continuous movement to the end of the slide. The blood will be drawn along over the slide. Finally, dry and label the slide, using a pencil on the frosted end.

14. To prepare a thick malaria smear, place a large drop of blood on a slide, spread it out to about the size of a dime, and let the sample dry for at least 2 hours.

15. Therapeutic phlebotomy is often used in the treatment of polycythemia. The prefix *poly-* means "excessive" or "a lot"; the root word *cyte* means "cell"; and the suffix *-emia* means "blood." Thus polycythemia is excessive red blood cell production. Therapeutic phlebotomy is also used for hemochromatosis. "Heme" refers to the blood, and "chroma" to color. In hemochromatosis, the skin takes on a bronze color because of excess iron in the blood.

CERTIFICATION EXAM PREPARATION

1. b	8. d
2. d	9. a
3. c	10. c
4. b	11. b
5. a	12. c
6. a	13. d
7. b	14. b

CHAPTER 15

STUDY QUESTIONS

1. Random urine specimens can be collected at any time. They are used to screen for obvious abnormalities in the concentration of proteins, glucose, and other significant constituents of urine.

2. A first-morning specimen is collected after the patient wakes up. It is a very concentrated specimen. A timed specimen is collected over a 24-hour period to provide a single large specimen. Typically, the first-morning sample is discarded in a timed specimen.

3. To collect a midstream clean-catch specimen, the patient should cleanse the area surrounding the urethra, begin voiding into the toilet, bring the container into the urine stream until sufficient urine has been collected, and then void the remainder of the urine into the toilet.

4. Fecal specimens are collected to look for intestinal infection and screen for colorectal cancer.

5. Semen specimens are collected to determine whether viable sperm are present, either to test for fertility or to assess the success of a vasectomy. Semen may also be collected as a forensic specimen from a rape victim.

6. Nasopharyngeal specimens are collected to diagnose whooping cough, croup, pneumonia, and other upper respiratory tract infections.

7. The SE test is used to help diagnose cystic fibrosis.

8. In CSF collections, three tubes are collected. Tube 1 is delivered to the chemistry laboratory; tubes 2 and 3 are delivered to the microbiology and hematology laboratories. Which department receives which tube is set by the policies of the institution.

9. Amniotic fluid is collected to analyze the presence of certain genetic disorders, such as Down syndrome. It can be analyzed for lipids (to indicate lung development), bilirubin (associated with hemolytic disease), and proteins (associated with other abnormalities, such as spina bifida).

10. A throat culture is collected from the back of the mouth around the tonsils and uvula with a swab. A nasopharyngeal culture is collected through the nose.

11. a. Pleural fluid is found in the lungs and thoracic cavity.

    b. Synovial fluid is found in the knee joint.

    c. Cerebrospinal fluid is found in the brain and spinal cord.

    All of these specimens are collected by a physician only.

12. A 24-hour collection may detect low levels of certain proteins and hormones.

13. The methods for inducing sweat in an SE test use iontophoresis and the drug pilocarpine. Sweat is collected on a sterile filter paper, which must be covered with paraffin and handled with forceps or sterile gloves. The chloride level is obtained via weight and analysis of electric charge.

CERTIFICATION EXAM PREPARATION

1. a	6. a
2. c	7. a
3. c	8. a
4. b	9. b
5. d	10. b

CHAPTER 16

STUDY QUESTIONS

1. Tubes with anticoagulant should be inverted gently and completely 5 to 10 times immediately after the sample is drawn.

2. Tests affected by glycolysis include glucose, calcitonin, phosphorus, aldosterone, and a number of enzymes.

3. No more than 2 hours should pass between collection of the sample and separation of cells from plasma or serum.

4. Specimens that must be maintained at 37°C during transport and handling should be warmed in a heel warmer before and after collection. Some tests require warming of the sample in a 37°C incubator before testing.

5. Chilling a specimen slows metabolic processes and keeps analytes stable during transport and handling.

6. Minimum documentation to be included with each specimen delivered to the laboratory should include the patient's name, the patient's hospital number and room number, the specimen type, the date and time of delivery to the drop-off area, and the name of the person depositing the specimen.

7. Disadvantages of pneumatic tube systems include unreliability of the system, speed of delivery, potential for specimen damage during transport, and cost of the alternative.

8. An accession number is a unique identifying number used for cataloging a sample in the laboratory.

9. A centrifuge must carry a balanced load; otherwise, the rotor of the centrifuge may spin out of center, which can damage the centrifuge and cause samples to break.

10. Aliquots are small portions of a specimen transferred into separate containers for distribution to a variety of laboratory departments. All tubes into which aliquots are placed should be labeled before filling and then capped before delivery to the appropriate department. Aliquots are removed with any one of several types of disposable pipetting systems.

11. To remove a stopper from a tube, place a 4- $\times$ 4-inch gauze pad over the top and pull the stopper straight up, twisting it if necessary. Do not rock it from side to side or pop it off.

12. Stat specimens should be transported to the laboratory immediately after being drawn, whereas routine specimens should be delivered to the laboratory within 45 minutes of being drawn.

13. Tubes must be transported in an upright position to allow complete clot formation, prevent sample contamination due to prolonged contact with the stopper, and reduce the formation of aerosol during uncapping.

14. Delivery of specimens in a timely manner will ensure the quality of test results. Glycolysis and other chemical changes increase as time passes.

15. One light-sensitive analyte is bilirubin. To transport, the specimen must be protected from light—the tube must be wrapped in aluminum foil, or an amber-colored tube must be used. Other light-sensitive analytes include vitamin B_{12}, carotene, folate, and urine porphyrin.

CERTIFICATION EXAM PREPARATION

1. c
2. c
3. b
4. b
5. d

6. d
7. c
8. c
9. b

CHAPTER 17

STUDY QUESTIONS

1. Point-of-care testing (POCT) is the performance of analytic tests immediately after obtaining a sample at the "point of care," such as the bedside, clinic, intensive care unit or emergency department, physician's office, nursing home, assisted living center, or patient's home.

2. Advantages to point-of-care testing include shorter turnaround times for obtaining test results, allowing more prompt medical attention, faster diagnosis and treatment, potentially decreased recovery time, and decreased costs to the laboratory. Disadvantages include misleading test results due to improperly following manufacturer's directions, inadequate training of personnel, improper maintenance, and poor record keeping.

3. Quality assurance and controls are essential for use of POCT instruments. The laboratory is usually responsible for documentation and maintenance of POCT instruments, and proper and adequate training for all personnel performing these procedures is critical to successfully implement POCT.

Strict adherence to guidelines regarding calibration, running controls, performing maintenance, and record keeping is a must for a POCT program. Failure in any one of these areas can result in misleading test results and negative consequences for the patient.

4. Hematology tests that can be performed as POCT include anemia and polycythemia evaluation and coagulation monitoring. (See the chapter discussion on specific tests and how to perform them.)

5. Chemistry tests that can be performed as POCT include glucose, cardiac troponin T, cholesterol, blood gases, and electrolytes. (See the chapter discussion on specific tests and how to perform them.)

6. The five waves that make up an ECG are P, Q, R, S, and T.

7. a. The heart activity corresponding to the P wave is atrial depolarization.

   b. The heart activity corresponding to the QRS complex is ventricular depolarization.

   c. The heart activity corresponding to the ST segment is ventricular repolarization.

8. To perform a dipstick urinalysis test, make sure the fresh urine specimen is at room temperature and thoroughly mixed; completely and briefly immerse the urine strip into the urine specimen; remove excess urine from the strip by tapping the side of the strip on the container; and compare the color change on the strip to the reference color chart on the bottle at the appropriate time.

9. It is extremely important to follow the manufacturer's directions when performing POCT because manufacturers tend to vary in their methods of testing. If their specific method of testing is not followed, inaccurate test results can occur.

10. a. Anemia may be evaluated using a handheld hemoglobin analyzer or a hematocrit reading.

    b. Warfarin therapy may be monitored by using the prothrombin time test.

    c. Cholesterol may be evaluated by using color card testing or instrumentation.

    d. Arterial blood gases may be evaluated by using handheld analyzers.

11. The common electrolytes that can be measured by POCT include sodium, potassium, calcium, chloride, and bicarbonate.

12. The normal ECG pattern consists of a tracing with five prominent points where the graph changes direction. These are known as P, Q, R, S, and T. The sections joining these points are known as segments, complexes, or intervals. Each part of the graph corresponds to a particular portion of the cardiac cycle and can be analyzed to determine how the heart is functioning.

13. Important parameters that can be determined from the ECG include the time intervals between different phases of the cardiac cycle, which indicate conduction efficiency, and the size of the electrical signals, which may be correlated with increase or decrease of heart muscle mass. The duration of the cardiac cycle can be read directly from the ECG, because each small square represents a known unit of time.

14. The dipstick tests most commonly performed on random urine specimens include protein, pH, glucose, ketones, bilirubin, urobilinogen, blood, leukocyte esterase, nitrite, and specific gravity.

15. A dipstick urine test is commonly used to determine pregnancy, measuring the presence of HCG. This hormone, produced by the placenta after implantation of a fertilized egg, is present in urine.

16. The adherence guidelines for a POCT program to be successful are calibration, running controls, performing maintenance, and record keeping. Not adhering to the guidelines can result in inaccurate test results and negative consequences for the patient.

17. The microcuvette tests and measures the hemoglobin value and is essential in determining the response to therapy.

18. ACT is the activated coagulation time. Blood collected in a prewarmed tube is incubated at 37°C for 1 minute and then inspected by tilting the tube to determine whether a clot has formed. If a clot does not form at 1 minute, the tube is examined every 5 seconds until a clot forms.

19. The analytes obtained in the ABG are P_{O_2}, P_{CO_2}, and pH, and the common electrolytes tested are sodium, potassium, calcium, chloride, and bicarbonate.

20. The electrode placements for the precordial leads of an ECG are as follows:

V_1, fourth intercostal space in the right margin of the sternum

V_2, fourth intercostal space in the left margin of the sternum

V_3, between position 2 and position 4

V_4, fifth intercostal space at the left midclavicular line

V_5, fifth intercostal space at the anterior axillary line

V_6, fifth intercostal space at the midaxillary line

CERTIFICATION EXAM PREPARATION

1. c		6. d
2. b		7. c
3. b		8. a
4. c		9. a
5. d		10. d

CHAPTER 18

STUDY QUESTIONS

1. Quality assurance is a set of methods used to guarantee quality patient care, including the methods used for patient preparation and collection and transportation protocols. These methods ensure better care, help reduce errors in and improve the quality of test results, and save money. Quality assurance programs are mandated by the Joint Commission.

2. Quality control refers to the quantitative methods used to monitor the quality of procedures to ensure accurate test results. Quality control is part of quality assurance, which is a larger set of methods that guarantees quality patient care through a specific program, including both technical and nontechnical procedures.

3. The Joint Commission's role is to mandate quality assurance programs, requiring that a systemic process be in place to monitor and evaluate the quality of patient care.

4. Documentation processes include a procedure manual for laboratory procedures, a floor book detailing schedules and other information, the identification of variables that may affect patient care and test results, and continuing education for all members of the laboratory staff.

5. A procedure manual contains protocols and other information about all the tests performed in the laboratory, including the principle behind the test, the purpose of performing it, the specimen type the test requires, the collection method, and the equipment and supplies required.

6. A delta check helps identify patient identification errors. This check compares previous patient results with current results and alerts laboratory personnel to the possibility of error if the difference ("delta") between the two sets of results is outside the limit of expected variation.

7. The patient's physical condition at the time of the collection has a significant effect on the sample quality. If a phlebotomist must draw from a patient who smokes, the phlebotomist must document this factor. Since smoking can affect the variables of many tests, the phlebotomist's documentation of this factor will aid in the interpretation of test results.

8. Each aliquot must be properly labeled as to the source and the additives present.

9. The purpose of quality phlebotomy is to ensure that a systemic process is in place to monitor and evaluate the quality of patient care, as mandated by the Joint Commission.

10. The philosophy and purpose of total quality management (TQM) are to focus on continuous improvements in the quality of services provided by the laboratory. The role of this program is to set guidelines and to evaluate and change its due process and standards as needed to reflect its philosophy.

11. The procedure manual lists all of the procedures, processes, protocols, and handling and transport guidelines for each phlebotomy procedure. The floor logbook lists patients, their room numbers, specimens collected, phlebotomists' initials, the dates and times of collection, and their outcomes.

12. Preanalytic variables exist in requisition handling, equipment, identification, preparation and specimen collection, transport, and processing. Variables are problems and errors that can arise in any of these areas. Variables for each area vary.

13. One negative outcome of improper patient identification is a patient's death. The wrong medication can be administered based on erroneous tests results. To ensure proper patient identification, the phlebotomist *must* ask the patient his or her name and date of birth and then compare such information with the requisition slip. If the patient is an inpatient, the same is done, but the patient's identification number is also matched with the requisition slip.

14. Variables of which phlebotomists must be aware vary based on the procedure they are performing. Such variables may include patient identification, delta check, patient preparation for specimen collection, specimen collection, transport, time constraints, processing, and separation time. Prevention or control of each will differ with each variable. Examples of control procedures include asking the patient to state his or her name and checking that against the ID band, removing the tourniquet as quickly as possible to prevent hemolysis, and delivering the sample to the laboratory quickly to prevent sample degradation.

CERTIFICATION EXAM PREPARATION

1. d
2. d
3. c
4. b
5. c

6. b
7. c
8. a
9. d

CHAPTER 19

STUDY QUESTIONS

1. Health care costs have increased due to the gradual inflation in the price of all goods and services, the growing sophistication of medical technology, the need for highly trained operators of health care delivery, the fast pace of drug discovery and development, and an increase in the number of tests ordered by doctors.

2. OSHA creates administrative laws; these laws are given the force of law by the statutory laws that created OSHA.

3. A plaintiff is a person claiming to have been harmed by a defendant in a court of law.

4. To be liable for an action means that you are legally responsible for it and can be held accountable for its consequences. Scenarios include reusing a needle, thereby infecting a patient with a disease; probing for a vein and damaging a nerve; failing to perform a physician-ordered test, and having the patient suffer harm as a result. There are many more ways in which a phlebotomist could be held liable for his or her actions.

5. Negligence is the failure to perform an action consistent with the accepted standard of care.

6. Malpractice is the delivery of substandard care that results in harm to a patient.

7. The phlebotomist fails to safeguard patient privacy when he or she reveals test results or any information about the patient to anyone not directly involved in that patient's care; discusses a patient's care in a public place; releases medical information concerning a patient to anyone not specifically authorized to acquire it; leaves patient records out where anyone can glance at them.

8. Phlebotomists can adopt several measures to protect them from malpractice suits, such as precise and detailed documentation, clear patient communication, and following procedures and protocols accurately. Some phlebotomists opt to purchase their own liability insurance.

9. Effective communication includes giving clear information to the patient in order to obtain consent, explaining the procedure for the patient to fully understand what will happen, and always getting a clear "Yes" or "I understand" response from the patient.

10. A criminal action is taken when a public law is violated. There is a jury trial in the presence of a district attorney. A phlebotomist can be prosecuted under criminal action for assault or battery, using dirty needles, or patient misidentification. If a patient dies as a consequence of a wrongful action by the phlebotomist, the charge against the phlebotomist can be manslaughter.

    A civil action is the violation of private law. A civil action is taken when the accused injures the plaintiff. A civil action suit for a phlebotomist can result from reusing needles, careless probing, or an accidental stick.

11. Professional liability is being legally responsible for your actions and failure to act. Phlebotomists are bound to act within the realm of their training; they are professionally liable if they do not. Phlebotomists can perform venipunctures, deliver specimens, and assist the physician and nurse in specimen collection. Phlebotomists cannot perform a tracheostomy or amniocentesis, collect a CSF, or perform other procedures for which they have not been trained.

12. The plaintiff *must* prove duty, dereliction, injury, and direct cause in a malpractice suit.

13. The statement "a phlebotomist who does so is derelict in his or her duty" means that the phlebotomist has not followed the set standards of care. For example, if a phlebotomist has trouble with a venipuncture procedure and fails to call for help as he or she was trained to do, the phlebotomist is being derelict in duty.

14. The key defense against a malpractice suit is to show that the standards of care were followed. Clear, precise documentation is vital in proving no misconduct occurred.

15. Liability insurance covers monetary damage that must be paid if the defendant loses a liability suit. Phlebotomists should carry liability insurance in case they are accused in a civil action and the health care institution will not cover such charges.

16. The phlebotomist maintains doctor-patient integrity by allowing test results to be given to the patient by the physician.

17. When a case cannot be settled easily, the case will go to a jury trial and judgment.

18. A phlebotomist may commit a negligent act if he or she does not follow the standards of care for the procedure being performed. Examples include performing more than two attempted draws before calling for assistance, leaving the equipment tray on the bed or other place it may be overturned, and failing to return the bed rail to its raised position, if it was raised initially.

CERTIFICATION EXAM PREPARATION

1. c		7. a	
2. a		8. d	
3. c		9. d	
4. d		10. b	
5. c		11. d	
6. b			

APPENDIX E

MOCK CERTIFICATION EXAM ANSWERS

1. C	28. B	55. D	82. D
2. A	29. C	56. B	83. C
3. C	30. A	57. C	84. A
4. A	31. C	58. D	85. D
5. A	32. C	59. C	86. C
6. D	33. B	60. D	87. C
7. B	34. A	61. D	88. D
8. A	35. A	62. C	89. D
9. B	36. B	63. C	90. B
10. C	37. A	64. B	91. D
11. D	38. C	65. D	92. C
12. D	39. D	66. D	93. B
13. B	40. B	67. B	94. B
14. C	41. C	68. C	95. B
15. B	42. D	69. C	96. D
16. C	43. D	70. C	97. A
17. C	44. B	71. C	98. B
18. D	45. D	72. A	99. D
19. D	46. D	73. C	100. A
20. C	47. D	74. D	101. B
21. A	48. D	75. B	102. B
22. D	49. C	76. A	103. B
23. D	50. B	77. D	104. A
24. D	51. D	78. A	105. C
25. A	52. D	79. D	106. B
26. C	53. D	80. C	107. A
27. D	54. D	81. C	108. D

109. C	132. A	155. B	178. B
110. D	133. C	156. B	179. C
111. B	134. D	157. B	180. A
112. C	135. B	158. C	181. A
113. C	136. B	159. D	182. C
114. B	137. A	160. D	183. B
115. A	138. D	161. C	184. A
116. B	139. C	162. A	185. C
117. A	140. B	163. B	186. D
118. D	141. D	164. B	187. A
119. B	142. D	165. D	188. B
120. D	143. B	166. D	189. A
121. B	144. A	167. A	190. A
122. A	145. C	168. B	191. C
123. A	146. D	169. C	192. A
124. A	147. B	170. B	193. B
125. B	148. B	171. C	194. B
126. D	149. D	172. B	195. D
127. C	150. C	173. C	196. B
128. A	151. C	174. D	197. C
129. A	152. B	175. C	198. A
130. B	153. C	176. B	199. D
131. C	154. D	177. C	200. C

Glossary

abdominal cavity Body cavity containing the stomach, intestines, spleen, liver, gall bladder, pancreas, and kidneys.

abduction Movement that takes a body part farther away from the central axis.

accepted standard of care Consensus of medical opinion on what is adequate patient care in a particular situation.

accession number Unique identifying number used for cataloging a sample in the laboratory.

accreditation Official approval of a program from a professional organization.

acquired immunodeficiency syndrome (AIDS) Syndrome caused by human immunodeficiency virus infection.

additive Chemical added to evacuated tubes.

adduction Movement that brings a body part closer to the central axis.

adhesion The process in which platelets stick to endothelial cells.

administrative law Law created by administrative agencies.

adrenal cortex Outer portion of the adrenal gland.

adrenal medulla Inner portion of the adrenal gland, which secretes the catecholamines epinephrine and norepinephrine.

adrenocorticotropic hormone (ACTH) Hormone released by the pituitary to stimulate release of adrenal cortex hormones.

aerobic bacteria Bacteria that need oxygen.

aerosol Mist of droplets.

afferent Nerve cell bringing sensory information to the central nervous system.

agglutination Sticking together.

aggregation Process in which additional platelets stick to endothelial cells and platelets.

agonist Muscle performing a movement.

Airborne Infection Isolation Precautions Precautions that are used with patients known or suspected to have serious illnesses transmitted by airborne droplet nuclei.

airborne transmission Spread of infection either by airborne droplet nuclei or by dust particles that contain microorganisms.

albumin Principal protein in blood plasma.

aldosterone A mineral corticoid hormone.

aliquot Portion of a sample.

allergic contact dermatitis Allergic reaction following skin contact with an allergen.

allergy Inappropriately severe immune reaction to an otherwise harmless substance.

alternate site testing (AST) See *point-of-care testing.*

alveolus Sac within the lung at which gas exchange occurs.

amino acid derivative One of three hormone types.

amniocentesis Collection of amniotic fluid for detection of inherited diseases and other abnormalities.

amphiarthrosis Partially movable joint.

anaerobic bacteria Bacteria that live without oxygen.

analyte Substance being analyzed.

anaphylaxis Severe immune reaction in which the airways may swell and blood pressure may fall.

anatomic and surgical pathology area One of the two main branches of the clinical laboratory, responsible for analyzing cells and tissues.

anatomic position Reference position for description of the body.

ancillary blood glucose test Bedside test to determine blood glucose level, performed by dermal puncture.

antagonist Muscle opposing a movement.

anterior Front.

antibody Protein made by B cells to fight infection.

anticoagulant Additive that prevents blood clotting.

antidiuretic hormone (ADH) Hormone released by the pituitary that regulates water reabsorption by the kidney.

antigen Marker on the surface of foreign cells; substance that provokes an immune response.

antiseptic Substance that prevents infection.

aorta Artery leaving the heart at the left ventricle, supplying the systematic circulation.

aortic semilunar valve See *left atrioventricular (AV) valve.*

approval Official acceptance from a professional organization.

arachnoid One of three membranes surrounding the brain.

arterial blood gas (ABG) testing Tests to determine the concentrations of oxygen and carbon dioxide in arterial blood and the pH of the blood.

arterial line Vascular access device that is placed in an artery.

artery Largest of the blood vessels carrying blood away from the heart.

arteriole Smaller of the blood vessels carrying blood away from the heart.

arteriospasm Rapid contraction of the arterial wall.

arteriovenous (AV) shunt Artificial connection between an artery and a vein.

articular cartilage Smooth cartilage lining the bearing surface of bones.

assault An unjustifiable attempt to touch another person, or the threat to do so.

atrium An upper chamber of the heart.

autoimmunity Condition in which the immune system attacks the body's own tissues.

autologous donation Donation of a patient's own blood for use at a later time.

autonomic motor system Group of neurons controlling smooth muscle and glands.

B cell Antibody-producing cell.

bacteremia Blood infection by a bacterium.

bacteriostatic Agent that prevents growth of bacteria.

basal state The body's state after 12 hours of fasting and abstention from strenuous exercise.

basilic vein Prominent vein in the antecubital fossa.

basophil A type of granulocyte.

battery Intentional touching of another person without consent.

bicuspid valve See *left atrioventricular (AV) valve.*

bile Fat-emulsifying fluid released by the gall bladder; formed from bilirubin.

Bili light UV light treatment for elevated bilirubin.

bilirubin Substance produced by the normal breakdown of red blood cells that may accumulate in the blood.

bilirubin, uric acid, phosphorus, and potassium (BURPP) Group of tests that may be elevated by use of povidone-iodine.

biotinidase deficiency Inherited metabolic disorder.

bleeding time (BT) test Test that measures the length of time required for bleeding to stop after an incision is made.

blood bank Department that deals with blood for transfusions.

bloodborne pathogen (BBP) Infectious agent carried in the blood.

blood culture (BC) Test for the presence of micro-organisms in the blood.

blood type Presence and type of antigens on the surface of red blood cells.

Bowman's capsule Cup of cells surrounding the glomerulus in the nephron.

brachial artery Large artery in the antecubital fossa.

brainstem A region at the base of the skull vital for basic life processes.

bronchiole Smaller tube within the lungs connecting bronchi and alveoli.

bronchus One of the paired tubes leading to the lungs from the trachea.

Broviac Type of central venous catheter.

bulbourethral gland Gland supplying fluid for semen.

butterfly See *winged infusion set.*

calcaneus Heel bone.

calcitonin Thyroid hormone that lowers calcium levels in body fluids.

capillary blood gas (CBG) testing Alternative to arterial blood gas testing.

capillary tube Small plastic tube used primarily for hematocrit tests.

Caraway pipet See *micropipet.*

carbohydrase Carbohydrate-digesting enzyme.

cardiac cycle Set of events in one complete heartbeat.

cardiac muscle Heart muscle.

cardiac troponin T (cardiac TnT) Part of a protein complex in cardiac muscle that aids the interaction of actin and myosin; elevated in heart attack.

cardiopulmonary resuscitation (CPR) Emergency manual means to maintain breathing and circulation.

case law Law determined by court decisions.

catheterized urine sample Urine sample collected via a catheter inserted into the bladder.

CD4+ cell See *helper T cell.*

cellular immunity T-cell mediated immunity.

central nervous system (CNS) Brain and spinal cord.

central venous catheter (CVC) Most common vascular access device, inserted into one of the large veins emptying into the heart.

central venous line See *central venous catheter.*

centrifuge Separation of components of a sample based on density by using a machine that spins a sample at a very high speed.

cephalic vein Prominent vein of the antecubital fossa.

cerebellum Highly folded outgrowth at the rear of the brain, involved in coordination.

cerebral cortex Highly folded outer layer of the brain.

cerebrospinal fluid (CSF) Fluid within the brain and spinal cord.

cerebrum Outermost layer of the brain, including the cerebral cortex.

certification Verification that an individual has demonstrated proficiency in a particular area of practice.

cervix Narrow opening between the vagina and the uterus.

chain of custody (COC) Protocol that ensures the sample is always in the custody of a person legally entrusted to be in control of it.

chain of infection Continuous link among the infection source, the means of transmission, and the susceptible host.

chemical hygiene plan Plan that describes all safety procedures, special precautions, and emergency procedures used when working with chemicals.

chemistry panel Group of chemistry tests.

chyme Fluid mass of food within the gastrointestinal tract.

cilium Cell extension on bronchi responsible for movement of mucus.

civil action A suit in civil court.

Clinical and Laboratory Standards Institute (CLSI) Nonprofit organization that sets standards and guidelines under the Clinical Laboratory Improvement Act of 1988 (formerly National Committee for Clinical Laboratory Standards).

clinical laboratory Hospital branch that analyzes samples from a patient at the request of the physician or other health care personnel.

Clinical Laboratory Improvement Act of 1988 (CLIA '88) Federal law that mandated regulation of all facilities that performed patient testing.

clinical pathology area One of the two main branches of the clinical laboratory, responsible for analyzing blood and other body fluids.

clot activator Additive that stimulates clotting.

coagulation Clotting.

cold agglutinin An antibody often formed in response to infection with *Mycoplasma pneumoniae.*

collateral circulation Accessory supply of blood to a region by more than one artery.

collecting duct Tube that collects urine at the end of the nephron.

College of American Pathologists (CAP) Accrediting agency; accreditation by CAP is required for Medicare or Medicaid reimbursement.

combining form Combination of the word root and the combining vowel.

combining vowel Vowel added to a word root to make pronunciation easier.

common pathway Part of the coagulation cascade.

common vehicle transmission Transmission by means of contaminated items, such as food, water, medications, devices, and equipment.

compartment syndrome Condition in which collection of fluid in a confined space prevents blood flow.

complement Proteins that form part of the immune response.

complete blood count (CBC) Automated test used to test for conditions that affect the number and ratio of cell types in the blood.

conduction system System of conductive cells in the heart that trigger contraction.

connective tissue Tissue with few cells and a large amount of extracellular material, often serving to connect other tissues.

Contact Precautions Precautions used for patients known or suspected to have serious illnesses that are easily transmitted by direct patient contact or by contact with items in the patient's environment.

contact transmission Transfer of microorganisms from an infected or colonized person to a susceptible host by body surface–to–body surface contact or through contact with a contaminated object.

continuing education units Credits for participation in a continuing education program.

continuous quality improvement (CQI) Goal of total quality management.

coronary artery Artery supplying heart muscle.

corticosterone A glucocorticoid hormone.

cortisol A glucocorticoid hormone.

cortisone A glucocorticoid hormone.

cranial cavity Cavity enclosing the brain.

criminal action A charge of criminal conduct; contrast with civil action.

cryofibrinogen Abnormal type of fibrinogen that precipitates when cold.

cryoglobulin Abnormal serum protein that precipitates when cold.

culture and sensitivity (C&S) test Test to detect and identify microorganisms and to determine the most effective antibiotic therapy.

cytokine Chemical messenger; includes interferon and interleukin.

cytoplasm Jelly-like cell contents not including the nucleus.

cytotoxic T cell Lymphocyte that recognizes antigens and directly destroys both foreign cells and infected host cells.

damages Monetary compensation for pain, suffering, and legal costs.

delta check Quality assurance procedure that helps discover identification errors by comparing previous patient results with current results.

Department of Transportation (DOT) label Label indicating the type of hazard, the United Nations hazard class number, and a specific identifying number.

depolarization Contraction of the heart.

dereliction Breach of the duty of care.

dermis Skin layer underlying outer epidermis.

diarthrosis Freely moving joint.

diastole Relaxation portion of the cardiac cycle.

differential count (diff) Determination of the proportions of the various blood cell types.

disinfectant Agent used to clean a surface other than living tissue.

disseminated intravascular coagulation (DIC) Condition in which blood clots form abnormally in the circulatory system.

distal Farther away from the midline or site of attachment.

distal convoluted tubule Twisted tubule through which fluid flows in the nephron.

diurnal variation Normal daily fluctuations in body chemistry related to hormonal cycles, sleep-wake cycles, and other regular patterns of change.

dorsal Toward the back.

dorsalis pedis artery Artery in the foot.

droplet nuclei Particles smaller than 5 μm that remain suspended in the air for long periods.

Droplet Precautions Precautions used for patients known or suspected to have serious illnesses transmitted by large particle droplets.

droplet transmission Spread of infection through airborne droplets.

dura mater One of three membranes surrounding the brain.

efferent Nerve cell carrying motor information away from the central nervous system.

8-hour specimen See *first-morning specimen.*

electrocardiogram (ECG or EKG) Output tracing of electrocardiography.

electrocardiography Method for recording the electrical activity of the heart.

electrolytes Ions in the plasma or interstitial fluid.

embolism Obstruction in a blood vessel.

emesis Nausea and vomiting.

endocardium Inner layer of the heart.

eosinophil A type of phagocytic granulocyte.

epicardium Outer layer of the heart.

epidermis The outermost skin layer.

epididymis Coiled tube in which sperm mature and are stored.

epinephrine Hormone responsible for arousal and "fight or flight"; also called adrenaline.

epinephrine tolerance test Test that determines the patient's ability to mobilize glycogen from the liver in response to a dose of the hormone epinephrine.

epithelial tissue Groups of cells arranged in a sheet, usually functioning as a barrier or exchange surface.

erythrocyte Red blood cell.

esophagus Tube at the rear of the throat down which food travels to the stomach.

eutectic mixture of local anesthetic (EMLA) Topical anesthetic cream.

estrogen Hormone controlling the female reproductive cycle.

event report Prompt and complete documentation of the circumstances of an incident.

Expanded Precautions (EPs) Precautions targeted at patients known or suspected to be infected with a highly transmissible pathogen.

exposure control plan Comprehensive document outlining all procedures and policies for preventing the spread of infection.

extension Extending a body part farther away from the body midline.

external arteriovenous (AV) shunt AV shunt consisting of a cannula with a rubber septum through which a needle may be inserted for drawing blood.

external respiration Exchange of gases in the lungs.

extrinsic pathway One of two pathways in coagulation.

fallopian tube Tube through which an egg reaches the uterus.

fasting specimen Specimen drawn after a 12-hour complete fast.

feathered edge Blood smear characteristic in which cells farther from the original drop appear to thin out.

feedback loop Interactive systems designed to maintain homeostasis.

femoral artery Artery in the groin area above the thigh.

fever of unknown origin (FUO) Fever without a known cause.

fibrin Fibrous plasma protein that forms clots.

fibrin degradation products (FDPs) Breakdown products of fibrin that can be monitored clinically.

fibrinogen Inactive form of fibrin, the clotting protein.

fibrinolysis Process in which fibrin is broken down slowly; prevents blood clots from growing and becoming problematic.

first-morning specimen Urine sample collected immediately after a patient wakens.

fistula Permanent internal connection between an artery and a vein.

"flea" Metal filing used to mix blood with additives in small tubes.

flexion Bringing a body part closer in toward the body midline.

flow cytometry Analytic technique used to identify cellular markers on the surface of white blood cells.

follicle-stimulating hormone (FSH) Hormone released by the pituitary that acts on ovaries and testes.

fomite Contaminated object.

forensic Related to legal proceedings.

formed element Cellular portion of the blood.

frontal plane A vertical plane dividing the body into front and back.

galactosemia A metabolic disease.

gauge Number describing the diameter of a needle's lumen.

Globally Harmonized System (GHS) of Classification and Labeling of Chemicals Internationally agreed upon labeling system; each label contains information on the identity of the chemical, chemical manufacturer or other responsible party, appropriate hazard warnings communicated through visual symbols, explanations of the hazards involved in exposure to the chemical, and first-aid measures to take in the event of exposure.

glomerulus Ball of capillaries in the nephron that absorb fluid from the blood.

glucagon Hormone released by the pancreas that promotes the breakdown of glycogen back into glucose.

glucagon tolerance test Test that determines the patient's ability to mobilize glycogen from the liver in response to a dose of the hormone glucagon.

glucocorticoid Hormone that influences glucose metabolism.

glucose tolerance test (GTT) Test for both diabetes mellitus and other disorders of carbohydrate metabolism.

glycolysis Metabolic sugar breakdown within cells.

gonad Testis or ovary.

granulocyte A type of white blood cell; includes neutrophils, eosinophils, and basophils.

Groshong A type of central venous catheter.

ground substance Material surrounding connective tissue cells.

growth hormone (GH) Hormone released by the pituitary that regulates the rate of growth throughout the body.

half-life The time for half the ingested amount of drug to be metabolized.

health care–associated infection Infection contracted by a patient during a hospital stay.

health maintenance organization (HMO) Health care delivery system that functions as full-service outpatient clinics, providing all or almost all medical specialties under one roof.

helper T cell A type of cell that regulates the immune response.

hematoma Reddened, swollen area in which blood collects under the skin.

hematopoiesis Blood formation.

hemochromatosis Excess of iron in the blood.

hemoconcentration Increase in the ratio of formed elements to plasma, usually caused by leaving the tourniquet on too long.

hemolysis Destruction of red blood cells.

hemolyzed Characteristic of a sample in which red blood cells have been broken.

hemostasis Process by which the body stops blood from leaking out of a wound.

heparin lock Tube temporarily placed in a peripheral vein; used to administer medicine and draw blood.

hepatitis B virus (HBV) Virus that causes the liver disease hepatitis B; spreads through contact with human blood or body fluids.

Hickman A type of central venous catheter.

high-efficiency particulate air (HEPA) A type of air filter.

homeostasis Maintenance of a constant internal environment.

homocystinuria Inherited metabolic disorder.

hormone Chemical substance released into circulation by one group of cells that affects the function of other cells.

human chorionic gonadotropin (hCG) Hormone produced by the placenta after implantation of a fertilized egg.

human immunodeficiency virus (HIV) Causative agent for acquired immunodeficiency syndrome (AIDS).

human leukocyte antigen (HLA) See *major histocompatibility complex.*

humoral immunity Antibody-based immunity.

hyperglycemia High level of blood sugar (glucose).

hyperventilation Rapid, shallow breathing.

hypoglycemia Low level of blood sugar (glucose).

hypothalamus Portion of brain principally responsible for control of the endocrine system.

hypothyroidism Condition caused by too little secretion of thyroid hormones.

iatrogenic anemia Anemia caused by excessive blood draws.

icteric Related to jaundice.

immunization Deliberate provocation of an immune response to stimulate immune memory.

immunochemistry Branch of biochemistry concerned with immune responses and systems; immunochemistry tests use antibodies to detect a range of substances in the blood.

immunoglobulin Antibody.

immunohematology See *blood bank.*

implanted port Chamber located under the skin and connected to an indwelling line.

infection Invasion by and growth of a microorganism in the human body that causes disease.

inferior Below.

inflammation Coordinated nonspecific defense against infection or irritation, which combines increased blood flow and capillary permeability, activation of macrophages, temperature increase, and the clotting reaction to wall off the infected area.

informed consent Consent to a procedure with full understanding of the risks and the right to refuse to undergo the procedure.

inpatient Patient admitted to the hospital.

insulin Hormone released by the pancreas that promotes uptake of glucose by the body's cells.

interferon Type of cytokine.

interleukin Type of cytokine.

internal arteriovenous (AV) shunt AV shunt consisting of a fistula that uses the patient's tissue, a piece of bovine tissue, or a synthetic tube.

internal respiration Exchange of oxygen and carbon dioxide at the cellular level.

interneuron Neuron connecting two other neurons.

interstitial fluid Fluid between cells.

intrinsic pathway One of two pathways in coagulation.

iontophoresis Induction of sweat by application of a weak electric current.

iontophoretic pilocarpine test Detection of salt levels in sweat; used as part of the diagnosis for cystic fibrosis.

irritant contact dermatitis Direct irritation of the skin by contact with a chemical irritant.

ischemia Lack of oxygen.

isolation Separation of an infection source from susceptible hosts, thereby breaking the chain of infection.

jaundice Yellowing of the skin due to accumulation of bile.

(The) Joint Commission Organization that sets standards regarding systems to monitor and evaluate the quality of patient care.

kernicterus Brain damage caused by bilirubin entering the brain.

lactose tolerance test (LTT) Test that determines whether the lactose-digesting enzyme lactase is present in the gut.

larynx Muscular structure at the top of the trachea that regulates voice pitch; "voicebox."

lateral Toward the side.

latex sensitivity Response to latex proteins in gloves and other medical equipment that usually leads to contact dermatitis.

left atrioventricular (AV) valve Valve that separates the left atrium from the left ventricle.

leukemia Malignant neoplasm in the bone marrow, causing increased production of white blood cells.

leukocyte White blood cell.

liability insurance Insurance that covers monetary damages that must be paid if the defendant loses a liability suit.

liable To be legally responsible for an action or inaction.

ligament Tissue holding bone to bone.

lipase Fat-digesting enzyme.

lipemic Related to increased fats in the serum.

loop of Henle Loop within the nephron important in regulating salt in the urine.

Luer adapter Device for adapting a butterfly needle to an evacuated tube.

lumen Hollow tube within a needle.

luteinizing hormone (LH) Hormone released by the pituitary that acts on ovaries and testes.

lymph node One of many chambers located along the lymphatic vessels.

lymphedema Accumulation of interstitial fluid in tissues due to a blocked lymphatic vessel.

lymphocyte A type of white blood cell that circulates between the lymphatic system and the circulatory system.

lymphoma Tumor of a lymph gland.

lymphostasis Lack of movement of lymph fluid.

major histocompatibility complex (MHC) Set of surface proteins detected by the immune system that are used to distinguish self from non-self tissue.

malpractice Delivery of substandard care that results in harm to a patient.

maple syrup disease Inherited metabolic disorder.

marrow Interior of the bone where hematopoiesis occurs.

medial Toward the middle.

median antecubital vein Prominent vein in the antecubital fossa.

median cubital vein One of the three prominent veins on the anterior surface of the forearm.

megakaryocyte Cell precursor of a platelet.

melanocyte-stimulating hormone (MSH) Hormone released by the pituitary that increases melanin pigment production in skin cells.

memory cell B cell specialized to respond quickly upon the second encounter with an antigen.

memory T cell T cell that is primed to respond rapidly if an antigen is encountered again later in life.

meninges Collective term for the three membranes surrounding the brain.

microcollection tube Small tube used to collect dermal puncture samples; also called a "bullet."

microhematocrit tube See *capillary tube.*

micrometer Unit of measure equal to one millionth of a meter; a caliper for making precise measurements that has a spindle moved by a finely threaded screw.

micropipet Large glass capillary tube.

midstream clean catch Most common procedure for collecting any type of urine specimen.

mineralocorticoid Hormone that influences electrolyte balance.

mitochondrion Cellular organelle that creates ATP, an energy carrier for cell processes.

mitral valve See *left atrioventricular (AV) valve.*

modified Allen test Test for collateral circulation.

molecular diagnostics Department that analyzes deoxyribonucleic acid within a variety of tissues.

monocyte Large phagocytic cell.

mononuclear leukocyte A white blood cell, including lymphocytes and monocytes.

motor neuron Nerve cell that stimulates muscle contraction or gland secretion.

multisample needle Double-ended needle designed to be used with an evacuated tube system.

myelin Fatty insulation on neurons.

myocardial infarction (MI) Heart attack; loss of blood supply to the heart muscle.

myocardium Middle layer of the heart.

nasopharyngeal (NP) culture Used to diagnose whooping cough, croup, pneumonia, and other upper respiratory tract infections.

Natelson pipet See *micropipet.*

National Fire Protection Association (NFPA) label Label that warns fire fighters of the location of hazardous materials in the event of a fire.

natural killer (NK) cell A lymphocyte that kills infected cells.

needle adapter Translucent plastic cylinder connecting a multisample needle to an evacuated tube.

negligence Failure to perform an action consistent with the accepted standard of care.

nephron Functional unit of the kidney that filters blood plasma to form urine.

nerve Bundle of neurons.

neuromuscular junction Region on the muscle surface that receives stimulus from a neuron.

neuron Nerve cell that stimulates muscle contraction or gland secretion.

neurotransmitter Chemical released by neuron to stimulate or inhibit action of muscle, gland, or other neuron.

neutrophil A type of phagocytic granulocyte.

nonstriated involuntary muscle Smooth muscle; muscle controlling movement of substances through tubes.

norepinephrine Hormone responsible for arousal and "fight or flight"; also called noradrenaline.

nosocomial infection Infection acquired during a hospital stay.

nucleus The membrane-bound organelle in a cell that contains the chromosomes.

nursing home Long-term care facility.

occluded Blocked.

occult blood specimen Fecal specimen for detection of blood in the stool.

Occupational Safety and Health Administration (OSHA) Organization responsible for regulations governing workplace safety.

oral glucose tolerance test (OGTT) Test for diabetes mellitus.

order of draw Prescribed sequence in which tubes with different additives should be filled during a multitube collection.

osteoblast Bone-forming cell.

osteochondritis Painful inflammation of the bone or cartilage.

osteoclast Bone-remodeling cell.

osteomyelitis Bone infection.

out-of-court settlement Settlement in which the two parties reach an agreement without the intervention of a judge or jury.

outpatient Patient treated at a hospital without being admitted as an inpatient.

ovary Site of egg production.

ovulation Release of an egg.

oxyhemoglobin Hemoglobin to which oxygen is bound.

oxytocin Hormone released by the pituitary that stimulates smooth muscle contraction in the uterus during labor, and in the mammary glands during nursing.

P wave Part of the normal electrocardiogram tracing.

palpation Probing or feeling.

parathormone See *parathyroid hormone (PTH)*.

parathyroid hormone (PTH) Hormone released by the parathyroid gland that regulates the amount of calcium and phosphorus in circulation.

partial pressure of carbon dioxide (PCO_2) Amount of carbon dioxide dissolved in the blood.

partial pressure of oxygen (PO_2) Amount of oxygen dissolved in the blood.

pathogen Infectious organism.

peak level Highest serum level of a drug.

pelvic cavity Cavity enclosing the bladder, rectum, ovaries, and testes.

penis Male urethra and copulation organ.

peptide One of three hormone types.

pericardial cavity Cavity surrounding the heart.

pericardium Sac surrounding the heart.

peripheral nervous system (PNS) Nerve cells outside the brain and spinal cord.

peripherally inserted central catheter (PICC) Vascular access device threaded into a central vein after insertion into a peripheral (noncentral) vein.

peristalsis Wavelike muscular contraction propelling food along the gastrointestinal tract.

peritoneal cavity Cavity within the abdominal cavity enclosing the abdominal organs with the exception of the kidneys.

personal protective equipment (PPE) Fluid-resistant gowns, masks, respirators, face shields, shoe covers, and gloves.

petechia A small red spot appearing on the skin that is caused by a tourniquet that is too tight.

phagocyte A cell that eats bacteria and cellular debris.

pharynx Throat.

phenylketonuria (PKU) Inherited metabolic disease.

phlebotomy Practice of drawing blood.

physician office laboratory (POL) Physicians in a group practice that may employ a phlebotomist to collect patient samples.

pia mater One of three membranes surrounding the brain.

plaintiff Person claiming to have been harmed by the defendant.

plasma Fluid portion of the blood.

plasma cell B cell specialized for producing antibodies.

plasma membrane Outer enclosure of a cell.

plasmin Protein that breaks down fibrin.

plasminogen Inactive form of plasmin.

platelet Cell fragment important in clotting.

pleural cavity Cavity enclosing the lungs.

pneumatic tube system Sample transport system in which samples are carried in a sealed container within a network of tubes.

point-of-care testing (POCT) Performance of analytic tests immediately after obtaining a sample; also called alternate site testing.

polycythemia Excessive production of red blood cells.

polymer gel An inert, synthetic additive used to separate cells from plasma during centrifugation; also called thixotropic gel.

polymorphonuclear (PMN) leukocyte See *neutrophil*.

posterior Rear.

preanalytic variable Variable that occurs before performing analysis of the specimen.

preferred provider organization (PPO) Group of physicians and hospitals who offer their services to large employers to provide health care to employees.

prefix Word part preceding the root.

primary hemostasis Combination of the vascular phase and the platelet phase.

private law Law which, when violated, leads to a civil action.

procedure manual Book that contains protocols and other information about all the tests performed in the laboratory, including the principle behind the test, purpose of performing it, specimen type the test requires, collection method, and equipment and supplies required.

professional services Hospital branch that, at the request of the physician, provides services that aid in the diagnosis and treatment of the patient; includes the clinical laboratory.

progesterone Hormone controlling the reproductive cycle.

prolactin Hormone released by the pituitary that increases milk production in the mammary glands.

prone Lying belly downward.

prostate Gland supplying fluid for semen.

protease Protein-digesting enzyme.

protected health information (PHI) Any part of a patient's health information that is linked to information that identifies the patient.

protective environment (PE) Isolation of immuno-compromised patients to prevent exposing them to infection.

prothrombin Inactive form of thrombin.

proximal Closer to the midline or site of attachment.

proximal convoluted tubule Twisted tubule through which fluid flows in the nephron.

public law Law which, when violated, leads to a criminal action.

pulmonary arteries Arteries connecting heart to lungs.

pulmonary circulation System carrying blood between heart and lungs.

pulmonary semilunar valve Valve that separates the right ventricle from the pulmonary arteries.

pulmonary trunk Short artery connecting the right ventricle to the left and right pulmonary arteries.

pulmonary vein Vein returning blood to the left atrium.

pulmonic valve See *pulmonary semilunar valve.*

QRS complex Part of the normal electrocardiogram tracing.

Q–T interval Part of the normal electrocardiogram tracing.

quality assurance (QA) Set of methods used to guarantee quality patient care.

quality control (QC) Quantitative methods used to monitor the quality of procedures.

quality phlebotomy Set of policies and procedures designed to ensure the delivery of consistently high-quality patient care and specimen analysis.

radial artery Artery supplying the hand.

radioactive hazard symbol Symbol used to mark areas where radioactivity is used.

random specimen Specimen that may be collected at any time.

rapid group A *Streptococcus* Test for the rapid detection of group A *Streptococcus* bacteria.

reagent Test chemical.

reference laboratory Independent laboratory that analyzes samples from other health care facilities.

reflux Flow of blood from the collection tube back into the needle and then into the patient's vein.

repolarization Relaxation and recovery of the heart after contraction.

requisition Form specifying which tests must be run or which samples to collect.

reservoir Person carrying an infectious agent without being sick.

respiratory steady state State required for arterial blood gas collection, in which blood gas concentrations are steady.

reticulocyte Immature red blood cell.

right atrioventricular (AV) valve Valve separating atrium and ventricle on the right side of the heart.

right lymphatic duct Terminus of the lymphatic system, which empties into the venous system.

root Main part of a word.

safety data sheet (SDS) Sheet that provides information on the chemical, its hazards, and procedures for cleanup and first aid.

sagittal plane A vertical plane dividing the body into left and right.

saline lock See *heparin lock.*

scalp artery Artery used for arterial blood collection in infants.

sclerosed Hardened.

scope of practice Set of procedures, actions, and processes that a trained and licensed individual is permitted to perform.

scrotum Sac containing the testes.

secondary hemostasis Coagulation.

section Slice through.

segmented neutrophil (segs) See *neutrophil.*

semen Ejaculated fluid containing sperm, sugars, and other substances.

seminal vesicle Gland supplying fluid for semen.

sepsis Bacterial infection.

septicemia Blood infection by any pathogenic microorganism.

serum Plasma without its clotting factors.

72-hour stool specimen Specimen used for quantitative fecal fat determination.

severe combined immune deficiency (SCID) Inherited disorder marked by almost total lack of B and T cells.

sharps Needles, lancets, broken glass, and other sharp items.

short turnaround time (stat) Requisition requiring immediate attention and processing.

sickle cell anemia Inherited disorder of the hemoglobin molecule.

sinoatrial node Pacemaker of the heart.

skeletal muscle Muscle under voluntary control; moves the skeleton.

smooth muscle Muscle not under voluntary control; regulates passage of fluid through tubes.

sodium polyanethol sulfonate (SPS) An anticoagulant.

somatic motor system Group of neurons controlling the skeletal muscles.

sphincter Ring of muscle regulating passage of food through the gastrointestinal tract.

sphygmomanometer Blood pressure measuring device.

spinal cavity Cavity enclosing the spine.

ST segment Part of the normal electrocardiogram tracing.

Standard Precautions Infection control method that uses barrier protection and work control practices to prevent direct skin contact with blood, other body fluids, and tissues from other people.

standards Established requirements used in an accredited program.

stat A requisition requiring immediate attention and processing.

statutory law Law created by a legislative body.

steroid hormone One of three hormone types.

striated involuntary muscle Cardiac muscle.

striated voluntary muscle Skeletal muscle.

stroke Loss of oxygen supply to a portion of the brain.

stylus Recording pen of the electrocardiogram machine.

suffix Word part following the root.

superior Above.

supine Lying on the back.

suprapubic aspiration Sample collected via a needle inserted through the abdominal wall into the bladder.

sweat electrolytes (SE) Salt present in normal sweat that is used as part of the diagnosis for cystic fibrosis.

synapse, synaptic cleft Space between two neurons into which a neurotransmitter is released.

synarthrosis Fixed joint.

syncope Fainting.

synovial cavity Fluid-filled joint cavity.

systemic circulation System carrying blood between heart and the body (except for lungs).

systole Contraction portion of the cardiac cycle.

T cell Lymphocyte that controls the immune response.

T wave Part of the normal electrocardiogram tracing.

tendon Tissue holding muscle to bone.

terminal lymphatic Closed-end lymph tube.

testosterone Principal male sex hormone.

thalamus Major relay station for incoming sensory information.

therapeutic drug monitoring (TDM) Timed specimens that are tested for levels of a medication.

therapeutic phlebotomy Removal of blood from a patient's system as part of the treatment for a disorder.

thermoregulation Control of body temperature.

thixotropic gel Inert additive used to separate cells from plasma during centrifugation.

thoracic cavity Chest cavity.

thoracic duct Terminus of the lymphatic system, which empties into the venous system.

thrombin Protein that activates fibrinogen to form fibrin.

thrombocyte See *platelet.*

thrombosis Clot formation within a blood vessel.

thymosin Hormone released by the thymus gland that helps to maintain the immune system.

thyroid-stimulating hormone (TSH) Hormone released by the pituitary to stimulate release of thyroxine by the thyroid.

thyroxine (T$_4$) Thyroid hormone that regulates the basal metabolic rate.

timed specimens Series of samples often collected over 24 hours and combined to provide a single, large specimen.

tissue Group of cells with similar structure and function.

tissue plasminogen activator (t-PA) Enzyme that converts plasminogen to plasmin.

tort Injury to one person for which another person who caused the injury is legally responsible.

total quality management (TQM) Entire set of approaches used by an institution to provide customer satisfaction.

tourniquet Strip of material used to reduce circulation and increase prominence of veins.

trachea Cartilage-reinforced "windpipe" connecting pharynx and bronchi.

tract Bundle of neurons within the central nervous system.

transverse plane A horizontal plane dividing the body into top and bottom.

tricuspid valve See *right atrioventricular (AV) valve.*

triiodothyronine (T$_3$) Thyroid hormone that regulates the basal metabolic rate.

triple lumen See *central venous catheter.*

trough level Lowest serum level of a drug.

tube advancement mark Mark on a needle adapter indicating how far the tube can be pushed in without losing vacuum,

tube holder See *needle adapter.*

tunica adventitia Outer layer of blood vessels.

tunica intima Inner layer of blood vessels.

tunica media Middle layer of blood vessels.

2-hour postprandial test Test that compares the fasting glucose level with the level 2 hours after consuming glucose; used to test for diabetes mellitus.

umbilical artery Artery used for arterial collection in infants.

unintentional tort Unintentional injury that is the basis for most medical malpractice claims.

ureter Tube that delivers urine from kidney to bladder.

urethra Tube carrying urine from the bladder.

urgent care center Outpatient clinic that provides walk-in services to patients who cannot wait for a scheduled appointment with their primary health care provider.

uterus Site of egg implantation and fetal development.

vagina Passage in a female in which sperm and semen are deposited during intercourse.

vas deferens Tube in a male through which sperm reach the urethra.

vascular access device (VAD) Tube that is inserted into either a vein or an artery; used to administer fluids or medications, monitor blood pressure, or draw blood.

vascular spasm Contraction of the smooth muscle lining the vessel.

vector Carrier of disease.

vein Vessel carrying blood toward the heart.

vena cava Vein returning blood to the right atrium.

venous thrombosis Formation of a blood clot within a vein.

ventral Toward the belly.

ventricle Lower chamber of the heart, or space within the brain and spinal cord in which cerebrospinal fluid circulates.

venule Small vein.

villus Finger-like projection of the intestine.

whole blood Blood before it is separated.

winged infusion set Small needle and flexible tube for delicate veins.

Index

Fire hazards, 32–33, 33f, 33t

Fires
classes of, 33
prevention of, 32–33, 33f

First-aid procedures, 33–34
bleeding aid, 34
CPR, 34
for shock, 34

First morning specimen, urine, 223–224

Fiscal and information services, in hospital organization, 15

Flow cytometry, 20

Follicle-stimulating hormone (FSH), 87

Fomite, defined, 41

Food and Drug Administration (FDA), U.S., 211–213
on CLIA-waived tests, 244
gloves regulated by, 35

Fractures, 75

Freezers, as QA variable, 263–264

G

Galactosemia, screening for, 186

Geriatric patients, 181, 188–189
common disorders of, 188–189
mental impairment of, 189
physical changes in, 188
special considerations for, 189

Glands. *See also* Endocrine system
bulbourethral, 88–89
in digestive process, 81
endocrine, 85–86, 86f, 87–88
prostate, 88–89, 89f
of skin, 76, 77f
thymus, 86f, 87

Globally Harmonized System (GHS) of Classification and Labeling of Chemicals, 29

Glomerulus, 83–84, 83f

Gloves
as PPE, 45
Standard Precautions for, 46

Glucocorticoids, 88

Glucose, common tests for, 17t

Glucose monitoring
bedside, 246
capillary collection for, 152

Glucose tolerance test (GTT), 208–209, 209t

Glycolysis
inhibited by sodium fluoride, 120–121
tests affected by, 234

Goggles, 43

Gold-top tubes, 122, 122f

Gonads, 86f, 88

Gout, 75, 75b

Gowns
fluid-resistant, 43
Standard Precautions for, 46

Granulocytes, 104

Gray-top tubes, 122, 122f

Green-top tubes, 122, 122f

Green-gray–top tubes, 122, 122f

Groshong central venous line, 190

Growth hormone (GH), 87

H

Hand
blood draw from, 133t, 136
veins of, 170, 170f

Hand collection, procedure for, 170, 171–173t

Hand hygiene, 38, 42–46, 262, 262f
procedure for, 43
Standard Precautions for, 46
when to perform, 43, 43b

Handwashing
competency checklist for, 282
proper technique for, 43, 44–45t

Health care–associated infection (HAI), 39

Health care costs, 268

Health care structure, 12, 14–16, 14f

Health fairs, 23

Health Insurance Portability and Accountability Act (HIPAA) of 1996, 9, 274–275

Health maintenance organizations (HMOs), 23

Hearing loss, in geriatric patients, 188

Heart, 96–97
anatomy of, 97f
circulation through, 97–99
contraction of, 99
disorders of, 99–100, 101t

Heart attack, 99-100. *See also* Myocardial infarction

Heel puncture, 184–185

Heel-warmer packet, 263

Helicobacter pylori (H. pylori), POC test for, 252

Helper T cells, 110

Hemostasis
coagulation phase, 106, 107f
platelet phase, 106
vascular phase, 106

Hematocrit (Hct), at POC, 245

Hematology tests, 19–20, 20t
CBC, 19–20, 20t
coagulation tests, 19, 19b, 19f
at POC, 245, 245f

Hematomas
in arterial puncture, 199
blood drawn from, 176
complications with, 169
during venipuncture, 174

Hematopoiesis, 73

Hemochromatosis, 213

Hemochron system, 246f

Hemoconcentration
in blood donor collection, 213
with improper tourniquet use, 133t, 135, 170

Hemogard top, 239

Hemoglobin (Hgb)
disorders of, 108t
at POC, 245, 245f

Hemoglobin A$_{1C}$, at POC, 246

Hemolysis
causes of, 176, 176b
with improper tourniquet use, 133t, 136
tests affected by, 176, 177b
as venipuncture complication, 176, 176b, 177b

Hemophilia, 19

Hemorrhage, with arterial puncture, 199

Hemostasis, 19, 95, 106–107, 107f
disorders of, 108t
fibrinolysis, 107
primary, 69b

Heparin, as tube additive, 120

Heparinized needle, for arterial puncture, 196–197

Heparinized syringe, for arterial puncture, 196–197

Heparin lock, 190, 191f

Heparin therapy, monitoring of, 245–246

Hepatitis B surface antigen, 21t

Hepatitis B virus (HBV)
OSHA standard for, 49
survival in dried blood of, 40–41

Hickman central venous line, 190

High-efficiency particulate air (HEPA), 42, 42f

Histology, 16

Homeostasis, 67

Homocystinuria, screening for, 186

Honesty, importance of, 4, 24b

Hormones, 87. *See also* Endocrine system

Hospital organization, 14–16, 14f
fiscal and information services in, 15
nursing services in, 15
professional services in, 15
support services in, 15

Hospitals
infectious agents in, 39
and Patient Care Partnership, 269–270b

Hub, of needle, 117

Human body. *See* Body systems

Human chorionic gonadotropin (hCG), 21t

Human chorionic gonadotropin (hCG) test, urine specimen for, 223–224

Human immunodeficiency virus (HIV)
OSHA standard for, 49
POC test for, 252

Human leukocyte antigens (HLAs), 110

Humoral immunity, 110

Hydrogen breath test, for lactose intolerance, 209

Hypersecretion, in endocrine system, 88, 88b

Hypodermic needle, 117–118

Hyposecretion, in endocrine system, 88, 88b

Hypothalamus, 85–86

Hypothyroidism, screening for, 186

I

Iatrogenic anemia, 152, 177

ICD-9-CM code, 129

Ice, in arterial puncture, 200–202t, 201

ID bands, for patients, 131

Identification (ID), patient, 128
for geriatric patients, 189
of newborns, 184
problems with, 167–168
as QA variable, 258, 260f
in routine venipuncture, 131–132, 133, 133t

Identifiers, 131

Immune system, 95, 109–110
disorders of, 110
nonspecific immunity, 109–110
specific immunity, 110

Immunoglobulins, in plasma, 103

Immunohematology department, 16–17

Immunology department, 21

Immunology tests, common, 21, 21t